RNA Interference: Challenges and Therapeutic Opportunities

RNA Interference: Challenges and Therapeutic Opportunities

Editor: Sam Kennedy

MURPHY & MOORE
www.murphy-moorepublishing.com

www.murphy-moorepublishing.com

MURPHY & MOORE

Cataloging-in-Publication Data

RNA interference : challenges and therapeutic opportunities / edited by Sam Kennedy.
p. cm.
Includes bibliographical references and index.
ISBN 978-1-63987-495-8
1. RNA interference. 2. Gene therapy. 3. Gene silencing. I. Kennedy, Sam.
QH450.26 .R53 2022
572.88--dc23

Murphy & Moore Publishing,
1 Rockefeller Plaza,
New York City, NY 10020, USA

ISBN 978-1-63987-495-8 (Hardback)

Contents

Preface VII

Chapter 1 **RNAi-Induced Immunity** 1
Wenyi Gu

Chapter 2 **Preclinical Development of RNAi-Inducing Oligonucleotide Therapeutics for Eye Diseases** 10
Tamara Martínez, Maria Victoria González, Beatriz Vargas, Ana Isabel Jiménez and Covadonga Pañeda

Chapter 3 **Perspectives on RNA Interference in Immunopharmacology and Immunotherapy** 38
Zhaohua Hou, Qiuju Han, Cai Zhang and Jian Zhang

Chapter 4 **Utility of Potent Anti-Viral MicroRNAs in Emerging Infectious Diseases** 63
Zhabiz Golkar, Donald G. Pace and Omar Bagasra

Chapter 5 **RNA Interference as a Tool to Reduce the Risk of Rejection in Cell-Based Therapies** 77
Constanca Figueiredo and Rainer Blasczyk

Chapter 6 **RNAi — Implications in Entomological Research and Pest Control** 91
Nidhi Thakur, Jaspreet Kaur Mundey and Santosh Kumar Upadhyay

Chapter 7 **Management of Insect Pest by RNAi — A New Tool for Crop Protection** 121
Thais Barros Rodrigues and Antonio Figueira

Chapter 8 **RNA Interference - Natural Gene-Based Technology for Highly Specific Pest Control (HiSPeC)** 141
Eduardo C. de Andrade and Wayne B. Hunter

Chapter 9 **In Search of New Methodologies for Efficient Insect Pest Control: The RNAi "Movement"** 160
Anna Kourti, Luc Swevers and Dimitrios Kontogiannatos

Chapter 10 **RNA Interference - A Powerful Functional Analysis Tool for Studying Tick Biology and its Control** 185
Remil Linggatong Galay, Rika Umemiya-Shirafuji, Masami Mochizuki, Kozo Fujisaki and Tetsuya Tanaka

Chapter 11 **Current Status for Application of RNA Interference Technology as Nucleic Acid Drug** **220**
Tomoko Takahashi, Yuko Nakano and Kumiko Ui-Tei

Permissions

List of Contributors

Index

Preface

Every book is a source of knowledge and this one is no exception. The idea that led to the conceptualization of this book was the fact that the world is advancing rapidly; which makes it crucial to document the progress in every field. I am aware that a lot of data is already available, yet, there is a lot more to learn. Hence, I accepted the responsibility of editing this book and contributing my knowledge to the community.

RNA interference (RNAi) is a genetic regulatory mechanism that occurs in eukaryotic cells and regulates the activity of genes. Its main function is to suppress, silence or deactivate genes. RNAi can occur either naturally or artificially. It occurs naturally through the production of pre-miRNA. RNAi can also be induced experimentally by using double-stranded RNA (dsRNA). The synthetic dsRNA may be of two types: small hairpin RNA (shRNA) or short interfering RNA (siRNA). An enzyme known as DICER is necessary in both natural and artificial pathways for the formation of miRNA from pre-miRNA or for the formation of siRNA from shRNA. This book traces the progress of this field and highlights some of its key concepts and applications. It studies, analyses and upholds the pillars of RNA interference and its utmost significance in modern times. This book includes contributions of experts and scientists which will provide innovative insights into this field.

While editing this book, I had multiple visions for it. Then I finally narrowed down to make every chapter a sole standing text explaining a particular topic, so that they can be used independently. However, the umbrella subject sinews them into a common theme. This makes the book a unique platform of knowledge.

I would like to give the major credit of this book to the experts from every corner of the world, who took the time to share their expertise with us. Also, I owe the completion of this book to the never-ending support of my family, who supported me throughout the project.

Editor

1

RNAi-Induced Immunity

Wenyi Gu

Abstract

RNA interference has a close relationship with the host defense system including adaptive immunity. It is not only involved in regulating immune cells at different stages of the immune response but also directly induces or enhances antigen presentation and subsequent immune responses. We have previously reported that a small hairpin RNA (shRNA) targeted the downstream site of a dominant cytotoxic T lymphocyte (CTL) epitope of human papillomavirus (HPV) type 16 oncogene E7 can stimulate an immune response against E7 expressing tumors in C57BL/6 mice. This results in the elimination of tumor growth *in vivo*, whereas an shRNA that targets the upstream site does not. Our recent data further confirm the long half-life of the 5'-mRNA fragment after shRNA degradation and its involvement in protein synthesis. This chapter summarizes these findings and provides some updated explanations for the findings.

Keywords: RNAi, shRNA, immune response, HPV E7, miRNA

1. Introduction

RNA interference (RNAi) is a conserved gene-regulation mechanism in all eukaryotic cells, where small RNAs including small interfering RNA (siRNA), small hairpin RNA (shRNA), and micro-RNA (miRNA, miR) interact with message RNAs (mRNAs) in a sequence-specific manner and cause the cleavage or translational blockage of a gene [1, 2]. Because of its specificity and efficiency, it has been widely utilized as a routine tool for gene functional studies in biology laboratories worldwide. In addition, since RNAi blockage is very specific and at the transcriptional level, RNAi-based gene therapy (RNAi therapy) is thought to hold a great potential for treating many diseases, especially viral infections and genetic disorders. Synthesized siRNA is thus regarded as a specialized drug for gene therapies. So far, promising results have been obtained with RNAi therapy in various diseases and many are being tested in clinical trials, including viral infections, cancers, and genetic or inflammatory disorders [3-7]. As cancers and other emerging diseases such as dementia and super-bug infections become major public health issues, RNAi therapy can offer a new solution and has the additional ability to overcome drug resistances.

Beside the fundamental gene-silencing and gene-regulating roles of RNAi, which will also regulate the gene functions of immune cells and thus the immune responses, RNAi pathway itself has an additional function and involvement in inducing adaptive immunity. This function has not been well-studied, and the mechanism is not clear. Its relationship with the immune system in terms of antigen reactivation and antigen presentation is still a new area to be investigated. Indeed, in plants and primitive species, RNAi is a part of the defense system against viral infections. However, in mammals, RNAi seems not directly involved in the immune system, probably due to the development of an advanced and sophisticated immune system. This chapter summarizes the evidence of RNAi-induced immunity against tumors and provides some updated possible explanations for the findings. The possible link between miRNA and its degraded products with the immune system has been also discussed. Exploring the relationship between RNAi and the immune system may lead to new discoveries in RNAi biology and approaches for more effective cancer immunotherapy or treatment for viral and intracellular pathogen infections.

2. The discovery of RNAi-induced adaptive immunity against tumors

In 2009, we reported a discovery about RNAi-induced immunity [7]. We investigated two shRNAs encoded by lentiviral vectors on their ability to suppress tumor cell growth and stimulate antitumor immunity *in vivo*. One shRNA targeted the downstream site of a dominant cytotoxic T lymphocyte (CTL) epitope of the oncogene E7 of human papillomavirus (HPV) type 16 (termed downstream shRNA), while another shRNA targeted the upstream site of this epitope (termed upstream shRNA). Both shRNAs were equally effective at silencing E7 gene expression (in mRNA and protein levels) and led to the inhibition of tumor cells growth *in vitro* and *in vivo* [7]. In spite of this, TC1 tumor cells (expressing HPV E6 and E7) treated with downstream shRNA stimulated an immune response against E7 in C57BL6 mice and resulted in elimination of tumor growth *in vivo*, whereas cells treated with the upstream shRNA did not. When untreated TC1 tumor cells were injected to the same mice (challenging tumors), the group of downstream shRNA exhibited a total inhibition of challenging tumor growth, whereas no inhibition was observed in the upstream shRNA group. This ability of downstream shRNA was absent in $Rag^{-/-}$ mice (lack of T- and B-cells), suggesting adaptive immune response or T-cell response was required. To prove that the immune response was antigen-specific, we carried out a same animal experiment by immunizing C57BL/6 mice with TC-1 cells treated with these shRNAs but challenged with another tumor cell line C2, which has the E7 expression and H-2b genetic background as C57BL/6 mice. Again, we observed that only mice immunized with downstream shRNA treated cells had a loss of tumor formation, indicating tumor clearance was specific to E7. Our data indicate that a more effective treatment can be developed for cervical cancer by combining RNAi treatment with immunotherapy. Our results also reveal that RNAi may be widely used as an antitumor immunity stimulator or enhancer (Fig 1).

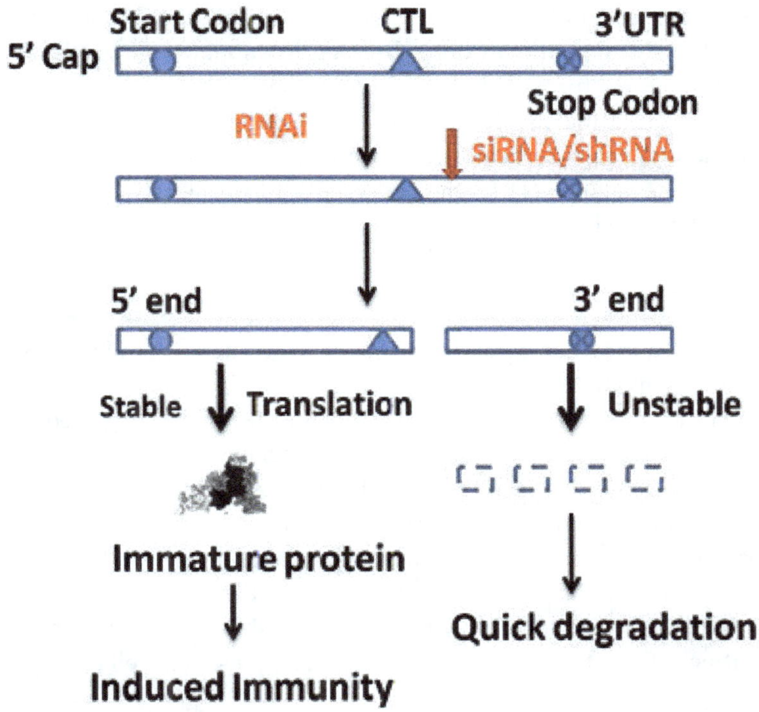

Figure 1. Schematic diagram shows RNAi targeting site and 5' mRNA fragment. It is known that in cervical cancer HPV E7 and mouse lymphoma EG7/OVA (ovalbumin) models, the shRNA targets the downstream site of the CTL epitope that produce the 5' fragment of mRNA. This makes immature proteins and further induces an immune response.

To prove the applicability of immune response to general tumor antigens, we tested a model antigen ovalbumin (OVA) expressed in EG7 cells that are a mouse thymoma cell line with C57BL6 genetic background. We chose the major CTL epitope of OVA, SIINFEKL, as the target site and designed two upstream shRNAs OVA-1 and -2 and a downstream shRNA OVA-3. The shRNA-treated EG7 cells were used to immunize the mice, which were subsequently challenged with untreated EG7 cells. We observed that only mice inoculated with OVA-3-shRNA treated cells had significantly reduced tumor formation but not with OVA-1 and -2 shRNAs.

3. Confirmation of mRNA fragments and truncated proteins in treated cells

To determine if the RNAi-induced immune response was actually from degraded products of RNAi, we designed a series of primers that would amplify RNA fragments inside and outside the targeting sites of upstream shRNA (E6-1) and downstream shRNA (E7-1, Fig 2A). If an inside fragment was present while the outside fragment was absent, it would indicate that the mRNA had been cleaved by shRNA at the target site. The cells were treated with E6-1 and E7-1 shRNAs and incubated for 2–4 days before real-time RT-PCR was carried out. As expected, the shortest PCR fragment, R3, was observed in all samples (Fig 2B). The full-length R1 PCR fragment was only observed in untreated TC1 cells or cells infected with the lentiviral vector control (PLL, Fig 2B). In cells treated with both E7-1 and E6-1, R1 was not found, indicating that shRNA-mediated cleavage was occurring. Of most interest was the R2 fragment which was found in all samples except cells treated with E6-1. These results suggest that R2 or R3 short fragments of E6-1 and E7-1 existed in the cells, at least temporarily at the time we isolated RNA. These short-form mRNAs may act as templates for short-form proteins (truncated proteins) and trigger antigen presentation to CD8+ T-cells and a CTL immune response to E7.

Apart from our data, a previous study reported that degradation of the 3' mRNA fragment resulting from siRNA-mediated cleavage was blocked for some mRNAs, leaving an mRNA fragment that could act as a template for cDNA synthesis. They suggested that this could give rise to false negative results and that this phenomenon may be avoided by the careful design of RT-qPCR primers for each individual siRNA experiment [8]. This report further confirms that mRNA fragments from RNAi do sometimes exist in the cells. In addition, it was noticed by researchers that un-degraded fragments of an siRNA-targeted mRNA may cause false positive effects of microarray analysis [9]. To avoid this, they developed a qRT-PCR protocol, which allowed for the determination of the optimal time point for mRNA analyses, indicating mRNA fragments after RNAi can be present in cell for a certain time.

What is the functional role of these mRNA fragments after RNAi? Our data demonstrated that they can be involved in translational machinery and produce truncated proteins. To experimentally prove this, we utilized the OVA-expressing EG7 cell model again. The cells were treated with downstream and upstream shRNAs and further treated with the protease inhibitor MG132 to reduce protein degradation before immunoblotting was performed. The blots were probed with an antibody against the N terminus of OVA protein. The predicted size of a truncated protein produced by the cleavage of OVA-2 shRNA was 14.7 kDa. We observed a protein band about 15-kDa in cells treated with the OVA-2 shRNA but not in untreated and OVA-1 or OVA-3 shRNA treated cells. It proves that truncated proteins can be produced in cells by the translation of mRNA fragment cleaved by shRNA. The predicted truncated product by shRNA-OVA3 was not observed due to cross-reacting proteins on the blot [7].

Our recent data (unpublished) showed that the cleaved 5′ and 3′ fragments of human papillomavirus type 16 (HPV-16) E6/7 mRNA after shRNA treatment were unevenly degraded. The 5′ mRNA fragment was more abundant and displayed a greater stability than the corresponding 3′ fragment in the treated cells. Further analysis revealed that the 5′ fragment was polysome-associated, indicating its active translation, and this was further confirmed by using tagged E7 protein to show that C-terminally truncated proteins were produced in treated cells (Singhania et al. submitted).

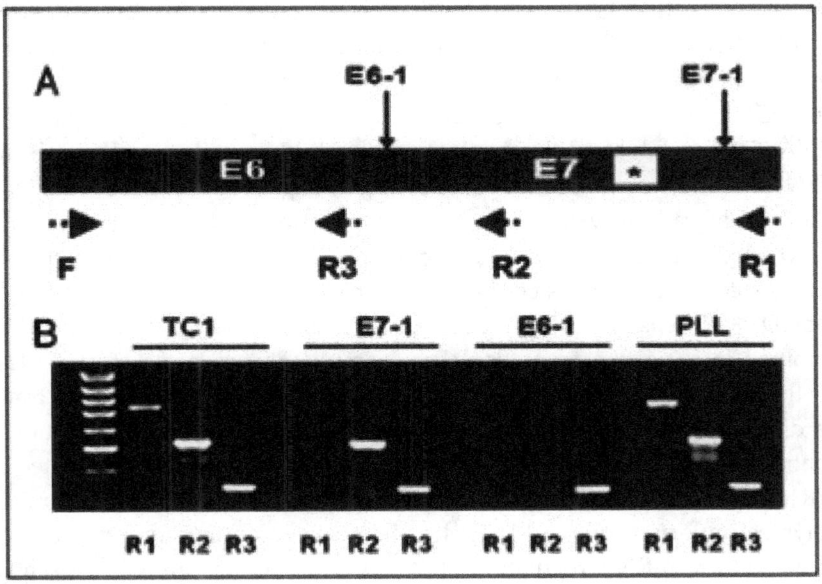

Figure 2. The shRNA targeting sites and primer design for HPV E6/E7 mRNA (Adapted from Gu et al 2009). (A) The shRNA and primer sites on E6/E7 mRNA. (B) The PCR products on an agarose gel. Notes: TC1, the untreated cell control. PLL, lentiviral vector control. *: indicates the site of CTL epitope. F: forward primer, R: reverse primer.

4. Possible models for explaining RNAi-induced immunity

It is well established that miRNAs play an important role in regulating innate and adaptive immune responses as a part of their gene-regulating roles. Evidence has accumulated that miRNAs are involved in the adaptive immune responses by regulating T-cells, B-cells, and antigen-presenting cells (APCs). For example, miR-214 was reported to target phosphatase and tensin homolog (PTEN) and increase proliferation and the activation of T-cells [10], while miR-150, -155, and let-7 have been shown to be involved in the development of T-cells into memory cells [11]. In addition, miR-184 was shown to inhibit nuclear factor of activated T-cells-1 (NFAT-1) in the activation of CD4 T-cell in the early stage of adaptive immune responses [12] and miR-181-a could promote CD4 and CD8 double positive T-cell development [13]. For B-cells, miR-155 is required for their normal function such as production of isotype-switched, high-affinity antibodies and for memory responses [14]. It has also been demonstrated that miR-155 is induced by B-cell receptor (BCR) [15]. However, overexpression of miR-155 can immortalize B-cells and lead to transformation, for instance, EBV was shown to have induced miR-155 expression and transformed B-cells [16, 17]. In addition, miR-150 is important in B-cell development [18] and so is miR-17 [19, 20].

For dendritic cells (DCs), a recent review summarized the need of miRNAs in their lineage commitment from bone marrow progenitors and for the development of subsets such as plasmacytoid DCs and conventional DCs [21]. Liu et al. (2010) used software to predict and then conducted experiments to confirm that three members of the miR-148 family, miR-148a, miR-148b, and miR-152 are negative regulators of the innate immune response and antigen-presenting capacity of DCs. They showed that miR-148/152 expression was upregulated in DCs on maturation and activation induced by TLR3, TLR4, and TLR9 agonists. These miRNAs in turn inhibited the production of cytokines including IL-12, IL-6, TNF-alpha, and IFN-beta and upregulation of MHC class II expression and DC-initiated antigen-specific T-cell proliferation by targeting Calcium/calmodulin-dependent protein kinase II alpha (CaMKIIα) [22]. In addition, miR-150 and miR-223 has been shown to play an important regulatory role in Langerhans cells (LCs) by cross-presenting a soluble antigen to antigen-specific CD8(+) T-cells [23, 24]. Beside APCs such as DC and LC, miRNA is shown to be directly involved in antigen presentation. For example, Bartoszewski et al. (2011) demonstrated that the mRNA of human endoplasmic reticulum (ER) antigen peptide transporter 1 (TAP1) is a direct target of miR-346. They showed that the 3'-UTR (un-translational region) of TAP1 contains a 6-mer seeding region for miR-346 and the ER stress-associated reduction of TAP1 mRNA and protein levels could be reversed by inhibitory miRNA of miR-346 [25]. As TAP plays an important role in MHC class I-associated antigen presentation, their data provide an insight for miRNA-regulating MHC class-I-associated antigen presentation during ER stress.

The above-highlighted results clearly indicate miRNA's regulatory role in many aspects of adaptive immunity. However, is it possible that miRNA also takes part in host immunity through mRNA fragments produced after RNAi just like shRNA described in section 2 and 3? Normally, miRNAs target the 3' UTR and lead to the translation block or degradation of the targeted mRNAs. So when they degrade mRNAs, it is supposed to produce long 5' mRNA fragments and may also produce truncated proteins. If this is true, the translated defective proteins could be treated as truncated protein and be processed by proteasome. If there is a CTL epitope in the defective structure, it could be coupled with the MHC class I molecule and presented to T-cells by DCs through antigen cross-presentation, as described above with shRNA. This could be a link between RNAi pathway and antigen presentation or adaptive immune response.

In the shRNA case discussed above, the target should be at the downstream of a CTL epitope to induce immunity. When miRNAs target 3' UTR, a site certainly at the downstream site of any possible CTL epitopes, it is assumed to have the ability to produce truncated proteins and so to induce immune responses. Therefore, an important question for miRNA biology is whether miRNAs can routinely induce immune responses by degrading mRNA at 3' UTR and generating 5' mRNA fragments or truncated proteins that contain CTL epitopes? So far, there is no answer for this question. Another critical question is: what is the difference between blocking and degrading mRNA by miRNAs at 3' UTR? Does this relate to antigen presentation of different proteins?

Because it has been shown that miRNA can act as siRNA and shRNA can be produced in the same pathway as miRNA [26], it is important and interesting to investigate if miRNA can induce the same immune response as shRNA. The systems of HPV 16 E7/TC1 and

OVA/EG7 can be used as good models to investigate this. As miRNAs are routinely transcribed and involved in interacting with mRNA, this mechanism can be considered as a routine way in cells to generate CTL containing truncated proteins. However, because most mRNAs in cells are for self-proteins, their CTL epitopes will not be presented to T-cells. This leaves the question of whether this is a mechanism just for cells that express viral genes (such as HPV E7 in TC1 and C2 as above) or for cells expressing foreign genes/antigens (such as OVA in EG7)? The next question is: can this be generalized to any tumor antigens including self-antigens? This is an interesting subject to investigate and will facilitate our understanding of how RNAi pathways interact with and are involved in adaptive immune responses (antigen presentation) to utilize them for cancer immunotherapy.

Although some miRNA are highly conserved between lower animals and higher animals, mammals have far more miRNAs compared to nonmammals. This suggests that during evolution, as gene regulation became so complex and important in higher animals, miRNA or RNAi pathway gradually specialized into gene regulation. At the same time, as the adaptive immune system became well developed and highly specialized, these two systems got separated, but as described above, they still have some links. Future investigations leading to insight into these links will provide answers to the above questions.

5. Conclusion

In summary, RNAi-induced immunity opens a new perspective in which to explore the relationship between RNAi pathways and the immune system, especially its involvement in antigen presentation in the adaptive immune response. For RNAi biology, it will provide an insight into the understanding of function roles of RNAi (including miRNA and siRNA) in host defense. In the field of gene therapy for cancers, RNAi can be used as an approach to silence oncogenes as well as a strategy to enhance immunity against cancer antigens (at least viral infection related cancers) and further explored as a novel cancer immunotherapy. Finally, for intracellar pathogens, it can be used as a strategy for developing new vaccine through RNAi reactivating their antigens to the immune system.

Author details

Wenyi Gu*

Address all correspondence to: w.gu@uq.edu.au

Australian Institute of Bioengineering and Nanotechnology, University of Queensland, QLD, Australia

References

[1] Sharp, P.A., *RNA interference--2001.* Genes Dev, 2001. 15(5): p. 485-90. doi:10.1101/gad.880001.

[2] Elbashir, S.M., et al., *Duplexes of 21-nucleotide RNAs mediate RNA interference in cultured mammalian cells.* Nature, 2001. 411(6836): p. 494-8. doi:10.1038/35078107.

[3] Jacque, J.M., K. Triques, and M. Stevenson, *Modulation of HIV-1 replication by RNA interference.* Nature, 2002. 418(6896): p. 435-8. doi:10.1038/nature00896.

[4] Harper, S.Q., et al., *RNA interference improves motor and neuropathological abnormalities in a Huntington's disease mouse model.* Proc Natl Acad Sci U S A, 2005. 102(16): p. 5820-5. doi:0501507102.

[5] Putral, L.N., et al., *RNA interference against human papillomavirus oncogenes in cervical cancer cells results in increased sensitivity to cisplatin.* Mol Pharmacol, 2005. 68(5): p. 1311-9. doi:10.1124/mol.105.014191.

[6] Bitko, V., et al., *Inhibition of respiratory viruses by nasally administered siRNA.* Nat Med, 2004. doi:10.1038/nm1164.

[7] Gu, W., et al., *Both treated and untreated tumors are eliminated by short hairpin RNA-based induction of target-specific immune responses.* Proc Natl Acad Sci U S A, 2009. 106(20): p. 8314-9. doi: 10.1073/pnas.0812085106.

[8] Holmes, K., et al., *Detection of siRNA induced mRNA silencing by RT-qPCR: considerations for experimental design.* BMC Res Notes, 2010. 3: p. 53. doi: 10.1186/1756-0500-3-53.

[9] Hahn, P., et al., *RNA interference: PCR strategies for the quantification of stable degradation-fragments derived from siRNA-targeted mRNAs.* Biomol Eng, 2004. 21(3-5): p. 113-7. doi:10.1016/j.bioeng.2004.09.001.

[10] Jindra, P.T., et al., *Costimulation-dependent expression of microRNA-214 increases the ability of T cells to proliferate by targeting Pten.* J Immunol, 2010. 185(2): p. 990-7. doi: 10.4049/jimmunol.1000793.

[11] Almanza, G., et al., *Selected microRNAs define cell fate determination of murine central memory CD8 T cells.* PLoS One, 2010. 5(6): p. e11243. doi: 10.1371/journal.pone.0011243.

[12] Weitzel, R.P., et al., *microRNA 184 regulates expression of NFAT1 in umbilical cord blood CD4+ T cells.* Blood, 2009. 113(26): p. 6648-57. doi: 10.1182/blood-2008-09-181156.

[13] Liu, G., et al., *Pre-miRNA loop nucleotides control the distinct activities of mir-181a-1 and mir-181c in early T cell development.* PLoS One, 2008. 3(10): p. e3592. doi: 10.1371/journal.pone.0003592.

[14] Calame, K., *MicroRNA-155 function in B Cells.* Immunity, 2007. 27(6): p. 825-7. doi: 10.1016/j.immuni.2007.11.010.

[15] Yin, Q., et al., *B-cell receptor activation induces BIC/miR-155 expression through a conserved AP-1 element.* J Biol Chem, 2008. 283(5): p. 2654-62. doi: 10.1074/jbc.M708218200.

[16] Rahadiani, N., et al., *Latent membrane protein-1 of Epstein-Barr virus induces the expression of B-cell integration cluster, a precursor form of microRNA-155, in B lymphoma cell lines.* Biochem Biophys Res Commun, 2008. 377(2): p. 579-83. doi:S0006-291X(08)01984-0.

[17] Linnstaedt, S.D., et al., *Virally induced cellular microRNA miR-155 plays a key role in B-cell immortalization by Epstein-Barr virus.* J Virol, 2010. 84(22): p. 11670-8. doi:JVI.01248-10.

[18] Xiao, C., et al., *MiR-150 controls B cell differentiation by targeting the transcription factor c-Myb.* Cell, 2007. 131(1): p. 146-59. doi:10.1016/j.cell.2007.07.021.

[19] Koralov, S.B., et al., *Dicer ablation affects antibody diversity and cell survival in the B lymphocyte lineage.* Cell, 2008. 132(5): p. 860-74. doi:S0092-8674(08)00268-7.

[20] Mendell, J.T., *miRiad roles for the miR-17-92 cluster in development and disease.* Cell, 2008. 133(2): p. 217-22. doi:S0092-8674(08)00449-2.

[21] Smyth, L.A., et al., *MicroRNAs affect dendritic cell function and phenotype.* Immunology, 2015. 144(2): p. 197-205. doi:10.1111/imm.12390.

[22] Liu, X., et al., *MicroRNA-148/152 impair innate response and antigen presentation of TLR-triggered dendritic cells by targeting CaMKIIalpha.* J Immunol, 2010. 185(12): p. 7244-51. doi:10.4049/jimmunol.1001573.

[23] Mi, Q.S., et al., *Lack of microRNA miR-150 reduces the capacity of epidermal Langerhans cell cross-presentation.* Exp Dermatol, 2012. 21(11): p. 876-7. doi:10.1111/exd.12008.

[24] Mi, Q.S., et al., *Deletion of microRNA miR-223 increases Langerhans cell cross-presentation.* Int J Biochem Cell Biol, 2013. 45(2): p. 395-400. doi:10.1016/j.biocel.2012.11.004.

[25] Bartoszewski, R., et al., *The unfolded protein response (UPR)-activated transcription factor X-box-binding protein 1 (XBP1) induces microRNA-346 expression that targets the human antigen peptide transporter 1 (TAP1) mRNA and governs immune regulatory genes.* J Biol Chem, 2011. 286(48): p. 41862-70. doi:10.1074/jbc.M111.304956.

[26] Zeng, Y., R. Yi, and B.R. Cullen, *MicroRNAs and small interfering RNAs can inhibit mRNA expression by similar mechanisms.* Proc Natl Acad Sci, 2003. 100(17): p. 9779-9784. doi: 10.1073/pnas.1630797100.

2

Preclinical Development of RNAi-Inducing Oligonucleotide Therapeutics for Eye Diseases

Tamara Martínez, Maria Victoria González, Beatriz Vargas, Ana Isabel Jiménez and Covadonga Pañeda

Abstract

RNA interference (RNAi) is a posttranscriptional mechanism of gene regulation present in eukaryotic cells. Inducers of RNAi are small molecules of RNA that act in the cytoplasm where they are able to impair translation of a specific mRNA to protein, hence modifying gene expression. The discovery of this mechanism in mammals led to the development of a new class of therapeutics with the aim of exploiting this endogenous mechanism of action. In the last decade, great efforts have been put into understanding RNAi and translating this accumulated knowledge into the design of modern therapeutics. With several compounds in phase III clinical development, the field is getting closer to its first market authorization. Here we make a thorough overview of the field of RNAi therapeutics in ophthalmology, one of the fields in which RNAi has been most successful.

Keywords: RNAi, eye diseases, ophthalmology, drug development

1. Introduction

Short interference RNAs (siRNA) are small molecules of double-stranded RNA of around 21 base pair long that specifically downregulate the expression of a target gene [1]. This mechanism of endogenous gene expression regulation, present in most eukaryotic cells, has been thoroughly used to study gene function [2]. SiRNAs exert their function in the cytoplasm of the cell, where they assemble with a several proteins to yield the RNA-induced silencing complex (RISC), a multimeric RNA–protein complex that recognizes complementary messenger RNAs (mRNA) and promotes their degradation, thus blocking the synthesis of specific proteins. RNAi may be activated by endogenous siRNAs synthesized in the nucleus of the cell and generated by subsequent processing within the cell cytoplasm to yield siRNAs. Alternatively, siRNAs can be exogenously introduced to mimic the action of endogenous RNAi triggers [3]. Among the benefits of RNAi are the potential of transiently silencing any given gene at any stage of development and to affect gene expression in specific anatomical regions without affecting nontargeted regions. These benefits are being used as a basis to develop a new class of innovative drugs that may reach the market in the next five years; the present report highlights the advances made in RNAi therapeutics on the field of ophthalmology.

2. The special environment of the eye: advantages and disadvantages

The eye has traditionally been considered a good organ for proof-of-concept studies to assess the efficacy of innovative therapies. It has a very particular anatomy that allows the transformation of sensory information into electrical signals that can be thereafter interpreted by the brain. Transformation and partial processing of sensory information takes place in the retina, located at the back of the eye. The correct function of the eye requires light to travel through several anatomical structures in order to reach the photosensitive retina; hence, these structures have to be transparent or semi-transparent to allow passage of light. The environment of the eye is extremely specialized to ensure that transparency is maintained, and there are several mechanisms in place to ensure that this specialized environment is preserved. One of the anatomical characteristics of the eye to allow light to travel through its structures is restricting the blood flow to regions where transparency is not strictly required.

In addition, access to the innermost regions of the eye is controlled by several barriers; these barriers isolate the eye from external aggressions and pathogens to but also limit the access of therapeutics. The influence of the particular anatomical features of the eye on drug delivery is further explained in Section 4 of this review. The barriers of the eye do not only isolate this organ from external aggressions or substances but also limit the access of internal elements; as such, the immune system has only limited access to the eye making the eye a partially immune-privileged region. Finally, the aqueous humor, the clear liquid that fills the eye and maintains its shape and pressure, has a very low content in proteins compared to serum. Among the proteins that are significantly reduced compared to other tissues are RNases and elements of the complement cascade. The reduced concentration of RNases increases the half-life of RNAs used as therapeutics, and reduction in the elements of the complement cascade further decreases the likelihood of an unwanted immune reactions to drugs.

In order to preserve its integrity, the eye has efficacious barriers to block the entrance of pathogens and substances that could potentially affect its sensory function. The eye has developed specific features that ensure that light travels through its tissues; this specialization of tissues to preserve visual function is also observed by the immune system [4]. Immune responses change the local environment of tissues and are frequently associated to tissue inflammation. In order to avoid these potentially harmful changes, the eye has a relatively immune privileged status. This immune privilege status is maintained by several mechanisms. Absence of lymphatic and blood vessels in certain areas and abundance of immunosuppressive factors in the aqueous humor are among these mechanisms [5]. On the other hand, the eye needs to be able to respond to situations in which its integrity can be compromised such as viral or bacterial infections. The innate immune response is the first system activated in response to aggressions; it acts like a watchdog mechanism recognizing pathogen-associated molecular patterns (PAMP). Depending on the molecular characteristics and location of the PAMP, different effectors of the innate response are activated; these responses can be mediated by toll-like receptors (TLR) or independent of these receptors. Toll-like receptors discriminate self-motifs from non-self-motifs [6]. There are ten known TLRs, and they differ in their subcellular localization and in the type of non-self-pattern they recognize. TLR1, TLR2, TLR4, TLR5, and TLR6 recognize components of bacterial walls and are located in the cell surface, whereas TLR3, TLR7, TLR8, and TLR9 recognize oligonucleotides and are sequestered in intracellular compartment. TLR3 binds to single- and double-stranded RNA, TLR7 binds to single-stranded RNA, and TLR9 binds to unmethylated CpG motifs, usually found in bacterial DNA. In the eye, the expression pattern of each TLRs varies depending on the anatomical structure; all TLRs are present in the corneal and retinal pigment epithelia; TLR4 is the predominant TLR in the rest of the eye structures where it localizes in resident antigen presenting cells [7, 8]. TLR-independent response mechanisms to cytoplasmic oligonucleotides include dsRNA-binding protein kinase, the RNA helicase (RIG-I), and oligoadenylate synthase enzyme. These proteins are cytoplasmic dsRNA sensors belonging to the antiviral innate immune system, which plays an important role in antiviral defense in response to viral infection and replication [9].

The first proof-of-concept studies to demonstrate the viability of silencing genes in the eye showed that the injection of siRNAs into the subretinal space or vitreous cavity could indeed downregulate specific genes. In these experiments, the downregulation of genes of the vascular endothelial growth factor (VEGF) family with siRNAs correlated with the inhibition of ocular neovascularization [10, 11]. The first set of these experiments used an adenoviral vector that codified for an siRNA designed against VEGF1. The subretinal injection of this vector 36 h after the induction of coroidal neovascularization (CNV) by laser reduced the areas of neovascularization compared to areas of mice injected with vector codifying for a scrambled siRNA [10]. In a subsequent study, Campochiaro and coworkers [10] demonstrated that the inhibition of ocular neovascularization could also be achieved by injecting a VEGFR1 siRNA directly, without an expression vector, into the vitreous cavity. The siRNA used in this study had the so-called canonical design, which comprises a 21-nucleotide guide strand and a complementary passenger strand annealed to form an siRNA duplex with a 19-bp dsRNA stem and 2 nucleotide 3′ overhangs at both ends [11].

In 2008, Kleinman and coworkers published a study in *Nature* demonstrating that the effect of siRNAs on CNV was mediated by activation of TLR3 rather than an effect on target [12]. The results of these studies showed that the effect of the siRNAs on CNV was dose-dependent but not dependent on sequence. In addition, the authors demonstrated that a minimum length of the siRNA was required in order for the molecules to have an effect on CNV; this length was show to be at least 21 nucleotides. The study also showed that the internalization of the siRNAs was not required for the inhibition of CNV as cells of the retinal pigment epithelium (RPE) abundantly express TLR3 on the cytoplasmic surface. The authors used several sequences to point out that the inhibition of CNV was mediated through an off-target effect. Using docking models, the authors showed that TLR3 and siRNAs were indeed able to interact with each other but the interaction was unstable when siRNAs were shorter than 21 nucleotides. A subsequent study by the same group showed that activation of TLR3 by IVT siRNAs led to caspase-3-mediated degeneration of the RPE questioning the safety these compounds as therapeutics for back of the eye diseases [13]. The findings of Kleinman and coworkers boosted research on alternative designs that could successfully block immune recognition; among the most commonly used strategies are incorporation of delivery systems and 2′-ribose modifications.

Finally, exogenous RNAs are quickly degraded by RNases present in tissues and body fluids [14]. These enzymes cut RNA into smaller components that are subsequently incorporated into the route of degradation of nucleotides. RNAses are present at high concentrations both in tissues, such as in spleen, liver, and pancreas, and in biological fluids, such as in serum [15]. In the eye, the tear fluid is rich in nucleases but the presence of these enzymes is considerably lower in most eye tissues, thus allowing for increased half-life of the siRNAs used for therapeutic purposes.

3. Efficacy studies: Animal models to study the eye

Proof-of-concept studies are required in order to demonstrate that a particular drug has the proposed activity. siRNAs are designed using bioinformatics tools to target specific regions of the human genome. Therefore, assessing the activity of these molecules in animal models requires that the siRNA has biological activity in the species chosen to perform the proof-of-concept study. With the sequencing of the genome of most animal models used in biomedical research, evaluating the homology of a given sequence between two species is nowadays common practice, but this does not warrant finding a fully homologous siRNA for all targeted genes. In cases where homologous sequences cannot be found, a surrogate compound can be used to perform animal efficacy studies; this entails designing a compound that targets the exact same region as the human version but with the sequence of the gene of the animal species to be used. Several animal models can be used to assess the activity of a compound. Here we highlighted the animal models used in the developmental programs of products included in the ophthalmic siRNA pipeline.

3.1. Ischemic optic neuropathy

Ischemic optic neuropathy is a sudden loss of vision caused by interruption or decreased blood flow in the optic nerve. There is a disagreement as to its pathogenesis, clinical features, and management because ischemic optic neuropathy is not a unique disease, but a spectrum of different types [16]. Ischemic optic neuropathy can be primarily of two types: anterior (AION) caused by the interruption of blood flow in the optic nerve head and posterior (PION) involving the posterior part the optic nerve. Both types can be further classified into different subtypes. AION comprises arteritic (A-AION) caused by giant cell arteritis and nonarteritic (NA-AION) caused by other than giant cell arteritis. NA-AION is by far the most common type and typically affects individuals between 55 and 67 years of age. The incidence of AION has only been thoroughly studied in the USA where there are 2.3–10.3 cases per 100,000 inhabitants; for the nonarteritic type, the numbers are lower: 0.36 per 100,000 inhabitants. NA-AION is characterized by visual loss, optic disc swelling, sometimes with flame hemorrhages on the swollen disc or nearby neuroretinal layer, and sometimes with nearby cotton wool exudates. Visual loss is usually sudden and may progress over several hours to days and even weeks [17].

Animal modes of this disease are used to assess efficacy of pharmaceuticals in development for these conditions and include the optic nerve crush model and the photoembolic stroke model. The optic nerve crush model is a general model in which surviving of the ganglionar cells can be studied in response to a physical damage to the optic nerve [18]. In the photoembolic stroke model, a photosensitive dye, such as rose bengal, is injected intravenously, and laser is specifically applied to the optic nerve head to activate the dye. The activation of the dye results in damage to the endothelial cells of the optic nerve vascular system that ultimately leads to thrombosis of vessels and edema of the optic nerve head [19].

3.2. Glaucoma

Glaucoma is a group of progressive optic neuropathies characterized by vision impairment and degeneration of retinal ganglion cells that if left untreated can lead to blindness. Glaucoma is the second leading cause of global irreversible blindness, and it has been estimated that 60.5 million people were affected by primary open-angle glaucoma (POAG) and primary angle–closure glaucoma (PACG) globally in 2010, a number expected to increase to nearly 80 million by 2020 [20]. The degeneration of the optic nerve is thought to be produced as a result of changes in intraocular pressure (IOP), but specific molecular mediators of these changes have yet to be identified. Because glaucoma may be asymptomatic until a relatively late stage where the nerve damage has already occurred, early diagnosis and treatment are crucial for halting the progression of the condition [21]. Reduction of IOP is the only proven strategy to treat the disease; thus, first-line treatments are aimed toward achieving this goal. There are several compounds currently used to lower IOP, and although most of them are efficacious in lowering IOP, they all come with their own set of side effects and tolerance to the drug is a frequent phenomenon. Tolerance or reduced response of the drug requires change of drug regimen, frequently increasing the dose or combining the prescribed pharmaceutical with another drug [22, 23].

Depending on the specific phase of the disease one wants to model, several animal models can be used [24]. If studying the degeneration of the retina is the main objective, the models mentioned in the previous section can be used. For assessing the IOP lowering efficacy of pharmaceuticals, models with increased IOP are generally used. The increased IOP model induced by oral water overloading in rabbits is a very easy and physiologic model to screen compounds. The basis behind this model is to give the animal an oral overload of water that will result in a transient increase in IOP [25]. Although the specific mechanism behind the increase in IOP following water overloading is uncertain, the model has been extensively used to perform rapid screens of IOP-lowering compounds. The main advantage of this model over other existing models of increased IOP is that the anatomical structure and physiology of eye structures are preserved allowing a normal response to hypotensive drugs. Other models of increased IOP include laser photocoagulation, intracameral injection of latex microspheres, topical application of prednisolone, light-induced reduced outflow facility, subconjunctival injection of betamethasone, or episcleral vein occlusion [24].

3.3. Dry eye disease

Dry eye disease (DED) is a multifactorial disease of the tear-fluid and ocular surface that results in symptoms of discomfort, visual disturbance, and tear film instability. It is accompanied by increased osmolarity of the tear film and inflammation of the ocular surface [26]. Common symptoms of this condition include blurry vision, tearing, and ocular pain. There are several factors that contribute to the etiology of the disease, among them are insufficient tear secretion, excessive evaporation, and alteration in the composition of the tear film [27]. Temporary changes of the composition of the tear film can cause an acute form of DED; if changes persist, the condition can turn into chronic DED. Damage to the ocular surface is usually more severe in the chronic forms than in the acute types. DED is frequently associated to other conditions such as Sjögren's disease or lachrymal gland dysfunction, but it can also be caused by vitamin deficiency, contact lens wear, and use of several prescription drugs. Acute DED is handled with lubricants and avoiding preservatives in concomitant eye drops. If DED persists, treatment options include procedures that favor tear retention such as punctal occlusion, moisture chamber spectacles, contact lenses, or pharmacologic agents that stimulate tear secretion. More severe forms may require the use of anti-inflammatory therapy [28]. Although some advances have been made toward alleviating some of the symptoms of DED, pain associated to this condition is not usually addressed. Pain in the eye results from stimulation of sensory axons of the trigeminal ganglion neurons innervating the cornea [29]. Animal models to assess the efficacy of ocular analgesics are extremely complex in terms of interpreting efficacy outcomes [30]. One of the commonly used models to study pain is the capsaicin-induced ocular pain model developed by Gertrudis and colleagues [31]. This model is based on the evaluation of animal behavior after topical ocular administration of capsaicin, a selective agonist of transient receptor protein vaniloid type 1 (TRPV1). Capsaicin applied locally to the eye activates TRPV1 inducing palpebral closure. Latency to open the eye and time required for complete palpebral opening can be used as measurements of the discomfort caused by capsaicin. Reference products used in this model include analgesics, in particular, capsazepine, the antagonist of TRPV1 channels.

3.4. Ocular allergy

Ocular allergies constitute a heterogenic group of diseases with a broad spectrum of clinical manifestations and include mild forms such as seasonal allergic conjunctivitis (SAC) and perennial allergic conjunctivitis (PAC), and more severe manifestations such as vernal keratoconjunctivitis (VKC), atopic keratoconjunctivitis (AKC), and giant papillary conjunctivitis (GPC). The severe forms can be associated to complications such as corneal damage and may cause vision loss. SAC and PAC are commonly IgE-mast cell-mediated hypersensitivity reaction to external allergens, whereas AKC and VKC are characterized by chronic inflammation involving several immune cell types. In SAC and PAC, allergens, with the help of antigen presenting cells, trigger a Th2-predominant immune response that induces B cells to release IgE. In SAC and PAC, allergen-induced local release of IgE prompts infiltration and degranulation of mast cells in Ca^{2+}-dependent mechanism. Mast cells liberate preformed inflammatory mediators such as histamine and leukotriene 4 that subsequently attract eosinophils amplify the allergic response [32]. The prevalence of ocular allergies in the general population is estimated to be around 40% in the United States [33] and up to 35% in Europe and the Middle East [34], but it is probably underestimated in most epidemiologic studies [35]. The primary treatment for ocular allergies includes avoidance of allergens, cold compresses, and lubrication. In persisting cases, symptoms can be treated using topical and oral decongestants, antihistamines, mast-cell stabilizers, or anti-inflammatory agents [36]. Allergic conjunctivitis can be modeled in animals by exposing them to allergens in the presence of an adjuvant [37]. The model developed by Magone and coworkers uses Female Balb/C mice that are sensitized with short ragweed and alum and several days later animals receive a topical dose of short ragweed pollen in the eye. A prescreening of mice can be performed in order to select only those animals that respond to allergens.

3.5. Age-related macular degeneration with choroidal neovascularization

Age-related macular degeneration (AMD) is the leading cause of severe vision loss in individuals over 50 years of age [38, 39]. AMD is caused by a combination of genetic and environmental factors. Risk factors include hypertension, cardiovascular disease, smoking, and high BMI. Among the genetic factors that confer susceptibility to developing AMD are variants in genes encoding complement pathway proteins [40, 41].

The underlying cause for AMD is accumulation of drusen or residual material produced by the renewal process of the external part of the photoreceptors of the retina in the retinal pigment epithelium (RPE). The accumulation of this material in the RPE leads to the production of inflammatory mediators that cause photoreceptor degeneration in the macula and severe vision loss [42]. In the early stages of the disease, accumulated drusen are small; the size and amount of this material increase as the disease progresses and central vision deteriorates.

There are two types of AMD: dry or wet. Dry AMD is characterized by the degeneration of the RPE and photoreceptors along with changes in pigmentation of the RPE. In the wet form, or choroidal neovascularization (CNV), fragile blood vessels of the choriocapillaris grow into the RPE and frequently leak blood and fluid that accumulate between RPE and choriocapillaris. As a result of these abnormal growths, dense scars are formed in the macula, and the RPE can detach. The wet form is more severe than the dry form and sometimes dry AMD can develop into wet AMD [43].

The characteristic invasion of leaky blood to the RPE in wet AMD is mediated by VEGF. The discovery of the relationship between VEGF and changes in vasculature in AMD led to the development of different approaches aimed to decrease the levels of this growth factor. Antibodies targeting VEGF are currently the first-line treatment for wet AMD [44]. The hallmark of wet AMD is CNV; thus, this is the lesion most extensively modeled in animals to assess efficacy of compounds targeting this disease. The laser-induced CNV model is by far the most used animal model. This model, initially developed for nonhuman primates (NHP), was later adapted into rodents. The basis for this model is to induce a break in Bruch's membrane using a high-energy laser. The experimental CNV can be analyzed in vivo using fluorescein angiography or optical coherence tomography or postmortem studying the retina explants. The model has been successfully transferred and validated to rat and mouse, and in both species, the chain of events taking place after lesion induction resembles the events that tale place in humans with the disease. Other models include the injection of subretinal materials such as Matrigel, angiogenic substances, macrophages, lipid peroxides, or polyethylene glycol. Although these models are promising, they have yet to be appropriately validated in order to be used as a proof of concept tools [45].

3.6. Diabetic retinopathy

Diabetic retinopathy (DR) is an ocular complication of diabetes mellitus characterized by microaneurysms in the retinal vasculature that eventually lead to ischemia and macular edema. Changes in the retina can cause rapid vision loss, and this complication is the main cause of visual loss in working-age individuals [46, 47].

The initial phase of DR, known as nonproliferative DR, is characterized by the thickening of the capillary basement membrane and apoptosis and migration of pericytes. These microchanges cause microaneurysms and small leakages in the vessels that irrigate the retina. As the disease progresses, interaction between endothelial cells and pericytes weakens and the capillaries become permeable; subsequent accumulation of fluids in the macula leads to edema. The microaneurysms in the retinal capillaries cause occlusions that compromise blood flow through the retina and cause ischemia. Local hypoxia upregulates angiogenic factors that cause capillaries to grow into the retina, preretinal space, and vitreous cavity; stage known as proliferative DR [48]. Among the upregulated angiogenic factors, one of the most critical is VEGF; the newly formed vessels are structurally deficient and very responsive to this growth factor. As such, antibodies used to treat AMD are also used for the treatment of diabetic retinopathy. DR is usually treated with laser photocoagulation, a procedure that does not cure the disease but mitigates the damage. IVT steroids can also be used to reduce accumulation of fluids within the retina. If accumulation of blood in the vitreous humor physically impedes laser photocoagulation, a vitrectomy has to be performed in order to remove the blood accumulated in the vitreous prior to laser photocoagulation.

There are several animal models of diabetic retinopathy, each of them comes with its own set of advantages and disadvantages. One of the most extensively used is the streptozotocin (STZ)-induced diabetes model. Intravenous or intraperitoneal injection of STZ causes a rapid and selective destruction of β-pancreatic cells leading to hyperglycemia and development of type I diabetes. The model has been used successfully in several animal species including rat, mouse, rabbit, dog, and monkey. Nonproliferative DR develops in this model, but microaneurysms and neovascularization are seldom observed; hence, this model can be complemented with the laser-induced CNV model explained in the AMD section. Larger animal models can be generated by surgically removing the pancreas, but this model is significantly more complicated to generate than the STZ model and has the same drawbacks. Alternatively, animals can be fed a high-galactose diet, but the induction of diabetes is considerably slower [50].

4. Biodistribution studies

Despite the extraordinary potential that RNAi technology displays in the treatment of ocular conditions, the transition of siRNAs programs to the clinical setting still presents challenges. The *in vivo* efficacy of therapies based on siRNAs depends on the ability of a given siRNA to reach the cytoplasm of its target cell in sufficient quantities to achieve its desired biological effect. The intrinsic characteristics of siRNAs such as their sensitivity to degradation by endogenous enzymes, their relative large size, and its negative charge limit their ability to cross biological barriers and reach the cytoplasm. Approaches used to overcome the hurdles associated to the use of siRNAs range from delivery strategies to chemical modifications aimed towards improving the pharmacological properties of the therapeutic siRNAs.

Drug delivery into the eye is challenging due to the presence of static and dynamics barriers that protect the internal tissues. The eye consists of two anatomically differentiated regions: the anterior and posterior segments. The anterior segment includes the cornea, conjunctiva, iris, ciliary body, lens, and anterior and posterior chambers; this segment occupies approximately the anterior third of the eyeball. The posterior segment is of greater size and comprises the sclera, choroid, retina, and vitreous cavity. There are significant anatomical, molecular, and immune differences between the two segments; thus, strategies to deliver molecules to the eye will be very different depending on the targeted segment [51]. The anterior region of the eye is protected from exterior aggressions by the cornea and tear film. The former is a specialized tissue composed of five layers that constitutes the main physical barrier to external molecules; the latter is an enzyme-rich fluid that degrades many biological molecules, lubricates the eye surface, and washes away materials from the cornea. In addition, many components of the tear film impede adhesion of molecules to the eye surface further restricting the access of external molecules to the inside of the eye.

Topical ocular administration of drugs is a patient-friendly administration route typically used for the treatment of pathologies affecting the anterior segment of the eye. However, molecules applied as eye drops are quickly cleared from the ocular surface being the bioavailability of a compound administered via this route less than 5% of the initially applied dose. The standard volume of a commercial eye drop is approximately 40 μL whereas the normal volume of the tear fluid in the ocular surface is 7-9 μl. Once an eye drop is instilled in the inferior conjunctival sac, there is a transient increase of volume that activates the blinking reflex and increases the turnover of the tear film. Most of the content of the eye drop is spilled out by the blinking process or drained via the nasolacrimal duct, drastically reducing the amount of compound available to the eye.

The cornea is a specialized tissue covering the anterior part of the eye whose main functions are protecting against harmful agents and provide the eye with a refractive surface that allows the entrance of light. The human cornea is approximately 0.5–0.8 mm thick, and it is comprised of three layers: the outer five cell layer-epithelium, a thick stroma rich in type I collagen fibrils and glycosaminoglycans, and the innermost endothelium consisting in a single layer of cuboidal cells. The corneal epithelium is separated from the stroma by the Bowman's membrane, while the stroma and the corneal endothelium are separated by the Descemet's membrane. There are no blood vessels irrigating the cornea; this provides the required transparency for the transmission and refraction of light. Drugs can take two paths to penetrate the corneal epithelium: the intracellular path crossing through the cells or the paracellular path bypassing between cells. The cells of the corneal epithelium are tightly attached to each other with gap and tight junctions that restrict the diffusion of large molecules between them [52–54]. The cross-cellular pathway requires molecules to be able to cross cell membranes; thus, lipophilic molecules have an easier access through this route. The stroma is an aqueous matrix composed mainly of hydrated collagen and proteoglycans with few keratinocytes interspersed [55]. The hydophilicity/lipophilicity index determines the diffusion of molecules through this layer [56]. The remaining layers of the cornea do not significantly hamper the diffusion of molecules.

Contrary to the cornea, the conjunctiva is a highly vasculated tissue that covers the sclera and lines the inner surface of the eyelids. Its main functions are producing mucus and tears to lubricate the eye surface and preventing the entrance of pathogens. The human conjunctiva is composed of three layers: the outer epithelium, the substantia propia, containing nerves and blood vessels, and the submucosa layer, which provides a lightweight attachment to the underlying sclera [57]. The histology of the stratified outer epithelium varies among the different regions of the conjunctiva, but it is always its apical portion that controls the permeability of the conjunctiva. The conjunctiva offers an attractive route for drug delivery when compared to the cornea as it presents an extended exchange surface as well as a superior rate of permeation to large hydrophilic molecules. The sclera is structurally continuous with the cornea and extends posteriorly from the limbus. The composition of the sclera is similar to that of the corneal stroma, mainly collagen and mucopolysaccharides leaving numerous channels through which drugs can freely diffuse [58]. The sclera is poorly vascularized and significantly more permeable than the cornea but less permeable than conjunctiva. There are contradictory reports on the ability of charged molecules to cross the sclera. Some authors suggest that this layer is more permeable to negatively charged molecules [59, 60], whereas other studies suggest that positively charged molecules cross the sclera more easily [61, 62]. Ranta and colleagues suggested that the negative charge of mucopolysaccharides in the sclera prevented the diffusion of negatively charged molecules as a consequence of charge repulsion. Other studies have shown that negatively charged molecules are indeed able to cross the sclera, pointing out that size is the limiting factor in drug diffusion through this layer [52]. It should be noted, however, that scleral drug binding does not necessarily impair drug delivery to inner structures of the eye; it can also act as a drug-depot if the molecules are subsequently released [63].

Ophthalmic drugs topically administered to de eye can thus be absorbed through two pathways: crossing the cornea to reach the aqueous humor or through the conjunctival-scleral pathway reaching the uvea. The relative quantity that enters through each of the above-mentioned routes varies significantly depending on the size and hydrophilic/lipophilic ratio of the molecule. Generally, the conjunctival route is favored for large hydrophilic molecules, whereas small lipophilic drugs are mainly absorbed through the cornea. The ability of siRNAs to penetrate the cornea has been thoroughly demonstrated as well as the ability of these compounds to enter the cytoplasm of cells within the cornea. However, the capacity of siRNAs to cross the cornea is limited, as shown by the limited amount of siRNAs detected in the aqueous humor following eye drop instillation [64].

Increasing the amount of compound in the anterior part may be of interest for treating specific conditions. For this purpose, several strategies can be used in order to improve delivery: (a) increasing the residence time of the compound within the eye surface, (b) directing the molecule to a specific region to increase the concentration locally, and (c) increasing absorption by using physical methods. Increasing the contact time of the molecule with the eye surface can be achieved by the use of formulations or depots. Formulations that increase viscosity and/or mucoadhesion of ophthalmic solutions are generally believed to increase absorption into the eye. Polymers such as methylcellulose or polyvinyl alcohol can be added to solutions to increase viscosity and consequently increase residence and reduce clearance time. Mucoadhesion may be increased by formulating the oligonucleotides in polymers such as chitosans. These polymers have been used to deliver DNA vectors into the eye [65]. Encapsulation in liposomes and in thermosensitive gels has also been attempted as a means to increase the absorption and residence time of oligonucleotides in the eye [53]. In these studies, a 16-mer was formulated in liposomes, a thermosensitve 27% poloxamer gel, and HEPES; the results of these studies showed that the amount of compound reaching external tissues such as the conjunctiva or the cornea was higher when the compound was prepared in HEPES. By contrast, access to deeper regions of the anterior chamber such as the sclera or the iris benefited from the increased viscosity of the gel formulation [53]. One of the main drawbacks of biodistribution studies to assess the fate of a given siRNA in a formulation is that most of these studies focus on the fate of nanocarrier rather than on that of the oligonucleotide and the relative distribution of the molecule among the tissues of the eye. Therefore, thorough biodistribution, studies are required to address the specific characteristics required for improving delivery for specific conditions. Targeting has scarcely been used to deliver oligonucleotides into the eye; there are a few reports using dendrimers with the goal of increasing the intracellular concentration of therapeutic oligonucleotides in specific regions of the eye, but advances toward this goal are as of today very limited [66]. Physical methods such as iontophoresis have also been studied aiming to increasing the amount of molecule that crosses the cornea and/or the sclera. Although iontophoresis certainly increases the amount of transcorneal and transcleral delivery of oligonucleotides mainly to the anterior chamber but also to some degree to the posterior chamber, the use of this method has not been extensively used most likely because the equipment required to apply the required current would entail in-office administration, which would significantly complicate repeated administrations [67].

Drugs administered systemically enter the eye from the bloodstream crossing the capillaries of the choroid. The choroid is a vascular layer composed of capillaries and supported by Bruch's membrane, a connective membrane of 2–4 μm thickness. Bruch's membrane separates the choroid from the retina, forming the main barrier to permeation across the choroid-Bruch's bilayer [68]. The permeability of Bruch's membrane is relatively high; charge and size do not generally affect drug diffusion through this membrane unless molecules are very big; in this particular case, size can reduce the rate of permeation [52]. The choroid is a thin and permeable membrane that is rich in melanin. Melanin has the ability to bind and retain many drugs hampering their entrance to the retina and inner tissues. Other drug-binding proteins, depending on the kinetic of binding/unbinding retention of drugs by melanin, can completely block the entrance or act as a reservoir for slow release [69]. Studies to assess the binding of oligonucleotides to melanin have yielded different results suggesting that at least some oligonucleotides bind to melanin reducing the rate of entrance to the retina; this is however not the case for all oligonucleotides [52, 70].

The main restriction to free permeation of molecules from systemic circulation to the eye is the blood–retinal barrier (BRB). The BRB is composed of the inner BRB and the outer BRB. The former includes the vessels of the retina, whereas the latter is constituted by the retinal pigment epithelium (RPE). Both barriers possess cells with well-developed intercellular junctions that control the permeation of substances through them. Larger molecules, such as proteins and nucleic acids, are mostly able to permeate through the choroid but have limited ability to cross the inner BRB; thus, drugs need to exit the choroid and penetrate the eye crossing the outer BRB. Crossing through the outer BRB usually requires high systemic doses increasing the likelihood of systemic side effects [71]. Delivery to the posterior segment of systemic or topically applied drugs requires thus crossing several biological barriers. Therefore, invasive administration procedures are frequently used to deliver drugs to the posterior segment. In addition, the outflow mechanisms of the eye rapidly remove drugs from the posterior chamber; thus, reaching clinically meaningful concentrations is challenging. Most of the programs developing siRNAs for eye conditions target the back of the eye; consequently, the route of administration is IVT injection. The concentration of siRNAs administered IVT is highest in the vitreous body, but they are also found in the RPE, choroid, and retina. Depending on the stability of the siRNAs, the compound can also be found in systemic circulation.

There are numerous reports describing strategies that can be of benefit for increasing the concentration of drugs in the back of the eye. Several nonbiodegradable (Retisert™, Illuvien™, and Vitrasert®) and one biodegradable (Ozurdex™) intravitreal ocular inserts are currently used in the clinical practice for delivering small molecules to the back of the eye. It is expected that these advances be soon incorporated into the pipelines of larger molecules such as proteins and oligonucleotides.

5. Toxicology

siRNAs are chemically synthesized oligonucleotides and are considered New Chemical Entities (NCEs) by the US and European Regulatory Authorities since 2009 when the European Commission excluded siRNAs from the definition of advanced medicinal products [72]. Toxicology assessment of RNAi-based drugs should be carried out following guidelines for NCEs, and the complete toxicology battery is usually performed following the recommendations of the ICH M3 (R2) guideline [73]. The guideline recommends the assessment of toxicology in two species, a rodent and a nonrodent, at three dose levels and for a duration that should be similar or superior to the clinical trial to be carried out. This assessment should include acute or maximum tolerated toxicology studies and repeated-dose toxicity studies. Additionally, pharmacokinetics, safety pharmacology, genotoxicity, carcinogenicity, and specific toxicology studies should be carried out depending of the nature, indication, and route of administration of the product. On the other hand, some aspects of RNAi-based products are closer to new biological entities (NBEs) rather than NCEs; therefore, some of the requirements of the ICH S6 guideline also apply to the design of their developmental programs [74]. As such, a tailored toxicology assessment program should be designed combining the recommendations outlined in the above-mentioned guidelines and the accumulated experience of numerous compounds tested in preclinical and clinical development.

Toxicology of ocular products depends on their biodistribution and on their biological activity. Moreover, the disease process, age, sex, or eye pigmentation are other potential factors affecting the toxicity profile of the ocular drug assessed. Additionally, the bioavailability of the RNAi compound will depend mainly on the route of ocular administration (topical versus injected) and on the physicochemical characteristics of the drug.

Toxicities arising from oligonucleotides, including siRNAs, can be classified into hybridization-dependent toxicities and hybridization-independent toxicities. Hybridization-dependent toxicities can be caused by (a) exaggerated pharmacology: excessive activity on the intended target or by (b) off-target effect: modulating gene expression of an unintended target by an RNAi-mediated mechanism. Hybridization-independent toxicities are often associated to the chemistry of the siRNA. Identified hybridization-independent toxicities include prolongation of activating partial thromboplastin time (aPTT), complement activation, and immunostimulation [75, 76, 77].

5.1. General toxicology

Up to date, numerous siRNAs indicated for different eye conditions have entered clinical trials (Table 1); the administration route of four of these compounds is by IVT injection, whereas the remaining two compounds are topically administered in eye drops. The toxicology assessment of these products follows the traditional schedule for NCEs; this schedule entails general toxicology studies in two species, a rodent and a nonrodent species of variable length. Most programs up to date have used NHP as the nonrodent species; this is because siRNAs are species specific, and it is likely that the assessment of toxicology was performed in the only species in which the compound was pharmacologically active. The rabbit is very frequently used to assess toxicology of compounds under development for eye conditions. Many sponsors of programs using NHP or dog as nonrodent species chose to use the rabbit as second species, although this animal is not a rodent per se. Reasons behind this choice include the similarity of the volume of the eye to that of humans and the difficulty of administering controlled doses to smaller animals. This is particularly relevant when the compound is administered by IVT injection. This rationale has also been followed for developing siRNAs for eye conditions; only in one case, PF-04523655, rats were used as the rodent species, and the rest of the programs developing siRNAs for eye indications used the rabbit (New Zealand White rabbits or Dutch Belted rabbit) as second species for toxicology assessment.

Most programs developing siRNAs for eye conditions include acute/maximum tolerated dose and repeat-dose toxicology studies. The length of these studies is determined by the indication, stage of development, and envisioned duration of treatment. In addition, most programs do not only perform toxicology studies using the envisaged route of administration but also include studies using intravenous route to challenge the systemic exposure to the drug and assess potential dose limitations and target organs.

5.2. Genotoxicity

As mentioned in the previous section, both the ICH M3 (R2) and the ICH S6 guidelines apply to programs developing siRNAs [73]. The ICH S6 states that the range and type of genotoxicity studies routinely conducted for NCEs are usually not applicable to NBEs; pointing out that performance of these studies is only required when there is a cause of concern. The European Medicines Agency (EMA) issued a reflection paper on the assessment of the genotoxic potential of antisense oligodeoxynucleotides in January 2005. This paper recommends addressing at least two issues in regards to oligonucleotides which may indicate a cause of genotoxic concern: (a) analyzing the potential of incorporation of phosphorothioated (PS) oligonucleotides into the DNA and (b) addressing the potential of triplex formation of oligonucleotides with the DNA fiber [78]. Several years of experience with siRNAs indicate that full-length molecules are very unlikely to interact with the DNA. Thus, the potential cause of concern may arise from the genotoxic potential of metabolites or chemical contaminants. The metabolism of nonmodified oligonucleotides yields naturally occurring nucleotides that are subsequently incorporated to the natural degradation pathways of endogenous nucleic acids; thus, toxicities derived from these degradation products are not expected. Modified oligonucleotides, on the other hand, incorporate very frequently backbone modifications to reduce nuclease activity and improve other pharmaceutical properties of the molecule. The most commonly used backbone modification is the replacement of a nonbridging oxygen on the backbone between two ribonucleotides with a sulfur to create a PS linkage [79]. Extensive genotoxicity studies performed with Vitravene, a PS antisense oligonucleotide administered by IVT injection, indicate that oligonucleotides with a PS backbone do not pose genotoxic potential [80, 81]. These results are in line with those obtained in the analysis of over 30 compounds studied in the standard battery, all of which have yielded negative results. Other modified nucleotides could potentially be incorporated into nucleotide pools and be thereafter used to synthesize DNA. The standard battery of tests would detect eventual damaging potential of theses degradation products.

The EMA reflection paper also recommends assessing the potential of triplex formation with the DNA fiber. For this to happen, siRNA molecules would have to enter the nucleus of the cell and their structure should include an uninterrupted homopurine stretch of at least 10–12 base pairs that should be homologous a given region of the DNA. In silico design of siRNAs usually addresses these issues and candidates with the ability of forming triplex are avoided prior to lead selection.

5.3. Carcinogenicity

Standard carcinogenicity studies are generally not required for NBEs, but these studies may be required for siRNAs depending on their chemical structure, clinical dosing, patient population, or biological activity. If the in vitro test genotoxic studies indicate that there is cause of concern for carcinogenic potential, further studies should be required in relevant models.

For RNAi products under development for eye conditions, the systemic bioavailability of these products is usually very low, and a waiver to perform these studies may be justified. Strategies should be discussed in a case-by-case base with the competent health authorities.

5.4. Reproductive and developmental toxicity

The assessment of reproductive and developmental toxicity is required to support the use of a given pharmaceutical in pregnant women, women of childbearing potential, or children. These studies are regulated by the ICH S5 guideline [82], which recommends assessing the effect of drugs on all phases of the reproductive cycle. These recommendations apply to siRNA-based products. Nevertheless, due to the unique features of these compounds, a case-by-case approach should be followed for each product, and the requirements for these studies should be discussed with the competent authorities. The target, indication, chemical modifications, and systemic bioavailability of the RNAi-based drugs are features that may influence in the nature of the required studies.

Because the toxicity of siRNAs can be caused by exaggerated pharmacology whenever reproductive toxicity studies are required, they should be performed in a pharmacologically active species. Standard reproductive toxicity species in rodents or rabbits can give information on toxicity related to chemical structure. However, if the compound is not active in these species or if the biological activity is not deemed to be equivalent to the foreseen activity in humans, the assessment of reproductive risk may be conducted using an active analog or in a nonrodent species in which the compound has biological activity. If the former strategy is chosen, the toxicity and toxicokinetic profile of the surrogate should be taken into account when interpreting the results. If the compound is only active in NHPs, studies should only be performed in cases where there is cause for concern. In these particular cases, the number of animals should be optimized, and a combined enhanced pre-and postnatal developmental study can be performed as recommended for NBEs. In NHP studies, the assessment of reproductive toxicology is usually studied by histopathologic examination of the reproductive organs as part of the general toxicology studies of at least three months. The timing of reproductive and developmental studies depends on when women of childbearing potential are to be included in clinical trials. If NHPs are required for the assessment, the timing is more flexible due to the length and complexity of the studies [83].

5.5. Local tolerance

Local tolerance studies are required for all topically administered drugs. In most cases, the potential adverse events caused by local tolerance issues are evaluated in the single or repeated-dose toxicology studies, reducing the number of animals required for the program.

5.6. Safety pharmacology

According to ICH S7A, safety pharmacology studies can be reduced or eliminated for locally applied products as well as for NBEs that achieve highly specific receptor targeting [84]. For siRNAs under development for ophthalmology indications, separate safety studies are not usually required; instead, functional safety end points are incorporated into the repeated-dose toxicity studies. If the results of the toxicology studies indicate that there is cause of concern, separate safety pharmacology studies should be performed.

6. Programs in development and future ahead

Table 1 summarizes the status of siRNA-based therapies under development for ocular conditions. As mentioned in Section 1, the eye offers multiple advantages for developing innovative therapies; therefore, studies in the eye pioneered the field of siRNA therapeutics. The first siRNA to enter clinical development for an ophthalmology indication was bevasiranib in 2004 shortly followed by sirna-027. Bevasiranib targeted VEGFA, whereas sirna-027 targeted VEGFR1. These compounds were being developed for the treatment of AMD as both showed a dose-dependent inhibition of experimental CNV in animal models that correlated with knockdown of their respective target genes [10, 85]. As mentioned in Section 1, in 2008 Kleinman and coworkers published a study demonstrating that the effect of siRNAs targeting VEGF and VEGFR on CNV was not mediated by an on-target effect but by activation of TLR3 [12]. The results of these studies indicated that the effect of the compounds on CNV was sequence-independent and mediated by siRNAs of 21 base pairs or longer. The study also showed that the internalization of the siRNAs was not required for the inhibition of CNV as cells of the RPE abundantly express TLR3 on the cytoplasmic surface. The authors used several sequences, including those of the siRNAs undergoing clinical trials at the time, to point out that the inhibition of CNV by both bevasiranib and sirna-027 was mediated through an off-target effect. A subsequent study by the same group showed that activation of TLR3 by IVT siRNAs led to caspase-3-mediated degeneration of the retinal pigment epithelium (RPE) questioning the safety of these compounds as therapeutics for back of the eye diseases [13].

The clinical development of bevasiranib was halted in 2007 and of sirna-027 in 2009 both as a result of not reaching or being unlikely to reach their respective efficacy end points in phase III trials.

The findings of Kleinman and coworkers boosted research on alternative designs that were not able to activate TLR3, and as result, a new generation of compounds is currently undergoing clinical trials. Currently, the most advanced siRNAs-based programs for ocular indications are Quark's QPI-007 and Sylentis' bamosiran (SYL040012). QPI-007 is a 19-nt modified siRNA-targeting caspase 2 currently in phase II/III for the treatment of nonarteritic anterior ischemic optic neuropathy (NAION) [86]. QPI-1007 has shown to be safe when IVT injected to animal models and humans. The ongoing phase II/III trial for this compound analyzes the potential of multiple IVT doses to improve visual acuity in patients suffering NAION [87, 88]. Bamosiran is a canonical-designed naked siRNA-targeting β2-adrenergic receptor (ADRB2) under development for the treatment of increased IOP associated to glaucoma [64, 89–91]. Glaucoma is a degenerative, chronic disease of the optic nerve that can lead to blindness if left untreated [92]. The mechanistic details of optic nerve degeneration observed in glaucoma are yet to be fully detailed, but it is well established that reduction of intraocular pressure avoids development of the disease. ADRB2 controls the production and release of aqueous humor. The aqueous humor is responsible for maintaining optimal IOP. Treatment with topic beta-blockers has shown to efficiently reduce intraocular pressure, but currently approved beta-blockers are small molecules and are thus able to reach systemic circulation and systemic organs were they cause unwanted effects. The rationale behind bamosiran is developing a locally active compound that efficiently knocks down ADRB2 in the eye but that is not able to reach systemic tissues reducing the likelihood of side effects. The compound is administered in eye drops and has been shown to be well tolerated in animal models and humans [64, 93]. Three different doses of bamosiran are currently being studied in an active controlled phase IIb trial. Previous clinical trials with this compound have shown promising results in healthy individuals and patients with ocular hypertension [91, 93].

SYL1001 is a naked 19-bp siRNA-targeting transient receptor potential vanilloid-1 (TRPV1) for the treatment of ocular pain. TRPV1 is a cation channel permeable to calcium activated by heat, low pH, and capsaicin among other signals. This receptor is present in several structures of the eye where it has been related, among other roles, to nociception [94]. SYL1001 has shown to be safe when administered in eye drops to animals and humans and to have analgesic effect in the capsaicin-induced eye pain model. The compound is currently undergoing a phase I/II for the treatment of ocular pain associated to dry eye disease, a condition for which no specific treatment currently exists [89].

PF-655 is a chemically stabilized siRNA-targeting RTP801, a stress-induced adaptor protein that inhibits mTOR function upstream to TSC1/TSC2 complex in response to a variety of stresses. Expression of RTP801 is upregulated in response to ischemia, hypoxia, and/or oxidative stress. Intravitreal injection of PF-655 in preclinical animal models of laser-induced CNV leads to silencing of RTP801 via a RNAi mechanism without TLR activation and reduction of CNV volume, vessel leakage, and infiltration of inflammatory cells into the choroid [95–97]. This compound has undergone phase II clinical trials for the treatment of diabetic macular edema and wet AMD. Treatment with PF-655 of patients with diabetic macular edema over a period of 12 months caused a dose-dependent improvement in visual acuity compared to the visual acuity observed in patients treated with laser photocoagulation [98]. A subsequent phase IIb trial was conducted with a new set of doses but terminated because the primary end point was not likely to be achieved. The compound was thereafter tested in combination with ranibizumab, a monoclonal antibody fragment that targets VEGF and is the current gold standards for treatment of the disease. The results of this study have not yet been disclosed. PF-655 has also been studied in patients suffering wet AMD. In this indication, the compound did not show improvement as a single agent or in combination with ranibizumab in mean visual acuity after 3 months of dosing.

Self-delivery rxRNAs (sd-rxRNAs) incorporate 2′-F and 2-′O-Me modifications and a sterol conjugate on the sense strand with the goal of improving stability and cellular uptake. These compounds have a 19-nt antisense strand and a sense strand usually shorter than 15 nt resulting in an asymmetric duplex with a phosphorothioated single-stranded tail on the antisense strand [99]. These compounds have been tested in vitro where they have shown to be able to induce target knockdown in different cell lines. In vivo analysis of their activity showed these compounds are readily taken-up by retinal cells and that the compound is evenly distributed throughout the mouse retina. Several of these compounds are under development for different eye conditions and are expected to enter clinical development shortly.

SYL116011 is a naked 19-bp siRNA targeting the calcium release-activated calcium modulator 1 (ORAI1). Store-operated Ca^{2+} entry (SOCE) is activated in response to depletion of endoplasmic reticulum Ca^{2+} pools. Activation of SOCE induces Ca^{2+} entry from extracellular compartments, and this is mediated by store-operated CRAC channels. CRAC channels are composed of calcium sensing proteins called STIM (stromal interaction molecule) and pore-forming subunits named ORAI [100]. Mammalian cells have three ORAI isoforms: ORAI1, ORAI 2, and ORAI3; although ORAI2 and 3 fulfill the same role as ORAI1, the Ca^{2+} currents generated by these proteins are around two- to threefold smaller than the ones generated by ORAI1 [101]. There is growing evidence that indicates that short-term and long-term activation of immune cells in allergic responses is mediated by influx of Ca^{2+} to immune cells from the extracellular compartment. Short-term responses include the degranulation of mast cells and the activation of effector cytolitic T cells. Indeed, mast cells lacking either STIM1 or ORAI1 show a considerable defect in degranulation [102, 103]. Long-term responses involve the modulation of gene expression that controls B and T cell proliferation and differentiation. SYL116011 is being developed for the treatment of ocular allergies and has shown to reduce immediate clinical signs in a mouse model of ragweed pollen-induced ocular allergy. The decrease in clinical signs was accompanied by a reduction in the number of infiltrating eosinophils in the conjunctiva and reduction of allergy biomarkers.

TT-211 is an AAV-encapsidated construct that expresses a single shRNA modeled into a miRNA backbone that inhibits the expression of VEGF-A for the treatment of wet AMD. VEGF-a protein is responsible initiating a signaling cascade that stimulates the growth of new blood vessels, a hallmark of wet AMD. TT-231 is a second-generation candidate designed to express three shRNAs, which target three different genes, VEGF receptor 2, PDGF-β, and human complement factor B, proteins that play a major role in the progression of wet AMD. Both these compounds are yet in a preclinical phase; IND filing is planned for 2017.

STP601 is a multitargeted siRNA cocktail nanoparticle formulation administered by IVT injection under development for treatment of wet AMD, proliferative diabetic retinopathy, and herpetic stromal keratitis. The cocktail includes three 25-mer siRNA duplexes targeting VEGF, VEGFR1, and VEGFR2. Inhibiting this clinically validated pathway at the endothelial cells lining the interior of the growing blood vessels is thought to halt the progression of AMD. This product is currently in preclinical stage.

AQA001 is a single-stranded long chain nonmodified ribonucleotide connected by a proline-derived linker that self-anneals to form a shot-hairpin structure within the molecule. The compound targeting periostin acts through an RNAi mechanism and is being developed for the treatment of diabetic retinopathy. The compound has shown positive result in a proof-of-concept study of CNV [104].

Name	Indication	Target	Route	Sponsor	Status
Bevasiranib	AMD with choroidal neovascularization	VEGFA	IVT	Opko Health	Halted in Phase III
Sirna-027	AMD with choroidal neovascularization	VEGFR1	IVT	Allergan	Halted in Phase III
QPI-1007	NAION	Caspase 2	IVT	Quark	Active, Phase II/III
	Primary Angle Closure Glaucoma				Active, Phase IIa
PF-655	AMD with choroidal neovascularization	RTP801	IVT	Quark/Pfizer	Completed, Phase II
	Diabetic macular oedema				Completed, Phase IIb
SYL040012	Glaucoma	β2 ADR	Eye Drop	Sylentis	Completed, Phase IIb
SYL1001	Ocular pain associated to dry eye disease	TRPV1	Eye Drop	Sylentis	Active, Phase IIa
Undisclosed	Retinal scaring	Undisclosed	Intraocular	RXi	Preclinical
Undisclosed	Corneal scaring	Undisclosed	Eye Drop	RXi	Preclinical
Undisclosed	Macular degeneration	Undisclosed	Intraocular	RXi	Preclinical
SYL116011	Ocular allergy	ORAI1	Eye Drop	Sylentis	Preclinical
TT-211	AMD	VEGF-A	IVT	Benitec	Preclinical
TT-231	AMD	VEGF-A, PDGFβ and CFB	IVT	Benitec	Preclinical
STP601	AMD and retinopathy	VEGF-VFGFR1-VEGF2	IVT	Sirnaomics	Preclinical
AQA001	Diabetic macular oedema	Periostin	IVT	Aqua Therapeutics	Preclinical

Table 1. siRNAs in development for ocular indication.

7. Conclusion

RNA interference is on the verge of becoming a new class of therapeutics [105]. The field of ophthalmology has played a major role in advancing siRNAs from laboratory tools to the clinic. In the last few years, significant advances have been made in the understanding of how these molecules enter and exert its action in the eye and in the identification of the main hurdles that still need to be addressed. The introduction of chemical modifications as well as the understanding of the immune activation in the eye has significantly improved the pharmaceutical properties of compounds for eye conditions. However, the following years will tell whether improvements on these molecules are enough to be of therapeutic value in the field of ophthalmology or not.

Author details

Tamara Martínez[#], Maria Victoria González[#], Beatriz Vargas, Ana Isabel Jiménez and Covadonga Pañeda[*]

*Address all correspondence to: cpaneda@sylentis.com

Sylentis SAU, Tres Cantos, Madrid, Spain

[#]These two authors contributed equally to the review.

References

[1] Zamore PD, Tuschl T, Sharp PA, Bartel DP. RNAi: double-stranded RNA directs the ATP-dependent cleavage of mRNA at 21 to 23 nucleotide intervals. Cell. 2000;101:25–33. DOI: 10.1016/S0092-8674(00)80620-0.

[2] Elbashir SM, Harborth J, Lendeckel W, Yalcin A, Weber K, Tuschl T. Duplexes of 21-nucleotide RNAs mediate RNA interference in cultured mammalian cells. Nature. 2001;411:494–8. DOI:10.1038/3507810735078107.

[3] Aagaard L, Rossi JJ. RNAi therapeutics: principles, prospects and challenges. Adv Drug Deliv Rev. 2007;59:75–86. DOI:10.1016/j.addr.2007.03.2005.

[4] Perez VL, Saeed AM, Tan Y, Urbieta M, Cruz-Guilloty F. The eye: a window to the soul of the immune system. J Autoimmun. 2013;45:7–14. DOI: 10.1016/j.jaut.2013.06.011.

[5] Stein-Streilein J. Immune regulation and the eye. Trends Immunol. 2008; 29:548–54. DOI: 10.1016/j.it.2008.08.002.

[6] Chang ZL. Important aspects of Toll-like receptors, ligands and their signaling pathways. Inflamm Res. 2010;59:791–808. DOI: 10.1007/s00011-010-0208-2

[7] Yu FS, Hazlett LD. Toll-like receptors and the eye. Invest Ophthalmol Vis Sci. 2006;47:1255–63. DOI: 10.1167/iovs.05-0956.

[8] Kumar MV, Nagineni CN, Chin MS, Hooks JJ, Detrick B. Innate immunity in the retina: Toll-like receptor (TLR) signaling in human retinal pigment epithelial cells. J Neuroimmunol. 2004;153:7–15. DOI: 10.1016/j.jneuroim.2004.04.018

[9] Sioud M. RNA interference and innate immunity. Adv Drug Deliv Rev. 2007 ;59:153–63. DOI: 10.1016/j.addr.2007.03.006.

[10] Reich SJ, Fosnot J, Kuroki A, Tang W, Yang X, Maguire AM, et al. Small interfering RNA (siRNA) targeting VEGF effectively inhibits ocular neovascularization in a mouse model. Mol Vis. 2003;9:210–6.

[11] Shen J, Samul R, Silva RL, Akiyama H, Liu H, Saishin Y, et al. Suppression of ocular neovascularization with siRNA targeting VEGF receptor 1. Gene Ther. 2006;13:225–34. DOI: 10.1038/sj.gt.3302641.

[12] Kleinman ME, Yamada K, Takeda A, Chandrasekaran V, Nozaki M, Baffi JZ, et al. Sequence- and target-independent angiogenesis suppression by siRNA via TLR3. Nature. 2008;452:591–7. DOI: 10.1038/nature06765.

[13] Kleinman ME, Kaneko H, Cho WG, Dridi S, Fowler BJ, Blandford AD, et al. Short-interfering RNAs induce retinal degeneration via TLR3 and IRF3. Mol Ther. 2011;20:101–8. DOI: 10.1038/mt.2011.212.

[14] Turner JJ, Jones SW, Moschos SA, Lindsay MA, Gait MJ. MALDI-TOF mass spectral analysis of siRNA degradation in serum confirms an RNAse A-like activity. Mol Biosyst. 2007;3:43–50. DOI: 10.1039/b611612d.

[15] Weickmann JL, Glitz DG. Human ribonucleases. Quantitation of pancreatic-like enzymes in serum, urine, and organ preparations. J Biol Chem. 1982 10;257:8705–10.

[16] Hayreh SS. Ischemic optic neuropathy. Prog Retin Eye Res. 2009;28:34–62. DOI: 10.1016/j.preteyeres.2008.11.002.

[17] Hayreh SS. Management of ischemic optic neuropathies. Indian J Ophthalmol. 2011;59:123–36. DOI: 10/4103/0301-4738.77024.

[18] Tang Z, Zhang S, Lee C, Kumar A, Arjunan P, Li Y, et al. An optic nerve crush injury murine model to study retinal ganglion cell survival. J Vis Exp. 2011;50:2685. DOI: 10.3791/2685.

[19] Bernstein SL, Guo Y, Kelman SE, Flower RW, Johnson MA. Functional and cellular responses in a novel rodent model of anterior ischemic optic neuropathy. Invest Ophthalmol Vis Sci. 2003;44:4153–62.

[20] Quigley HA, Broman AT. The number of people with glaucoma worldwide in 2010 and 2020. Br J Ophthalmol. 2006;90:262–7. DOI: 10.1136/bjo.2005.08-0875-7.

[21] Caprioli J, Varma R. Intraocular pressure: modulation as treatment for glaucoma. Am J Ophthalmol. 2011;152:340–4 e2. DOI: 10.1016/j.ajo.2011.05.029.

[22] Alward WL. Medical management of glaucoma. N Engl J Med. 1998;339:1298–307.

[23] Beckers HJ, Schouten JS, Webers CA, van der Valk R, Hendrikse F. Side effects of commonly used glaucoma medications: comparison of tolerability, chance of discon-

tinuation, and patient satisfaction. Graefes Arch Clin Exp Ophthalmol. 2008;246:1485–90. DOI: 10.1007/s00417-008-0875-7.

[24] Bouhenni RA, Dunmire J, Sewell A, Edward DP. Animal models of glaucoma. J Biomed Biotechnol. 2012;2012:692609. DOI: 10.1155/2012/692609.

[25] McDonald TO, Hodges JW, Borgmann AR, Leaders FE. The water-loading test in rabbits. A method to detect potential ocular hypotensive drugs. Arch Ophthalmol. 1969;82:381–4.

[26] The definition and classification of dry eye disease: report of the Definition and Classification Subcommittee of the International Dry Eye WorkShop (2007). Ocul Surf. 2007;5:75–92.

[27] Gayton JL. Etiology, prevalence, and treatment of dry eye disease. Clin Ophthalmol. 2009;3:405–12.

[28] Management and therapy of dry eye disease: report of the Management and Therapy Subcommittee of the International Dry Eye WorkShop (2007). Ocul Surf. 2007;5:163–78.

[29] Rosenthal P, Borsook D. The corneal pain system. Part I: the missing piece of the dry eye puzzle. Ocul Surf. 2012;10:2–14. DOI: 10.1016/j.jtos.2012.01.002.

[30] Johnson CB. New approaches to identifying and measuring pain. In: Scientific Assessment and Management of Animal Pain. OIE, OIE Technical Series; 2008. p. 131–44.

[31] Gonzalez GG, Garcia de la Rubia P, Gallar J, Belmonte C. Reduction of capsaicin-induced ocular pain and neurogenic inflammation by calcium antagonists. Invest Ophthalmol Vis Sci. 1993;34:3329–35.

[32] Bielory L. Allergic and immunologic disorders of the eye. Part II: ocular allergy. J Allergy Clin Immunol. 2000;106:1019–32. DOI: 10.1067/mai.2000.111238.

[33] Singh K, Axelrod S, Bielory L. The epidemiology of ocular and nasal allergy in the United States, 1988–1994. J Allergy Clin Immunol. 2010;126:778–83 e6. DOI: 10.1016/j.jaci.2010.06.050.

[34] Petricek I, Prost M, Popova A. The differential diagnosis of red eye: a survey of medical practitioners from Eastern Europe and the Middle East. Ophthalmologica. 2006;220:229–37. DOI: 10.1159/000093076.

[35] Leonardi A, Bogacka E, Fauquert JL, Kowalski ML, Groblewska A, Jedrzejczak-Czechowicz M, et al. Ocular allergy: recognizing and diagnosing hypersensitivity disorders of the ocular surface. Allergy. 2012;67:1327–37. DOI: 10.1111/all.12009.

[36] van Cauwenberge P, Bachert C, Passalacqua G, Bousquet J, Canonica GW, Durham SR, et al. Consensus statement on the treatment of allergic rhinitis. European Academy of Allergology and Clinical Immunology. Allergy. 2000;55:116–34.

[37] Magone MT, Chan CC, Rizzo LV, Kozhich AT, Whitcup SM. A novel murine model of allergic conjunctivitis. Clin Immunol Immunopathol. 1998;87:75–84.

[38] Rudnicka AR, Jarrar Z, Wormald R, Cook DG, Fletcher A, Owen CG. Age and gender variations in age-related macular degeneration prevalence in populations of European ancestry: a meta-analysis. Ophthalmology. 2011;119:571–80. DOI: 10.1016/j.ophtha.2011.09.027.

[39] Smith W, Assink J, Klein R, Mitchell P, Klaver CC, Klein BE, et al. Risk factors for age-related macular degeneration: pooled findings from three continents. Ophthalmology. 2001;108:697–704.

[40] Clemons TE, Milton RC, Klein R, Seddon JM, Ferris FL, 3rd. Risk factors for the incidence of advanced age-related macular degeneration in the Age-Related Eye Disease Study (AREDS) AREDS report no. 19. Ophthalmology. 2005;112:533–9. DOI:10.1016/j.ophtha.2004.10.047.

[41] Chen Y, Bedell M, Zhang K. Age-related macular degeneration: genetic and environmental factors of disease. Mol Interv. 2010;10:271–81. DOI: 10.1124/mi.10.5.4.

[42] Ding X, Patel M, Chan CC. Molecular pathology of age-related macular degeneration. Prog Retin Eye Res. 2009;28:1–18. DOI: 10.1016/j.preteyeres.2008.10.001.

[43] Sallo FB, Peto T, Leung I, Xing W, Bunce C, Bird AC. The international classification system and the progression of age-related macular degeneration. Curr Eye Res. 2009;34:238–40. DOI: 10.1080/02713680802714058.

[44] Keane PA, Tufail A, Patel PJ. Management of neovascular age-related macular degeneration in clinical practice: initiation, maintenance, and discontinuation of therapy. J Ophthalmol. 2011;2011:752543. DOI: 10.1155/2011/752543.

[45] Pennesi ME, Neuringer M, Courtney RJ. Animal models of age related macular degeneration. Mol Aspects Med. 2012;33:487–509. DOI: 10.1016/j.mam.2012.06.003.

[46] Scanlon PH, Aldington SJ, Stratton IM. Epidemiological issues in diabetic retinopathy. Middle East Afr J Ophthalmol. 2013;20:293–300. DOI: 10.4103/0974-9233.120007.

[47] Yau JW, Rogers SL, Kawasaki R, Lamoureux EL, Kowalski JW, Bek T, et al. Global prevalence and major risk factors of diabetic retinopathy. Diabetes Care. 2012;35:556–64. DOI: 10.2337/dc11-1909.

[48] Qian H, Ripps H. Neurovascular interaction and the pathophysiology of diabetic retinopathy. Exp Diabetes Res. 2011;2011:693426. DOI: 10.1155/2011/693426.

[49] Willard AL, Herman IM. Vascular complications and diabetes: current therapies and future challenges. J Ophthalmol. 2012;2012:209538. DOI: 10.1155/2012/209538.

[50] Mi XS, Yuan TF, Ding Y, Zhong JX, So KF. Choosing preclinical study models of diabetic retinopathy: key problems for consideration. Drug Des Devel Ther. 2014;8:2311–9. DOI: 10.2147/DDDT.S72797.

[51] Ghate D, Edelhauser HF. Ocular drug delivery. Expert Opin Drug Deliv. 2006;3:275–87. DOI: 10.1517/17425247.3.2.275.

[52] Pescina S, Govoni P, Antopolsky M, Murtomaki L, Padula C, Santi P, et al. Permeation of proteins, oligonucleotide and dextrans across ocular tissues: experimental studies and a literature update. J Pharm Sci. 2015;104:2190–202. DOI: 10.1002/jps.24465.

[53] Bochot A, Mashhour B, Puisieux F, Couvreur P, Fattal E. Comparison of the ocular distribution of a model oligonucleotide after topical instillation in rabbits of conventional and new dosage forms. J Drug Target. 1998;6:309–13. DOI: 10.3109/10611869808996838.

[54] Fattal E, Bochot A. Ocular delivery of nucleic acids: antisense oligonucleotides, aptamers and siRNA. Adv Drug Deliv Rev. 2006;58:1203–23. DOI: 10.1016/j.addr.2006.07.020.

[55] Barar J, Javadzadeh AR, Omidi Y. Ocular novel drug delivery: impacts of membranes and barriers. Expert Opin Drug Deliv. 2008;5:567–81. DOI: 10.1517/17425247.5.5.567.

[56] Prausnitz MR, Noonan JS. Permeability of cornea, sclera, and conjunctiva: a literature analysis for drug delivery to the eye. J Pharm Sci. 1998;87:1479–88.

[57] Ahmed I, Patton TF. Importance of the noncorneal absorption route in topical ophthalmic drug delivery. Invest Ophthalmol Vis Sci. 1985;26:584–7.

[58] Hamalainen KM, Kananen K, Auriola S, Kontturi K, Urtti A. Characterization of paracellular and aqueous penetration routes in cornea, conjunctiva, and sclera. Invest Ophthalmol Vis Sci. 1997;38:627–34.

[59] Cheruvu NP, Kompella UB. Bovine and porcine transscleral solute transport: influence of lipophilicity and the Choroid–Bruch's layer. Invest Ophthalmol Vis Sci. 2006;47:4513-22. DOI: 10.1167/iovs.06–0404.

[60] Maurice DM, Polgar J. Diffusion across the sclera. Exp Eye Res. 1977;25:577–82.

[61] Wen H, Hao J, Li SK. Influence of permeant lipophilicity on permeation across human sclera. Pharm Res. 2010;27:2446–56. DOI: 10.1007/s11095-010-0237-0.

[62] Lin CW, Wang Y, Challa P, Epstein DL, Yuan F. Transscleral diffusion of ethacrynic acid and sodium fluorescein. Mol Vis. 2007;13:243–51.

[63] Dubey S, Kalia YN. Understanding the poor iontophoretic transport of lysozyme across the skin: when high charge and high electrophoretic mobility are not enough. J Control Release. 2014;183:35–42. DOI: 10.1016/j.jconrel.2014.03.027.

[64] Martinez T, Gonzalez MV, Roehl I, Wright N, Paneda C, Jimenez AI. In vitro and in vivo efficacy of SYL040012, a novel siRNA compound for treatment of glaucoma. Mol Ther. 2014;22:81–91. DOI: 10.1038/mt.2013.216.

[65] de la Fuente M, Seijo B, Alonso MJ. Novel hyaluronic acid-chitosan nanoparticles for ocular gene therapy. Invest Ophthalmol Vis Sci. 2008;49:2016–24. DOI: 10.1167/iovs.07-1077.

[66] Marano RJ, Wimmer N, Kearns PS, Thomas BG, Toth I, Brankov M, et al. Inhibition of in vitro VEGF expression and choroidal neovascularization by synthetic dendrimer peptide mediated delivery of a sense oligonucleotide. Exp Eye Res. 2004;79:525–35. DOI: 10.1016/j.exer.2004.06.023.

[67] Berdugo M, Valamanesh F, Andrieu C, Klein C, Benezra D, Courtois Y, et al. Delivery of antisense oligonucleotide to the cornea by iontophoresis. Antisense Nucleic Acid Drug Dev. 2003;13:107–14. DOI: 10.1089/108729003321629647.

[68] Hussain AA, Starita C, Hodgetts A, Marshall J. Macromolecular diffusion characteristics of ageing human Bruch's membrane: implications for age-related macular degeneration (AMD). Exp Eye Res. 2010;90:703–10. DOI: 10.1016/j.exer.2010.02.013.

[69] Cheruvu NP, Amrite AC, Kompella UB. Effect of eye pigmentation on transscleral drug delivery. Invest Ophthalmol Vis Sci. 2008;49:333–41. DOI: 10.1167/iovs.07-0214.

[70] Pitkanen L, Ranta VP, Moilanen H, Urtti A. Binding of betaxolol, metoprolol and oligonucleotides to synthetic and bovine ocular melanin, and prediction of drug binding to melanin in human choroid-retinal pigment epithelium. Pharm Res. 2007;24:2063–70.DOI: 10.1007/s11095-007-9342-0.

[71] Rowe-Rendleman CL, Durazo SA, Kompella UB, Rittenhouse KD, Di Polo A, Weiner AL, et al. Drug and gene delivery to the back of the eye: from bench to bedside. Invest Ophthalmol Vis Sci. 2014;55:2714–30. DOI: 10.1167/iovs.13-13707.

[72] Srivatsa S. Regulatory challenges. Eur Biopharm Rev. 2012;Spring.

[73] ICH Harmonised Tripartite Guideline. Guidance on Nonclinical Safety Studies for the Conduct of Human Clinical Trials and Marketing Authorization for Pharmaceuticals M3(R2). 2009.

[74] Addendum to ICH Harmonised Tripartite Guideline preclinical safety evaluation of biotechnology-derived pharmaceuticals S6(R1). 2011.

[75] Kornbrust D, Cavagnaro J, Levin A, Foy J, Pavco P, Gamba-Vitalo C, et al. Oligo safety working group exaggerated pharmacology subcommittee consensus document. Nucleic Acid Ther. 2013;23:21–8. DOI: 10.1089/nat.2012.0399.

[76] Levin AA, Henry S. Toxicology of oligonucleotide therapeutics and understanding the relevance of the toxicities. In: Preclinical Safety Evaluation of Biopharmaceuticals: A Science-Based Approach to Facilitating Clinical Trials. John Wiley & Sons, Inc.; 2008. p. 537–75.

[77] Lindow M, Vornlocher HP, Riley D, Kornbrust DJ, Burchard J, Whiteley LO, et al. Assessing unintended hybridization-induced biological effects of oligonucleotides. Nat Biotechnol. 2012;30:920–3. DOI: 10.1038/nbt.2376.

[78] CHMP SWP reflection paper on the assessment of the genotoxic potential of antisense oligodeoxynucleotides, EMEA/CHMP/SWP/199726/2004. 2005.

[79] Eckstein F. Phosphorothioates, essential components of therapeutic oligonucleotides. Nucleic Acid Ther. 2014;24:374–87. DOI: 10.1089/nat.2014.0506.

[80] Henderson S. Preclinical safety evaluation of oligonucleotides. Developments in Life-Sciences 2008;9:4–8.

[81] Safety of intravitreous fomivirsen for treatment of cytomegalovirus retinitis in patients with AIDS. Am J Ophthalmol. 2002;133:484–98.

[82] ICH Harmonized Tripartite Guideline on detection of toxicity to reproduction for medicinal products & toxicity to male fertility S5(R2), CPMP/ICH136/95 modification. 2000.

[83] Cavagnaro J, Berman C, Kornbrust D, White T, Campion S, Henry S. Considerations for assessment of reproductive and developmental toxicity of oligonucleotide-based therapeutics. Nucleic Acid Ther. 2014;24:313–25. DOI: 10.1089/nat.2014.0490.

[84] ICH Harmonised Tripartite Guideline on the Safety Pharmacology Studies for Human Pharmaceuticals, CPMP/ICH/539/00-ICH S7A. 2000.

[85] Garba AO, Mousa SA. Bevasiranib for the treatment of wet, age-related macular degeneration. Ophthal Eye Dis. 2010;2:75–83. DOI: 10.4137/OED.S4878.

[86] Anderson J, Akkina R. CXCR4 and CCR5 shRNA transgenic CD34+ cell derived macrophages are functionally normal and resist HIV-1 infection. Retrovirology. 2005;2:53. DOI: 10.1186/1742-4690-2-53.

[87] Ahmed Z, Kalinski H, Berry M, Almasieh M, Ashush H, Slager N, et al. Ocular neuroprotection by siRNA targeting caspase-2. Cell Death Dis. 2011;2:e173. DOI: 10.1038/cddis.2011.54.

[88] Solano EC, Kornbrust DJ, Beaudry A, Foy JW, Schneider DJ, Thompson JD. Toxicological and pharmacokinetic properties of QPI-1007, a chemically modified synthetic siRNA targeting caspase 2 mRNA, following intravitreal injection. Nucleic Acid Ther. 2014;24:258–66. DOI: 10.1089/nat.2014.0489.

[89] Pañeda C, Martínez T, Wright N, Jimenez AI. Recent advances in ocular nucleic acid-based therapies: the silent era. In: Adio A, editor. Ocular Diseases. InTech; 2012. p. 157–86. DOI: 10.5772/48454

[90] Pañeda C. SYL040012, a siRNA for the treatment of glaucoma. Acta Ophthalmol. 2013;91:0–0. DOI: 10.1111/j.1755-3768.2013.4227.x.

[91] Pañeda C, Gonzalez V, Martínez T, Ruz V, Vargas B, Jiménez AI, editors. RNAi based therapies for ocular conditions. Proceedings of the 11th ISOPT 2014; 19–22 June 2014, Reykjavik. Medimond; 2014. p. 25–30.

[92] Weinreb RN, Khaw PT. Primary open-angle glaucoma. Lancet. 2004;363:1711–20. DOI: 10.1016/S0140-6736(04)16257-0.

[93] Moreno-Montanes J, Sadaba B, Ruz V, Gomez-Guiu A, Zarranz J, Gonzalez MV, et al. Phase I clinical trial of SYL040012, a small interfering RNA targeting beta-adrenergic receptor 2, for lowering intraocular pressure. Mol Ther. 2014;22:226–32. DOI: 10.1038/mt.2013.217.

[94] Martinez-Garcia MC, Martinez T, Paneda C, Gallego P, Jimenez AI, Merayo J. Differential expression and localization of transient receptor potential vanilloid 1 in rabbit and human eyes. Histol Histopathol. 2013;28:1507–16. 10.14670/HH-28.1507.

[95] Brafman A, Mett I, Shafir M, Gottlieb H, Damari G, Gozlan-Kelner S, et al. Inhibition of oxygen-induced retinopathy in RTP801-deficient mice. Invest Ophthalmol Vis Sci. 2004;45:3796–805. DOI: 10.1167/iovs.04-0052.

[96] Lee DU, Huang W, Rittenhouse KD, Jessen B. Retina expression and cross-species validation of gene silencing by PF-655, a small interfering RNA against RTP801 for the treatment of ocular disease. J Ocul Pharmacol Ther. 2012; 28:222–30. DOI: 10.1089/jop.2011.0116.

[97] Rittenhouse KD, Johnson TR, Vicini P, Hirakawa B, Kalabat D, Yang AH, et al. RTP801 gene expression is differentially upregulated in retinopathy and is silenced by PF-04523655, a 19-Mer siRNA directed against RTP801. Invest Ophthalmol Vis Sci. 2014;55:1232–40. DOI: 10.1167/iovs.13-13449.

[98] Nguyen QD, Schachar RA, Nduaka CI, Sperling M, Basile AS, Klamerus KJ, et al. Dose-ranging evaluation of intravitreal siRNA PF-04523655 for diabetic macular edema (the DEGAS study). Invest Ophthalmol Vis Sci. 2012;53:7666–74. DOI: 10.1167/iovs.12-9961.

[99] Byrne M, Tzekov R, Wang Y, Rodgers A, Cardia J, Ford G, et al. Novel hydrophobically modified asymmetric RNAi compounds (sd-rxRNA) demonstrate robust efficacy in the eye. J Ocul Pharmacol Ther. 2013;29:855–64. DOI: 10.1089/jop.2013.0148.

[100] Liao Y, Erxleben C, Abramowitz J, Flockerzi V, Zhu MX, Armstrong DL, et al. Functional interactions among Orai1, TRPCs, and STIM1 suggest a STIM-regulated heteromeric Orai/TRPC model for SOCE/Icrac channels. Proc Natl Acad Sci U S A. 2008;105:2895–900. DOI: 10.1073/pnas.0712288105.

[101] Prakriya M, Feske S, Gwack Y, Srikanth S, Rao A, Hogan PG. Orai1 is an essential pore subunit of the CRAC channel. Nature. 2006;443:230–3. DOI: 10.1038/nature05122.

[102] Holowka D, Calloway N, Cohen R, Gadi D, Lee J, Smith NL, et al. Roles for ca(2+) mobilization and its regulation in mast cell functions. Front Immunol. 2012;3:104. DOI: 10.3389/fimmu.2012.00104.

[103] Ma HT, Beaven MA. Regulators of Ca(2+) signaling in mast cells: potential targets for treatment of mast cell-related diseases? Adv Exp Med Biol. 2011;716:62–90. DOI: 10.1007/978-1-4419-9533-9_5.

[104] Nakama T, Yoshida S, Ishikawa K, Kobayashi Y, Zhou Y, Nakao S, et al. Inhibition of choroidal fibrovascular membrane formation by new class of RNA interference therapeutic agent targeting periostin. Gene Ther. 2014;22:127–37. DOI: 10.1038/gt.2014.112.

[105] Martinez T, Jiménez AI, Pañeda C. Short-interference RNAs: becoming medicines. EXCLI J. 2015;14:714–46. DOI: 10.17179/excli2015-297

3

Perspectives on RNA Interference in Immunopharmacology and Immunotherapy

Zhaohua Hou, Qiuju Han, Cai Zhang and Jian Zhang

Abstract

RNA interference (RNAi), mediated by short interfering RNA (siRNA), vector-derived short hairpin RNA (shRNA) and microRNA (miRNA), brings about revolutionary features to basic biomedical research and clinical application. New drugs based on RNAi have been developed for therapeutic applications. The family of RNAi molecules are efficient agents to modulate mammalian immune system, and many studies reported that these molecules could manipulate immune defence, surveillance and homeostasis. Both perfect match of siRNA/shRNA and non-perfect match of miRNA could be beneficial for designing RNAi-based drugs for treatment of tumour and viral infection. This chapter provides a view to control or utilize the immune regulation of various small RNAs that should help researchers to understand the successful clinical application of RNAi.

Keywords: RNA interference, siRNA, miRNA, immunopharmacology, immunotherapy

1. Introduction

RNA interference (RNAi) is a conserved mechanism against exogenous nucleic acid and transposon transcripts in plants and lower animals. No matter of transfected siRNA, vector-delivered shRNA or pre-miRNA (transcribed mainly by Pol II) , Dicer (DCLs) and Agronaute (AGO) family proteins efficiently process small RNAs into short double-stranded RNA(dsRNA). Further, dsRNAs assemble into the RNAi-induced silencing (protein) complex (RISC) to guide and cleave target mRNA, promote mRNA degradation or inhibit mRNA translation. The great potential of RNAi is to specifically repress the expression of disease-causing genes while avoiding undesirable effects.

It is well accepted that siRNA can be recognized by endosomal pathways, Toll-like receptor 3 (TLR3), TLR7, TLR8 and cytoplasmic pathways, retinoic acid-inducible gene I (RIG-I), melanoma differentiation-associated antigen 5 (MDA-5) and RNA-activated protein kinase (PKR), resulting in immune activation [1–5]. For example, it has been demonstrated that siRNA can cause activation of at least three key transcription factors, including NF-κB, interferon regulatory factor 3 (IRF-3) and IRF-7, and stimulate interferon (IFN) secretion. This activates T cells and dendritic cells (DCs) in the spleen in a TLR7-dependent manner [2,6]. Furthermore, 5′-triphosphate siRNA was demonstrated to activate RIG-I signal pathway, and then natural killer (NK) cells and DCs were activated [7,8]. In most circumstances, immune system stimulation is regarded as an unwanted side effect; therefore, siRNA-induced immune response should be controlled by using proper delivery system or chemical modification, although immune stimulation has been proved to be essential in cancer treatment and viral infection.

miRNAs are critical in regulating the development, differentiation, function and destiny of immune cells, including DCs, granulocytes, monocytes/macrophages, NK and natural killer T (NKT) cells and B and T lymphocytes. miRNAs influence both innate and adaptive immune defence and individual miRNAs may contribute their implications to various immune-mediated diseases. Furthermore, pattern recognition receptors (PRRs), kinases, adaptors, inflammatory factors and IFN could all be targets of miRNAs. Extra effort has been made to develop miRNA-based oligos or vectors for anti-infection purpose by manipulating corresponding immune genes.

In addition to silencing of targeted genes in a sequence-specific manner, components of RNAi technology often induce immune response. Several strategies were reported to design RNAi molecules with gene silencing and immune regulatory properties. Bifunctional molecules rely on the activation of PRRs such as TLR7/8, TLR9 or RIG-I, or just rely on down-regulation of target gene. This chapter summarizes RNAi-involved immune responses in the past 10 years and discusses the anticipated therapeutic application.

2. Chemically synthesized siRNA and vector-derived shRNA

2.1. RNAi drugs based on targeting specific immune genes

Immune disorders, both autoimmune diseases and immune defective or deficiency, are always caused by high-level overexpression of certain immune genes. A variety of immune inhibitory genes can serve as targets for RNAi-mediated gene silencing. Targeting specific immune suppressor could re-balance immune network and subsets.

Elevated activity of signal transducer and activator of transcription 3 (STAT3) has been found in several kinds of human tumours. Use of RNAi to knockdown STAT3 expression and inhibit its activation would reduce the tumour cell growth such as pancreatic cancer, colorectal cancer, melanoma and hepatocarcinoma cells. STAT 3 knockdown could induce bystanders immune response in vitro and in vivo, where CD4+, CD8+ and NKT cells were activated as well as the secretion of interferon-γ (IFN-γ), interleukin-12 (IL-12) and tumour necrosis factor alpha (TNF-α) was increased significantly [9–11]. siRNA-STAT3, synthetically linked to CpG (agonist of TLR9), was demonstrated to silence immune suppressor STAT3 gene in TLR9+ myeloid cells and B cells. This strategy of therapy leads to activation of various populations of immune cells, including DCs and macrophages, that ultimately induce potent anti-tumour immune responses [10,12]. Hossain DM et al. recently reported that CpG-siRNA-STAT3 conjugates could efficiently silence the target expression, and abrogate inhibition of CD8+ T cells in patients who received myeloid-derived suppressor cells (MDSCs) [13]. Researchers proved that immune-stimulation-inducing CpG(A)-STAT3-siRNA was non-toxic for normal human leukocytes [14]. In another experiment, Luo Z et al. [15] generated a nano-vaccine loaded with poly I:C (a TLR3 agonist) and STAT3 siRNA. Researchers found this kind of siRNA could promote the maturation of DC and reverse immunosuppression in the tumour micro-environment; the function of inhibitory cells in tumour-draining lymph nodes were inhibited; thus, anti-tumour immune responses were potently induced; and the survival were prolonged [15]. Therefore, STAT3 siRNAs are expected to be a promising immunomodulatory drugs to improve the treatment efficacy of cancer vaccines by abrogating tumour immunosuppression.

Suppressor of cytokine signalling 1 (SOCS1) is a negative regulator of antigen-presenting cell (APC)-based immune response. Silencing of SOCS1 gene expression by RNAi is essential for DCs to enhance Ag-specific anti-tumour immunity [16]. SOCS1-silenced bone marrow dendritic cells (BMDCs) were more potent in suppressing tumour growth [17]. When SOCS1 was silenced, maturation of DCs (i.e. expressions of CD80, CD40, CD86 and major histocompatibility complex II [MHC II]) was significantly accelerated. As a result, SOCS1 inhibition up-regulated the expression of IFN-γ and IL-12, and decreased IL-4 secretions, which induced Th1 cell differentiation and thereby affected the development of Th2 cell. The combined nanoparticle (NP) delivery, which can render both tumour antigen and siRNA-SOCS1 to BMDCs, simultaneously could enhance immunotherapeutic effects in BMDC-based cancer therapy [16,18]. DC-targeted delivery of SOCS1 siRNA has been shown to enhance antifungal immunity in response to *Candida albicans* in vitro and HIV-specific cytotoxic T cell in mice [16, 19]. This evidence suggests the use of SOCS1–siRNA, as a potent adjuvant to improve immune response.

A20 is usually regarded as an attractive target for siRNA-mediated gene knockdown in DCs because it is a negative feedback regulator of multiple pro-inflammatory signal transduction. Several reports demonstrated that RNAi-mediated A20 silencing in DCs enhanced expression of co-stimulatory molecules (CD80, CD86, CD40 and MHC class II) and pro-inflammatory cytokines (IL-6 and TNF-α). Tumour-infiltrating cytotoxic T lymphocytes (CTLs), T helper cells that produced IL-6 and TNF-α were also activated by siA20-DC. A20 silencing in DCs can enhance the immune response against self-tumour-associated antigens [20,21]. Furthermore, A20-silenced DCs were proved to overcome CD4+CD25+regulatory T (Treg) cell suppression [21,22]. A20-silenced DCs could skew naive CD4+ T cells towards Th1 cell, but not Treg, Th2 or Th17 cells. Because a high amount of IL-10 was produced in A20-silenced DCs, simultaneous down-regulation of IL-10 and A20 resulted in enhanced T cell stimulatory capacity in DCs. A20 down-regulation resulted in enhanced CTLs immune response by the NF-κB and AP-1 pathways [20,23]. RNAi of A20 has enabled DCs to gain a potent ability to activate CTLs and Th cells, and inhibit Treg, providing a novel strategy to promote a tumour immune response.

Programmed death ligand (PD-L) is another exciting target on the surface of antigen-presenting cells (APCs); PD-L/PD-1 interactions were related to functional impairment and exhaustion of tumour antigen-specific CD8+ T cells. Although PD-L antibody exerts a potent anti-tumour effect, previous reports [24] have demonstrated that PD-L1-siRNA-PEI were preferentially and avidly engulfed by tumour-associated CD11c+PD-L1+ tolerogenic DCs at ovarian cancer locations. This kind of nanoparticle uptake stimulated multiple TLRs signalling, mainly via myeloid differentiation factor 88 (MyD88). Then, regulatory DCs activated into potent stimulators of CTLs that led to significant anti-tumour immunity in mouse models of ovarian cancer. Most importantly, PD-L knockdown DCs showed superior potential to expand minor histocompatibility antigen (MiHA)-specific CD8+ effector and memory T cells from leukaemia patients early after donor lymphocyte infusion and later during relapse. Combined PD-L1 and PD-L2 knockdown resulted in improved proliferation of CD4+ T cells and enhanced cytokine production [25,26]. In addition, another report demonstrated the improved effector functions of tumour-specific CD4+ and CD8+ human T cells by siRNA-mediated silencing of PD-1 ligands, PD-L1 or PD-L2 [27]. These results suggest that siRNA-mediated knockdown of PD-L is a fascinating strategy to inhibit a negative regulatory mechanism of tumour-specific T cells.

siRNA-CD40, delivered by a novel delivery system with a poly-dA extension at the 5'-end of the siRNA sense strand that was stably incorporated into 1,3-β-glucan, was captured and incorporated into DCs through its receptor, Dectin [28]. This strategy could induce antigen-specific Tregs, resulting in the permanent acceptance of mouse cardiac allografts. CD40 knockdown significantly suppressed Th1-type cytokines and induced Th2-type cytokines in rats with myocarditis. Knockdown of CD40 in experimental autoimmune myocarditis (EAM) rats promoted Foxp3 gene expression and increased Treg cells [29].

In addition, when silencing of CD40 or CD80/CD86, DCs exhibited suppressed allostimulatory activity with impaired APC function. In the well-established collagen-induced arthritis (CIA) model, multigene-silenced DCs were capable of delaying onset of joint pathology. Therapeutic effects of gene-silenced DCs were mediated by the inhibition of collagen II-specific Ab production and suppression of T cell recall responses. Also, multigene-silenced DCs inhibited Th1 and Th17 response, demonstrating IFN-γ and IL-2 inhibition [30]. Thus, inhibition of specific co-stimulatory molecules of DCs reveals a promising approach of suppressing immune responses in autoimmunity. These findings highlight the potential of immunomodulation of siRNA-CD40, and have important implications for developing RNAi-based clinical therapy in the transplantation field.

It is well documented that tumours could secrete immunosuppressive molecules, including the cytokines transforming growth factor β (TGF-β) and IL-10. This creates an immunosuppressive environment, which inhibits anti-tumour immunity. The suppression of Treg cell, induced by targeting TGF-β1 using siRNA, can enhance the efficacy of a DC vaccine against a poorly immunogenic tumour in mice [31]. Nanoparticle-delivered TGF-β siRNA enhances vaccination against advanced melanoma, and the tumour micro-environment was modified with increased levels of tumour-infiltrating CD8+ T cells and decreased level of regulatory T cells [32]. siRNA targeting IL-10 receptor α (siIL-10RA) initiated the significant antigen-specific CD8+ T cell immune responses. Concordantly, the combination of knockdown of IL-10RA and TGF-βR in DCs showed significant up-regulation of MHC I, enhancing co-stimulatory molecules CD40, CD80, CD86 and chemokine CCR7 after lipopolysaccharide (LPS) stimulation. It induced the strongest anti-tumour effects in the TC-1 P0 (a cervical cancer model expressing the human papillomavirus [HPV]-16 E7 antigen) tumour model, and even in the immune-resistant TC-1 (P3) ones [33]. These data revealed that siRNA co-targeting immunosuppressive molecules enhance the potency of DC-based immunotherapeutics.

High-mobility group box 1 (HMGB1) is highly expressed in tumour cells and increased levels of HMGB1 in tumour cells are usually associated with a greater tumour angiogenesis, growth, invasion and metastasis. Knockdown of tumour cell-derived HMGB1 by shRNA did not affect tumour cell growth, while naturally acquired long-lasting tumour-specific IFN-γ- or TNF-α-producing CD8+ T cell responses were induced, and ability to induce Treg was attenuated. This led to naturally acquired CD8 T cell-dependent anti-tumour immunity [34].

Foxp3, a master gene that controls the development and function of Treg cells, contributes to pathogenesis of several different tumours. Owing to the intracellular localization of Foxp3, RNAi technology was employed to knockdown its activation to suppress Treg activity in vivo. Tsai et al. [35] performed a study targeting silencing Foxp3 gene expression by shRNAs-mediated RNAi using a lentivirus vector in a murine model of leukaemia. The lentiviral vector was used to overcome poor transfection efficiency. Lentiviral-mediated Foxp3 RNAi showed suppressive effects on tumour growth and prolonged the survival of tumour-transplanted mice. Furthermore, Foxp3 knockdown mediated by siRNA increased the ratio of Th1/Th2 in chronic hepatitis B patients; transcription factors T-bet and GATA-3 may be partly involved in this progress [36]. This strategy provides a novel view about how to decrease the number of Treg cells and weaken its function.

Selective knockdown of CCL22 and CCL17 expression in monocyte-derived DC (MoDC) by siRNA decreased the ratios of CD4+ to CD8+ as well as lowered the frequency of Tregs recruited by MoDC. Furthermore, intratumoural injection of MoDC, which was transfected with siCCL22 and siCCL17, significantly reduced the number of Tregs while inducing CD8+ T cells infiltration in thymic nude mice with human tumour xenografts [37]. Using siRNA to selectively silence chemokines may lead to a new strategy for DC vaccine development to improve cancer biotherapy.

High expression of indoleamine 2, 3-dioxygenase (IDO) in DCs leads to the suppression of T cell responses. Gene silencing by siRNA or shRNA of IDO in DC would up-regulate IL-12 and IFN-γ and inhibit apoptosis in CD8 and CD4 T cells as well as Treg cells; IL-10 expression was significantly down-regulated, thus finally restraining tumour growth. DC-based vaccine with IDO silence was demonstrated to augment and enhance the anti-tumour response against breast cancer, melanoma, bladder tumour and liver cancer [38–40]. A novel APC-targeted siRNA delivery system using mannosed liposomes (Man-lipo) with encapsulated siRNA-IDO

(Man-lipo-siIDO) was demonstrated to preferentially silence IDO in APCs and efficiently enhance anti-tumour immune response [41–43].

It was reported that natural killer group 2, member D (NKG2D) activation was involved in NK cell and CD8+ cell-mediated liver inflammation, and blockade of NKG2D by silencing of multiple NKG2D ligands on hepatocytes was considered efficient in liver disease intervention. Huang et al. [44] constructed a plasmid containing the three shRNA sequences (shRae1-shMult1-shH60). After hydrodynamic injection into mice, they found that the expression of all three NKG2D ligands on hepatocytes was down-regulated, and fulminant hepatitis mediated through NKG2D in NK cell was attenuated. Furthermore, simultaneous knockdown of multiple human NKG2D ligands (MHC class I polypeptide-related sequence B/A(MICA/B), UL16-binding protein 2 [ULBP2] and ULBP3) also significantly attenuated NK cell cytolysis. Simultaneous knockdown of multiple ligands of NKG2D is a potential therapeutic approach to treat liver diseases induced by NKG2D-expressing NK cells and CD8+ cells. Furthermore, inhibition of human leukocyte antigen-G (HLA-G) by siRNA boosted NK cell lytic function [45,46].

Among several molecules involved in immune response, the choice of targets should be carefully reviewed and validated comprehensively according to the emerging knowledge about their function.

2.2. Advantage of non-target immune effect of siRNA/shRNA drugs

siRNA/shRNA have the potential to recruit immune receptors specialized in RNA sensor, such as TLR3, TLR7/8 [2,3]. 5′-triphosphate siRNA (3p-siRNA) was demonstrated to be detected by RNA sensors RIG-I. These immunostimulatory siRNA or shRNA can non-specifically induce innate immune response, the so-called 'off-target' effects that have considerable implications for clinical application to cure cancer and infection disease.

IFN response is a common side effect of siRNAs and siRNAs with GU-rich sequences, which are very potent in inducing IFN-α response. A newly published report demonstrated that siRNA could induce IFN-α responses, and then induced the analgesic effects in the spinal cord. This off-target analgesia is dose- and sequence-dependent while non-GU-rich sequences also produced off-target analgesia at high doses, where pain relief by a designed siRNA may not be attributable to target gene knockdown but IFN response [47].

Early in 2004, Karikó et al. [48] demonstrated that siRNAs and shRNAs induce immune activation by signalling through TLR3 and activate sequence-independent inhibition of gene expression. Kleinman et al. [4] showed that non-targeted (against non-mammalian genes) and targeted (against vascular endothelial growth factor [VEGF] or VEGFR1) siRNAs suppressed choroidal neovascularization (CNV) via cell-surface TLR3 and its adaptor TIR-domain-containing adaptor-inducing interferon-β (TRIF), leading to the induction of IFN-α and IL-12. The effect of non-targeted siRNA to suppress dermal neovascularization in mice was as effective as vascular endothelial growth factor (VEGF) siRNA. This finding showed that two investigational siRNAs in clinical trials owe their anti-angiogenic effect in mice, which was not due to target knockdown but due to TLR3 activation. The efficiency of RNAi by siRNA is believed to be comparable with anti-VEGF antibodies. Kleinman's group then concluded that a 21-nucleotide (nt) non-targeted siRNA suppresses both hemangiogenesis and lymphangiogenesis in mouse models of neovascularization, induced by corneal sutures or hindlimb ischemia, as efficiently as a 21-nt siRNA targeting VEGF-A [1].

Among 15 siRNAs, Khairuddin et al. [49] identified an extremely immunostimulatory siRNAs, targeting the HPV, which exerted potent anti-tumoural function. This bifunctional siRNA could reduce growth of established TC-1 tumours in C57BL/6 mice, and its effect was TLR7 dependent, where ablation of TLR7 recruitment via 2′O-methyl modification of the oligo backbone reduced these anti-tumour effects. Flatekval et al. [40] designed either monofunctional siRNAs devoid of immunostimulation or bifunctional siRNAs with IDO silencing and immunostimulatory activities. They showed that bifunctional siRNAs were able to knock-down IDO expression and induce cytokine production through either endosomal TLR7/8 or RIG-I.

In the past 10 years, several studies reported that bifunctional 3p-siRNA (Exp:targeting Bcl2/TGF-β/Survivin/Glutaminase/IDO) with target silencing and an innate immunity stimulation via RIG-I activation could confer potent anti-tumour efficacy. This is illustrated for the first time by the work of Poeck et al. [8], who reported that bifunctional siRNAs, with 5′-triphosphate targeting Bcl2 (3p-siRNA), led to better melanoma tumour reduction than OH-siRNA or 5′-triphosphate siRNAs containing target mismatches. Poeck and his colleagues revealed that siRNA with 5′-triphosphate ends could be recognized by RIG-I and activate an innate immune cells such as DC; then, expression of IFNs was directly induced, leading to apoptosis in tumour cells. These bifunctional 3p-siRNAs with RIG-I activation and RNAi-mediated Bcl2 silencing could provoke massive apoptosis of tumour cells in lung metastases in vivo. This was the first report demonstrating that 3p-siRNA represents a single molecule-based approach in which RIG-I function activates immune cell and gene silencing, leading to a key molecular event. Researchers subsequently found that 3p-TGFβ1-siRNA combining RIG-I activation with gene silencing of TGF-β1 induced profound tumour cell apoptosis and revealed potent anti-tumour efficacy in pancreatic cancer. This kind of 3p-siRNA induces a Th1 cytokine profile, demonstrating IFN-γ induction and IL-4 inhibition. High level of IFN and CXCL10 recruited more activated CD8+ T cells to the tumour. Frequency of immunosuppressive CD11b+ Gr-1+ myeloid cells was reduced after 3p-TGFβ1-siRNA treatment [50].

In addition, 3p-siRNA against survivin gene was designed and generated. This finding demonstrated that 3p-survivin-siRNA inhibited lung cancer cell proliferation and induced a RIG-I-dependent type-I interferon response [7]. Recently, 5′-triphosphate siRNA combining glutaminase (GLS) silencing with RIG-I activation was demonstrated to induce more prominent anti-tumour responses than RIG-I ligand or GLS silencing capability alone. 3p-siRNA-GLS effectively induced intrinsic proapoptotic signalling, and GLS silence sensitized malignant cells to apoptosis induced by RIG-I activation. Moreover, cytotoxicity was enhanced, resulting from disturbed glutaminolysis induced by GLS silencing. Finally, RIG-I activation by 3p-siRNA-GLS blocked autophagic degradation, leading to dysfunction of mitochondria, whereas GLS silencing severely impaired reactive oxygen species (ROS) scavenging systems, leading to a vicious circle of ROS-mediated cytotoxicity [51]. Immature monocyte-derived DCs had been transfected with siRNA-bearing 5′-triphosphate-activated T cells [40].

In addition, 3p-siRNA can inhibit hepatitis B virus (HBV), Influenza A Virus and Coxsackievirus, by gene silencing and RIG-I activation. RNAi provides a promising approach for the specific treatment of HBV infection. Our laboratory has previously demonstrated that 3p-HBx-siRNA and shRNA-HBx not only directly inhibit HBV replication but also stimulate innate immunity against HBV, which are both beneficial for the inversion of HBV-induced immune tolerance [52]. In HBV-positive hepatoma HepG2.2.15 cells, 3p-HBx-siRNA combining RIG-I activation with HBx gene silencing induce stronger type I IFN response than non-target 3p-scramble-siRNA, indicating that a potent immunostimulatory effect may partly contribute to the reversal of immune tolerance through decreasing HBV load; 3p-HBx-siRNA more strongly inhibited HBV replication and promoted IFN production than HBx-siRNA in primary HBV(+) hepatocytes, and this effect was mediated by RIG-I activation [52]. This was consistent of the other two reports [53,54]. Our dually functional vector containing both an immunostimulatory single-stranded RNA (ssRNA) and an HBx-silencing shRNA could reverse HBV-induced hepatocyte-intrinsic immune tolerance; TLR7 signalling pathway was attributed to this progress [55].

Lin et al. [56] designed and tested a 3p-mNP1496-siRNA against influenza virus. They found that 3p-mNP1496-siRNA could activate the RIG-I-mediated IFN-β pathway and significantly reduce virus load and virus-induced pathogenesis. The inhibition effect was in an siRNA- and RIG-I-dependent manner, demonstrating siRNA playing dual antiviral roles: viral gene-specific silencing and non-gene-specific RIG-I activation. This strategy was also proved to elicit potent antiviral effects in coxsackievirus myocarditis, and virus-specific 3p-siRNA was superior to both conventional virus-specific siRNA and non-target 3p-siRNA in inhibiting viral replication and subsequent cytotoxicity [57].

In the attempt to inhibit the expression of woodchuck hepatitis virus (WHV), Meng et al. [58] found that innate immune responses could be enhanced by RNAi through the PKR- and TLR-dependent signalling pathways in primary hepatocytes. The immunostimulation by RNAi may contribute to the antiviral activity of siRNAs in vivo.

Furthermore, siRNA can also synergistically enhance DNA-mediated type III IFN (a newly characterized antiviral interferon) response in non-immune or primary immune cells. This enhancement is mediated by crosstalk signalling pathway between RIG-I (RNA sensor) and IFI16 (DNA sensor) [59].

Designing with GU sequences, addition of triphosphate motifs to siRNA, co-treatment with CpG oligos are believed to activate innate immunity when siRNA was applied in vitro and in vivo. Accumulating evidence suggests these bifunctional siRNAs could activate NK cells and CD8+ T cells in different models. Thus, specific clinical applications of RNAi can benefit from a concurrent activation of the immune system.

3. miRNA

It has been well discussed how miRNAs regulate signalling pathways, and the dynamics of the immune response, tolerance and homeostasis. Here we summarize and explore updated achievements of special miRNAs in immunopharmacology.

3.1. miRNAs as intrinsic targets in antiviral immunity

In addition to the conventional innate and adaptive immune responses, even in the earlier phase after virus invasion, the host cell suppresses viral replication by evolving the profile of special and constitutively expressed genes. These cell-intrinsic antiviral approaches based on host restriction factors may be no less important than in considerations of conventional immunity. At the same time, viruses also gain some countermeasures or adapt the unique phenotype of their hosts substantially to survive. Moreover, miRNAs may also be involved in the inextricably intertwined relationship between viruses and their hosts.

In 2005, a liver-specific miRNA, miR122, which is involved in cholesterol and lipid metabolism [60], was illustrated to be necessary for hepatitis C virus (HCV) accumulation in cultured liver cells [61]. Researchers found that miR122 directly binds to two close sites in the 5′ non-coding region of the HCV genome and promote HCV translation [62–64]. This miRNA kept conserved among all HCV subtypes [65,66]. Even in non-hepatic cell, miR122 could boost HCV replication [67]. Moreover, miR122 was further proved to be significantly reduced after IFN-β treatment, and miR122 mimics neutralized IFN-induced anti-HCV effect [68]. Epidemiological and genomic researches further suggested that the level of miR122 in individuals with HCV might be an 'indicator' for IFN therapy, and only those patients with high levels of miR122 responded well to IFN therapy [69,70]. Therefore, miR122 antagonist would also be called as IFN 'sensitizer' in HCV immune treatment.

Santaris Pharma designed and synthesized an LNA-based miR122 inhibitor, named Miravirsen (or SPC3649), to eradicate HCV. The product was first evaluated in preclinical studies in mice [71], cynomolgus monkeys [72], green African monkeys and chimpanzees [73,74]. Here the key concern is that whether miR122 inhibitor can effectively lower the level of free miR122 and inhibit HCV replication without disturbing normal cholesterol and lipid metabolism or without any potential chemical toxicity. Interestingly, although there was a reduction of cholesterol levels in plasma by nearly 40%, Miravirsen caused a dose-dependent reduction of miR122 and maintained ~5-week-long half-life in the liver of monkeys and chimpanzees [73, 74]. Moreover, in the high-dose treatment group, Miravirsen decreased HCV subtype 1a or 1b more than 2 orders of magnitude compared to control group. In all animal species, Miravirsen was reported to be safe, without serious adverse effects or dose-related toxicities in rats, monkeys and human [75,76].

In May 2008, Miravirsen was put into human clinical trials as the first miRNA-based drug (https://clinicaltrials.gov/ct2/show/NCT00979927). There was a significant, dose-dependent reduction and sustained decrease of HCV viremia after drug administration in human subjects, and several patients became even HCV undetectable during the study. At the same time, only infrequent and moderately adverse effects were caused to some volunteers and did not influence the trial process [77]. Because miR122 is only liver enriched in physiological conditions and there is high amount of miR122 in adult human liver, it may be an ideal target to design highly specific anti-HCV drugs with good resistance to HCV infected person, particularly to those who have no tolerance to traditional treatments. In the following years, miR196 [78], let-7b family [79] and some other miRNAs were then proved to influence HCV life cycle, providing new target to restrict hepatitis C infection and avoid chronic infection.

Besides HCV, some other kind of viruses also encode miRNAs or regulate the miRNAs expression in host cells to disturb the expression of many immune-associated genes directly and/or indirectly, so that they can be critical regulators for viral life cycle. For example, in HEK293T cell, prototype foamy virus I (PFV-1) encodes Tas protein to counteract cell-encoded miR32, which could inhibit PFV-1 gene expression and accumulation [80]. Kaposi's sarcoma-associated herpesvirus (KSHV)-induced miR132 could silence p300 expression, which is critical for the transcription initialization of many antiviral genes, to help themselves maintain long-time latency [81]. The hematopoietic-cell-specific miR142-3p potently restricts the replication of eastern equine encephalitis virus in myeloid-lineage cells by binding to the 3′-untranslated region (UTR) of viral genome [82]. Even Drosha, the enzyme that processes miRNA biogenesis and maturation, was an independent factor for limiting RNA virus replication along with canonical type I IFN system in particular cell type [83]. Above of all, it is much likely that miRNA mimics (for viral inhibitory miRNAs) or antagonists (for viral beneficial miRNAs) can be effective antiviral strategies as intrinsic immune drugs.

3.2. miRNA regulation antimicrobial and anti-tumour immunity

3.2.1. miRNA in antimicrobial innate immunity

Of the known PRRs, TLRs and RIG-like receptors (RLRs) have been well studied in mediating antimicrobial and inflammatory responses during infections, which may be targets of pathogens or host-encoded miRNAs.

The first PRR targeting miRNA let7i was reported in 2007 [84], which targeted TLR4 mRNA in a MyD88/NF-κB-dependent way during *Cryptosporidium parvum* infection, controlling the production of inflammatory factors. During *Bacillus Calmette-Guérin* (BCG) infection, miR124 exerts its function by targeting multiple components of the TLR signalling pathway, including TLR6, MyD88, TNF receptor-associated factor 6 (TRAF6) and TNF-α in mouse lung cell [85]. After HCV infection, miR373 was induced and negatively regulated the type I IFN signalling pathway by suppressing Janus kinase 1(JAK1) and IRF9 in hepatocytes [86]. Experimental evaluation using miR124 inhibitors or miR373 knockout up-regulated BCG-induced pro-inflammatory factors or type I IFN and so as to inhibit BCG or HCV more efficiently. Besides using host miRNAs, human cytomegalovirus (HCMV) targeted TLR2 by encoding its own miRNA, miR-UL112-3p, and reduced the expression of IL-1β, IL-6 and IL-8 upon stimulation with a TLR2 agonist [87]. Neutralizing this miRNA might recover normal cytokines production.

Besides immune inhibitory miRNAs, dengue virus (DENV)-induced miR30e* up-regulated IFN-β and the downstream IFN-stimulated genes (ISGs) by suppressing IkBα and promoting NF-κB-dependent IFN production [88]. The transfection of miR30e* would increase the expression of 2′-5′-oligoadenylate synthetase 1(OAS-1), myxovirus resistance A (MxA) and interferon-induced transmembrane protein (IFITM). In 2014, miR526 [89] was proved to enhance RIG-I-induced viral replication by suppression of the expression of cylindromatosis (CYLD), which suppresses RIG-I K-63-linked polyubiquitin. Moreover, Enterovirus 71(EV71) inhibited miR526 transcription in an IRF-dependent way and so as to attenuate virus-triggered type I interferon production. These studies suggested that recruitment or increase of miR30e* or miR526 would stimulate type I IFN expression and inhibit virus more quickly.

3.2.2. 'Immune miRs' as immunopharmaceutic agents

With the general knowledge of immunologically relevant miRNAs established in the past 10 years, many miRNAs have been intensively investigated using gain- and loss-of-function methods, showing how this novel class of small non-coding RNA participates in mammalian immunity. And individual immune miRNA might contribute its implications to various immune-mediated diseases.

The role of miR125b in immune signalling may be paradoxical. After stimulation with LPS, miR125b was down-regulated and TNF-α, one of miR125b targets, was overexpressed in RAW264.7, which is essential for antimicrobial activity. Moreover, during *M. tuberculosis* infection, the overexpression of miR125a significantly attenuated the antimicrobial effects in macrophages through targeting UV radiation resistance–associated gene (UVRAG) [90]. Nevertheless, in diffuse large B cell lymphoma (DLBCL), miR125a and miR125b directly target a negative NF-κB regulator tumour necrosis factor alpha-induced protein 3(TNFAIP3) and present a positive self-regulatory property to maintain prolonged NF-κB activity. Taken together, whether overexpression or inhibition of miR125b in an anti-infection therapeutic study depends on concrete circumstances.

miR146a also acts as a negative regulator in immune sensing. Both in mouse and human, miR146a was always exploited by virus to attenuate innate and adaptive antiviral immunity mainly in DC [91], lymphocyte [92] and hepatocytes by inhibiting interleukin-1 receptor-associated kinase 1(IRAK1), TRAF6 [93], son of sevenless homolog 1 (SOS1) [94] and STAT1 [95]. Silencing of miR146a via the delivery of sponge or antagomiR could restore the expression of inflammatory factors, augment type I IFN production and promote clearance of vesicular stomatitis virus (VSV) [96], dengue virus [97], enterovirus 71 (EV71) [94,98] and HBV [95]. Because miR146a was also abnormally expressed in hepatocellular carcinoma (HCC) and exerted negative anti-tumour effects by up-regulation of immunoinhibitory cytokines such as TGF-β, IL-17, VEGF, miR146a may also be a novel immunotherapeutic target for HCC [99].

Unlike miR146a, miR155 always promotes immune signal transduction, enhances immune function or speeds lymphocyte proliferation. Mice lacking miR155 have impaired CTL cell responses to infections with lymphocytic choriomeningitis virus and the intracellular bacteria *Listeria monocytogenes* because of insufficient activation of Akt pathway after TCR cross-linking [100]. miR155 knockout mice died soon after Erdman (a variant from severe acute respiratory syndrome [SARS]) infection and held higher level of colony-forming units (CFU) in lungs than wild-type mice [101]. During HIV infection, miR155 inhibited the HIV-activating effects of tripartite motif-containing protein 32 (TRIM32), and therefore, it might promote a return to latency in CD4+ reservoir cells [102]. In addition, in NK cells, miR155 might regulate T cell immunoglobulin-3 (Tim-3)/T-bet/STAT-5-signalling axis, and following cytokine expression that balanced antiviral response and immune injury during chronic HCV infection [103]. A remarkably ectopic up-expression of miR155 can be observed by delivering hepatotropic adeno-associated virus 8 (AAV8) vectors to the liver of mice, and then high level of miR155-enhanced GAP's protective capacity against parasite [104]. These studies imply miR155 as an immune-augmenting adjuvant in improving the antigenicity of vaccination.

miR223 was already proved to be of importance in myeloid progenitor cells proliferation and responsiveness to pathogenic stimuli in neutrophils by targeting myocyte-specific enhancer factor 2C (MEF2C), acting as a fine-tune regulator both in normal granulocytes generation and in preventing aberrant expansion and over-activated inflammatory responses. In recent years, miR223 was involved in inflammasome response by targeting NLR family pyrin domain containing 3 (NLRP3) in human [105]. Moreover, Epstein–Barr virus (EBV) encoded a mimic of hsa-miR223, called miR-BART15, targeting the same site within the NLRP3 3′-UTR to repress inflammasome activation. Furthermore, this miRNA can be secreted from EBV-infected B cells into exosomes to rheostat NLRP3 inflammasome activity in non-infected cells [106]. miR223 sponge would balance the amount of NLRP3 and 'absorb' EBV-miR-BART15 in macrophages and DCs.

It is noteworthy that two groups of miRNAs, which shaped NK-mediated cytotoxicity, have potent value for developing antiviral and anti-tumour biodrugs. First, NKG2D–NKG2D-L interaction plays a predominant role in 'NK cell–abnormal cell' recognition. MICB/A, ULBPs targeting miRNAs, are not only encoded by human genome as stress regulators but also synthesized by some virus (e.g. HCMV-miR-UL112 [107], EBV-miRBART2 [108], KSHV-miR-K12-7 [108] and BK virus (BKV)-miR-B1-3p, JC virus (JCV)-miR-J1-3p[109]), to escape from NK cell killing. Meanwhile, viral infected cell and tumour cell always express low MICA/B because of up-regulated MICB/MICA, targeting miRNAs such as miR20a, 93, 103, 106b [110] to maintain a compromised micro-environment. Furthermore, non-classical human leukocyte antigen G (HLA-G) is known as an inhibitory ligand, which suppresses the cytotoxic activity of T and NK cells. Studies demonstrated a strong post-transcriptional gene regulation of the HLA-G by miR148a, miR148b and miR152, and lower expression of these miRNAs in renal carcinoma [111] and placental choriocarcinoma cells [112]. Stable manipulation of these activating and inhibitory miRNAs may enhance NK and LAK cell-mediated cytotoxicity against infected and tumour cells. Therefore, it could be concluded that modulating the expression or inhibition of specific miRNAs could boost immune response during viral infections or against cancers.

3.3. miRNA in maintaining immune homeostasis

Because several miRNAs participate in immune cell development and differentiation, abnormal expression of miRNA may cause a disturbance of homeostasis by changing the ratio of helper and regulatory cell subsets, or perturb the functionality and survival of effect-

memory cells that lead to lymphoproliferative disease. Utilization of miRNA interference techniques may recover regular immune balance.

3.3.1. *miR17-92, miR146a and miR155 in Systemic Lupus Erythematosus (SLE)*

In 2007, a unique mouse strain, 'sanroque', presented a pattern of lupus pathology, revealing the core role of T follicular helper (Tfh) in systemic autoimmunity [113]. miR17-92 was found to regulate Tfh cell differentiation, which is essential for maintenance of the germinal centre formation and sustained antibody responses. Overexpression of this miRNA in T cells would enhance Tfh cell proliferation and survive an autoantibody production [112]. Similarly, miR155 increased IL-21-mediated STAT3 signalling in T cell [114], which might accelerate Tfh differentiation and maturation as well. Moreover, miR155 deficiency ameliorates autoimmune inflammation of SLE by targeting s1pr1 in mice [115]. Therefore, miR17-92 and miR155 might be a new target to restrain aggressive autoimmune response in SLE.

3.3.2. *miR29 and miR146 in type 1 diabetes*

Type 1 diabetes (T1D) is a chronic autoimmune disease that results from the persisting destruction of pancreatic β-cells by autoreactive CD8+ T cell and Th1 cytokines. Dicer 1 deletion in β-cell would disrupt normal β-cell development and survival, lead to impairment of insulin secretion and diabetes development [116], apparently suggesting that miRNAs network is necessary for normal glycometabolism. Recently, endogenous miR29b released from pancreatic β-cells within exosomes stimulated TNF-α secretion in spleen cells isolated from diabetes-prone non-obese diabetic (NOD) mice. Delivery of miR29b to mice activated myeloid cell and pDCs to induce IFN-α, TNF-α and IL-6 production [117]. Abnormal expression of miR146 is associated with high serum titers of glutamic acid decarboxylase antibody in T1D patients, indicating the involvement of miR146 in the sustained immune imbalance during T1D progress [118]. These findings raised the possibility of developing a new clue for T1D immunotherapy using miRNA-based agents.

3.3.3. *miR146a and miR155 in rheumatoid arthritis*

The role of miR146a in controlling Treg-mediated decrease of Th1 responses has been demonstrated [119]. In contrast, miR155 promoted Th1 and Th17 differentiation and cell formation and lowered T cell sensitivity to IFN-γ-driven proliferation by targeting C-MAF and IFNγRα [120]. Therefore, imbalance of miR146a and miR155 may be an epigenetic phenotype for autoimmune response. In rheumatoid arthritis (RA), decreased expression of miR146a contributes to an abnormal Treg phenotype and allows Th1/Th17 skewing while low level of miR155 failed to support effective Th2 immunity [121]. Systemic administration of miR146a has potential therapeutic intervention for preventing bone destruction by inhibited Th1 and Th17 cells, as well as IL-1β, IL-6 and TNF-α [122].

3.3.4. *miR15 and miR326 in multiple sclerosis*

Multiple sclerosis (MS) is manifested by chronic and progressive inflammatory demyelination of the central nervous system and is one of the main causes of regressive neurological diseases.

Study on MS animal model illustrated that mice with fewer Th17 cells were less susceptible to experimental autoimmune encephalomyelitis (EAE) [123]. Therefore, Th17-targeting biotherapeutic approaches may be a promising way to cure multiple sclerosis. Gang Pei' s laboratory [124] found that miR326 promoted Th17 differentiation by targeting Ets-1 (a negative regulator of Th17 polarization) and antagonizing miR326 by sponge vector that resulted in fewer Th17 cells and Th17 cytokines and remitting EAE symptom. Inversely, increased miR155 in primary human microglia up-regulated pro-inflammatory cytokine secretion and co-stimulatory surface marker expression suggested that miR155 inhibition in myeloid cell might be useful to suppress allogeneic T cell responses [125]. In conclusion, reverse pathological expressed miRNAs and re-balance dysregulated immune genes are of consideration to treat multiple sclerosis.

4. Conclusion

RNAi technology holds promise for treating various human diseases. It is becoming apparent that clinical outcome of cancer immunotherapy and infectious diseases can be improved by targeted strategies to abrogate tumour-induced immunosuppression. Anti-tumour strategies using siRNA/shRNA/miRNA for both silencing of oncogenes and recruiting of innate receptors were designed. The present researches highlighted the potential therapeutic applications of this new generation of siRNAs in immunotherapy.

Additionally, but importantly, siRNA/shRNA or miRNA drugs with regard to pharmacodynamic difficulties and unwanted side effects are even more complicated compared to low molecular weight drugs and hard to be delivered into immune cells. This requires more extensive procedure than any other traditional drugs. Considering clinical challenges for RNA-based nucleic acid drugs, including barriers and RNases, the advanced tissue-directed delivery systems with safety, high efficiency and specificity, long-term function and controllability are required. Although the exploration of such tiny regulators causally bring pharmacists a considerable effort to draw up individualized and tailor-made strategies, we believe that immunoregulation triggered by siRNA/shRNA/miRNA can be used to regulate the host immunity against cancers or viruses. The development of multifunctional RNAi molecules will greatly contribute to the future arsenal of tools to combat not only microbial pathogens but also hard-to-treat cancer.

Acknowledgements

This work was supported by the Natural Science Foundation of China (81172789, 81373222, 31200651), National Basic Research Program of China (No. 2013CB531503) and National Mega Project on Major Infectious Diseases Prevention and Treatment (2012ZX10002006), The Special Foundation of Taishan Overseas Distinguished Experts and Scholars, The Priority Research Program of Shandong Academy of Sciences, Natural Science Foundation of Shandong

Province (No.BS2015YY023), Natural Science Foundation of Shandong Academy of Sciences (No. 2014QN004) and Science and Technology Development Foundation of Shandong Analysis and Test Center.

Author details

Zhaohua Hou[1], Qiuju Han[2*], Cai Zhang[2] and Jian Zhang[2]

*Address all correspondence to: hanqiuju@sdu.edu.cn

1 Laboratory of Immunology for Environment and Health, Shandong Analysis and Test Center, Shandong Academy of Sciences, Jinan, China

2 Institute of Immunopharmaceutical Sciences, School of Pharmaceutical Sciences, Shandong University, Jinan, China

References

[1] Cho WG, Albuquerque RJ, Kleinman ME: Small interfering RNA-induced TLR3 activation inhibits blood and lymphatic vessel growth. Proc Natl Acad Sci U S A. 2009; 106: 7137–7142. DOI: 10.1073/pnas.08123171060812317106

[2] Forsbach A, Nemorin JG, Volp K: Characterization of conserved viral leader RNA sequences that stimulate innate immunity through TLRs. Oligonucleotides. 2007; 17: 405–417. DOI: 10.1089/oli.2007.0098

[3] Judge AD, Sood V, Shaw JR: Sequence-dependent stimulation of the mammalian innate immune response by synthetic siRNA. Nat Biotechnol. 2005; 23: 457–462. DOI: 10.1038/nbt1081

[4] Kleinman ME, Yamada K, Takeda A: Sequence- and target-independent angiogenesis suppression by siRNA via TLR3. Nature. 2008; 452: 591–597. DOI: 10.1038/nature06765

[5] Melchjorsen J, Jensen SB, Malmgaard L: Activation of innate defense against a paramyxovirus is mediated by RIG-I and TLR7 and TLR8 in a cell-type-specific manner. J Virol. 2005; 79: 12944–12951. DOI: 10.1128/JVI.79.20.12944-12951.2005

[6] Hornung V, Guenthner-Biller M, Bourquin C: Sequence-specific potent induction of IFN-alpha by short interfering RNA in plasmacytoid dendritic cells through TLR7. Nat Med. 2005; 11: 263-270. DOI: 10.1038/nm1191

[7] Wang K, Chen X, Yan F: 5'-triphosphate-siRNA against survivin gene induces interferon production and inhibits proliferation of lung cancer cells in vitro. J Immunother. 2013; 36: 294–304. DOI: 10.1097/CJI.0b013e318294183b

[8] Poeck H, Besch R, Maihoefer C: 5'-Triphosphate-siRNA: turning gene silencing and Rig-I activation against melanoma. Nat Med. 2008; 14: 1256–1263. DOI: 10.1038/nm.1887

[9] Alshamsan A, Hamdy S, Haddadi A: STAT3 knockdown in B16 melanoma by siRNA lipopolyplexes induces bystander immune response in vitro and in vivo. DOI: Transl Oncol. 2011; 4: 178–188. DOI: 10.1593/tlo.11100

[10] Herrmann A, Kortylewski M, Kujawski M: Targeting Stat3 in the myeloid compartment drastically improves the in vivo antitumor functions of adoptively transferred T cells. Cancer Res. 2010; 70: 7455–7464. DOI: 10.1158/0008-5472.CAN-10-0736

[11] Alshamsan A, Haddadi A, Hamdy S: STAT3 silencing in dendritic cells by siRNA polyplexes encapsulated in PLGA nanoparticles for the modulation of anticancer immune response. Mol Pharm. 2010; 7: 1643–1654. DOI: 10.1021/mp100067u

[12] Kortylewski M, Swiderski P, Herrmann A: In vivo delivery of siRNA to immune cells by conjugation to a TLR9 agonist enhances antitumor immune responses. Nat Biotechnol. 2009; 27: 925–932. DOI: 10.1038/nbt.1564

[13] Hossain DM, Pal SK, Moreira D: TLR9-targeted STAT3 silencing abrogates immunosuppressive activity of myeloid-derived suppressor cells from prostate cancer patients. Clin Cancer Res. 2015; 21: 3771–3782. DOI: 10.1158/1078-0432.CCR-14-3145

[14] Zhang Q, Hossain DM, Nechaev S: TLR9-mediated siRNA delivery for targeting of normal and malignant human hematopoietic cells in vivo. Blood. 2013; 121: 1304–1315. DOI: 10.1182/blood-2012-07-442590b

[15] Luo Z, Wang C, Yi H: Nanovaccine loaded with poly I:C and STAT3 siRNA robustly elicits anti-tumor immune responses through modulating tumor-associated dendritic cells in vivo. Biomaterials. 2015; 38: 50–60. DOI: 10.1016/j.biomaterials.2014.10.050

[16] Shi D, Li D, Yin Q: Silenced suppressor of cytokine signaling 1 (SOCS1) enhances the maturation and antifungal immunity of dendritic cells in response to Candida albicans in vitro. Immunol Res. 2015; 61: 206-218. DOI: 10.1007/s12026-014-8562-8

[17] Akita H, Kogure K, Moriguchi R: Nanoparticles for ex vivo siRNA delivery to dendritic cells for cancer vaccines: programmed endosomal escape and dissociation. J Control Release. 2010; 143: 311–317. DOI: 10.1016/j.jconrel.2010.01.012

[18] Heo MB, Cho MY, Lim YT: Polymer nanoparticles for enhanced immune response: combined delivery of tumor antigen and small interference RNA for immunosuppressive gene to dendritic cells. Acta Biomater. 2014; 10: 2169–2176. DOI: 10.1016/j.actbio.2013.12.050

[19] Subramanya S, Armant M, Salkowitz JR: Enhanced induction of HIV-specific cytotoxic T lymphocytes by dendritic cell-targeted delivery of SOCS-1 siRNA. Mol Ther. 2010; 18: 2028–2037. DOI: 10.1038/mt.2010.148

[20] Zhang X, Su Y, Song H: Attenuated A20 expression of acute myeloid leukemia-derived dendritic cells increased the anti-leukemia immune response of autologous cytolytic T cells. Leuk Res. 2014; 38: 673–681. DOI: 10.1016/j.leukres.2014.03.011

[21] Warashina S, Nakamura T, Harashima H: A20 silencing by lipid envelope-type nanoparticles enhances the efficiency of lipopolysaccharide-activated dendritic cells. Biol Pharm Bull. 2011; 34: 1348–1351. DOI: 10.1248/bpb.34.1348

[22] Song XT, Evel-Kabler K, Shen L: A20 is an antigen presentation attenuator, and its inhibition overcomes regulatory T cell-mediated suppression. Nat Med. 2008; 14: 258–265. DOI: 10.1038/nm1721

[23] Breckpot K, Aerts-Toegaert C, Heirman C: Attenuated expression of A20 markedly increases the efficacy of double-stranded RNA-activated dendritic cells as an anti-cancer vaccine. J Immunol. 2009; 182: 860–870. DOI: 10.4049/jimmunol.182.2.860

[24] Cubillos-Ruiz JR, Engle X, Scarlett UK: Polyethylenimine-based siRNA nanocomplexes reprogram tumor-associated dendritic cells via TLR5 to elicit therapeutic antitumor immunity. J Clin Invest. 2009; 119: 2231–2244. DOI: 10.1172/JCI3771637716 [pii]

[25] Hobo W, Maas F, Adisty N: siRNA silencing of PD-L1 and PD-L2 on dendritic cells augments expansion and function of minor histocompatibility antigen-specific CD8+ T cells. Blood. 2010; 116: 4501–4511. DOI: 10.1182/blood-2010-04-278739

[26] van der Waart AB, Fredrix H, van der Voort R: siRNA silencing of PD-1 ligands on dendritic cell vaccines boosts the expansion of minor histocompatibility antigen-specific CD8(+) T cells in NOD/SCID/IL2Rg(null) mice. Cancer Immunol Immunother. 2015; 64: 645–654. DOI: 10.1007/s00262-015-1668-6

[27] Iwamura K, Kato T, Miyahara Y: siRNA-mediated silencing of PD-1 ligands enhances tumor-specific human T-cell effector functions. Gene Ther. 2012; 19: 959–966. DOI: 10.1038/gt.2011.185

[28] Zhang Q, Ichimaru N, Higuchi S: Permanent acceptance of mouse cardiac allografts with CD40 siRNA to induce regulatory myeloid cells by use of a novel polysaccharide siRNA delivery system. Gene Ther. 2015; 22: 1–10. DOI: 10.1038/gt.2014.119

[29] Gong X, Han B, Zou Y: Attenuation of experimental autoimmune myocarditis by siRNA mediated CD40 silencing. Int Heart J. 2014; 55: 539–545. DOI: 10.1536/ihj.14-125

[30] Zheng X, Suzuki M, Ichim TE: Treatment of autoimmune arthritis using RNA interference-modulated dendritic cells. J Immunol. 2010; 184: 6457–6464. DOI: 10.4049/jimmunol.0901717

[31] Conroy H, Galvin KC, Higgins SC: Gene silencing of TGF-beta1 enhances antitumor immunity induced with a dendritic cell vaccine by reducing tumor-associated regulatory T cells. Cancer Immunol Immunother. 2012; 61: 425–431. DOI: 10.1007/s00262-011-1188-y

[32] Xu Z, Wang Y, Zhang L: Nanoparticle-delivered transforming growth factor-beta siRNA enhances vaccination against advanced melanoma by modifying tumor microenvironment. ACS Nano. 2014; 8: 3636–3645. DOI: 10.1021/nn500216y

[33] Ahn YH, Hong SO, Kim JH: The siRNA cocktail targeting interleukin 10 receptor and transforming growth factor-beta receptor on dendritic cells potentiates tumour antigen-specific CD8(+) T cell immunity. Clin Exp Immunol. 2015; 181: 164–178. DOI: 10.1111/cei.12620

[34] Liu Z, Falo LD, Jr., You Z: Knockdown of HMGB1 in tumor cells attenuates their ability to induce regulatory T cells and uncovers naturally acquired CD8 T cell-dependent antitumor immunity. J Immunol. 2011; 187: 118–125. DOI: 10.4049/jimmunol.1003378

[35] Tsai BY, Suen JL, Chiang BL: Lentiviral-mediated Foxp3 RNAi suppresses tumor growth of regulatory T cell-like leukemia in a murine tumor model. Gene Ther. 2010; 17: 972–979. DOI: 10.1038/gt.2010.38

[36] Yongsheng Y, Xiaoliang L, Zhenghao T: siRNA-mediated knockdown of FoxP3 promotes the ratio of T-helper 1 (Th1) to Th2 in chronic hepatitis B patients. Turk J Gastroenterol. 2011; 22: 587–593. DOI: 10.4318/tjg.2011.0251

[37] Kang S, Xie J, Ma S: Targeted knock down of CCL22 and CCL17 by siRNA during DC differentiation and maturation affects the recruitment of T subsets. Immunobiology. 2010; 215: 153–162. DOI: 10.1016/j.imbio.2009.03.001

[38] Zheng X, Koropatnick J, Chen D: Silencing IDO in dendritic cells: a novel approach to enhance cancer immunotherapy in a murine breast cancer model. Int J Cancer. 2013; 132: 967–977. DOI: 10.1002/ijc.27710

[39] Zheng X, Koropatnick J, Li M: Reinstalling antitumor immunity by inhibiting tumor-derived immunosuppressive molecule IDO through RNA interference. J Immunol. 2006; 177: 5639–5646. DOI: 10.4049/jimmunol.177.8.5639

[40] Flatekval GF, Sioud M: Modulation of dendritic cell maturation and function with mono- and bifunctional small interfering RNAs targeting indoleamine 2,3-dioxygenase. Immunology. 2009; 128: e837–848. DOI: 10.1111/j.1365-2567.2009.03093.x

[41] Chen D, Koropatnick J, Jiang N: Targeted siRNA silencing of indoleamine 2, 3-dioxygenase in antigen-presenting cells using mannose-conjugated liposomes: a novel strategy for treatment of melanoma. J Immunother. 2014; 37: 123–134. DOI: 10.1097/CJI.0000000000000022

[42] Yen MC, Lin CC, Chen YL: A novel cancer therapy by skin delivery of indoleamine 2,3-dioxygenase siRNA. Clin Cancer Res. 2009; 15: 641–649. DOI: 10.1158/1078-0432.CCR-08-1988

[43] Huang TT, Yen MC, Lin CC: Skin delivery of short hairpin RNA of indoleamine 2,3 dioxygenase induces antitumor immunity against orthotopic and metastatic liver cancer. Cancer Sci. 2011; 102: 2214–2220. DOI: 10.1111/j.1349-7006.2011.02094.x

[44] Huang M, Sun R, Wei H: Simultaneous knockdown of multiple ligands of innate receptor NKG2D prevents natural killer cell-mediated fulminant hepatitis in mice. Hepatology. 2013; 57: 277–288. DOI: 10.1002/hep.25959

[45] Zeng XC, Zhang T, Huang DH: RNA interfering targeting human leukocyte antigen-G enhanced immune surveillance mediated by the natural killer cells on hepatocellular carcinoma. Ann Clin Lab Sci. 2013; 43: 135–144.

[46] Chen LJ, Han ZQ, Zhou H: Inhibition of HLA-G expression via RNAi abolishes resistance of extravillous trophoblast cell line TEV-1 to NK lysis. Placenta. 2010; 31: 519–527. DOI: 10.1016/j.placenta.2010.03.008

[47] Tan PH, Gao YJ, Berta T: Short small-interfering RNAs produce interferon-alpha-mediated analgesia. Br J Anaesth. 2012; 108: 662–669. DOI: 10.1093/bja/aer492

[48] Kariko K, Bhuyan P, Capodici J: Small interfering RNAs mediate sequence-independent gene suppression and induce immune activation by signaling through toll-like receptor 3. J Immunol. 2004; 172: 6545–6549. DOI: 10.4049/jimmunol.172.11.6545

[49] Khairuddin N, Gantier MP, Blake SJ: siRNA-induced immunostimulation through TLR7 promotes antitumoral activity against HPV-driven tumors in vivo. Immunol Cell Biol. 2012; 90: 187–196. DOI: 10.1038/icb.2011.19

[50] Ellermeier J, Wei J, Duewell P: Therapeutic efficacy of bifunctional siRNA combining TGF-beta1 silencing with RIG-I activation in pancreatic cancer. Cancer Res. 2013; 73: 1709–1720. DOI: 10.1158/0008-5472.CAN-11-3850

[51] Meng G, Xia M, Xu C: Multifunctional antitumor molecule 5'-triphosphate siRNA combining glutaminase silencing and RIG-I activation. Int J Cancer. 2014; 134: 1958–1971. DOI: 10.1002/ijc.28416

[52] Han Q, Zhang C, Zhang J: Reversal of hepatitis B virus-induced immune tolerance by an immunostimulatory 3p-HBx-siRNAs in a retinoic acid inducible gene I-dependent manner. Hepatology. 2011; 54: 1179–1189. DOI: 10.1002/hep.24505

[53] Chen X, Qian Y, Yan F: 5'-triphosphate-siRNA activates RIG-I-dependent type I interferon production and enhances inhibition of hepatitis B virus replication in HepG2.2.15 cells. Eur J Pharmacol. 2013; 721: 86–95. DOI: 10.1016/j.ejphar.2013.09.050

[54] Ebert G, Poeck H, Lucifora J: 5' Triphosphorylated small interfering RNAs control replication of hepatitis B virus and induce an interferon response in human liver cells

and mice. Gastroenterology. 2011; 141: 696–706, 706 e691-693. DOI: 10.1053/j.gastro.2011.05.001

[55] Lan P, Zhang C, Han Q: Therapeutic recovery of hepatitis B virus (HBV)-induced hepatocyte-intrinsic immune defect reverses systemic adaptive immune tolerance. Hepatology. 2013; 58: 73–85. DOI: 10.1002/hep.26339

[56] Lin L, Liu Q, Berube N: 5'-Triphosphate-short interfering RNA: potent inhibition of influenza A virus infection by gene silencing and RIG-I activation. J Virol. 2012; 86: 10359–10369. DOI: 10.1128/JVI.00665-12

[57] Ahn J, Ko A, Jun EJ: Antiviral effects of small interfering RNA simultaneously inducing RNA interference and type 1 interferon in coxsackievirus myocarditis. Antimicrob Agents Chemother. 2012; 56: 3516–3523. DOI: 10.1128/AAC.06050-12

[58] Meng Z, Zhang X, Wu J: RNAi induces innate immunity through multiple cellular signaling pathways. PLoS One. 2013; 8: e64708. DOI: 10.1371/journal.pone.0064708

[59] Sui H, Zhou M, Chen Q: siRNA enhances DNA-mediated interferon lambda-1 response through crosstalk between RIG-I and IFI16 signalling pathway. Nucleic Acids Res. 2014; 42: 583–598. DOI: 10.1093/nar/gkt844

[60] Esau C, Davis S, Murray SF: miR-122 regulation of lipid metabolism revealed by in vivo antisense targeting. Cell Metab. 2006; 3: 87–98. DOI: 10.1016/j.cmet.2006.01.005

[61] Jopling CL, Yi M, Lancaster AM: Modulation of hepatitis C virus RNA abundance by a liver-specific MicroRNA. Science. 2005; 309: 1577–1581. DOI: 10.1126/science.1113329

[62] Jopling CL, Schutz S, Sarnow P: Position-dependent function for a tandem microRNA miR-122-binding site located in the hepatitis C virus RNA genome. Cell Host Microbe. 2008; 4: 77–85. DOI: 10.1016/j.chom.2008.05.013

[63] Henke JI, Goergen D, Zheng J: microRNA-122 stimulates translation of hepatitis C virus RNA. EMBO J. 2008; 27: 3300–3310. DOI: 10.1038/emboj.2008.244

[64] Randall G, Panis M, Cooper JD: Cellular cofactors affecting hepatitis C virus infection and replication. Proc Natl Acad Sci U S A. 2007; 104: 12884–12889. DOI: 10.1073/pnas.0704894104

[65] Machlin ES, Sarnow P, Sagan SM: Masking the 5' terminal nucleotides of the hepatitis C virus genome by an unconventional microRNA-target RNA complex. Proc Natl Acad Sci U S A. 2011; 108: 3193–3198. DOI: 10.1073/pnas.1012464108

[66] Li YP, Gottwein JM, Scheel TK: MicroRNA-122 antagonism against hepatitis C virus genotypes 1-6 and reduced efficacy by host RNA insertion or mutations in the HCV 5' UTR. Proc Natl Acad Sci U S A. 2011; 108: 4991–4996. DOI: 10.1073/pnas.1016606108

[67] Chang J, Guo JT, Jiang D: Liver-specific microRNA miR-122 enhances the replication of hepatitis C virus in nonhepatic cells. J Virol. 2008; 82: 8215–8223. DOI: 10.1128/JVI.02575-07

[68] Pedersen IM, Cheng G, Wieland S: Interferon modulation of cellular microRNAs as an antiviral mechanism. Nature. 2007; 449: 919–922. DOI: 10.1038/nature06205

[69] Sarasin-Filipowicz M, Krol J, Markiewicz I: Decreased levels of microRNA miR-122 in individuals with hepatitis C responding poorly to interferon therapy. Nat Med. 2009; 15: 31–33. DOI: 10.1038/nm.1902

[70] Murakami Y, Tanaka M, Toyoda H: Hepatic microRNA expression is associated with the response to interferon treatment of chronic hepatitis C. BMC Med Genomics. 2010; 3: 48. DOI: 10.1186/1755-8794-3-48

[71] Elmen J, Lindow M, Silahtaroglu A: Antagonism of microRNA-122 in mice by systemically administered LNA-antimiR leads to up-regulation of a large set of predicted target mRNAs in the liver. Nucleic Acids Res. 2008; 36: 1153–1162. DOI: 10.1093/nar/gkm1113

[72] Hildebrandt-Eriksen ES, Aarup V, Persson R: A locked nucleic acid oligonucleotide targeting microRNA 122 is well-tolerated in cynomolgus monkeys. Nucleic Acid Ther. 2012; 22: 152–161. DOI: 10.1089/nat.2011.0332

[73] Lanford RE, Hildebrandt-Eriksen ES, Petri A: Therapeutic silencing of microRNA-122 in primates with chronic hepatitis C virus infection. Science. 2010; 327: 198–201. DOI: 10.1126/science.1178178

[74] Elmen J, Lindow M, Schutz S: LNA-mediated microRNA silencing in non-human primates. Nature. 2008; 452: 896–899. DOI: 10.1038/nature06783

[75] van der Ree MH, van der Meer AJ, de Bruijne J: Long-term safety and efficacy of microRNA-targeted therapy in chronic hepatitis C patients. Antiviral Res. 2014; 111: 53–59. DOI: 10.1016/j.antiviral.2014.08.015

[76] Masaki T, Arend KC, Li Y: miR-122 stimulates hepatitis C virus RNA synthesis by altering the balance of viral RNAs engaged in replication versus translation. Cell Host Microbe. 2015; 17: 217–228. DOI: 10.1016/j.chom.2014.12.014

[77] Janssen HL, Kauppinen S, Hodges MR: HCV infection and miravirsen. N Engl J Med. 2013; 369: 878. DOI: 10.1056/NEJMc1307787

[78] Hou W, Tian Q, Zheng J: MicroRNA-196 represses Bach1 protein and hepatitis C virus gene expression in human hepatoma cells expressing hepatitis C viral proteins. Hepatology. 2010; 51: 1494–1504. DOI: 10.1002/hep.23401

[79] Cheng JC, Yeh YJ, Tseng CP: Let-7b is a novel regulator of hepatitis C virus replication. Cell Mol Life Sci. 2012; 69: 2621–2633. DOI: 10.1007/s00018-012-0940-6

[80] Lecellier CH, Dunoyer P, Arar K: A cellular microRNA mediates antiviral defense in human cells. Science. 2005; 308: 557–560. DOI: 10.1126/science.1108784

[81] Lagos D, Pollara G, Henderson S: miR-132 regulates antiviral innate immunity through suppression of the p300 transcriptional co-activator. Nat Cell Biol. 2010; 12: 513–519. DOI: 10.1038/ncb2054

[82] Trobaugh DW, Gardner CL, Sun C: RNA viruses can hijack vertebrate microRNAs to suppress innate immunity. Nature. 2014; 506: 245–248. DOI: 10.1038/nature12869

[83] Shapiro JS, Schmid S, Aguado LC: Drosha as an interferon-independent antiviral factor. Proc Natl Acad Sci U S A. 2014; 111: 7108–7113. DOI: 10.1073/pnas.1319635111

[84] Chen XM, Splinter PL, O'Hara SP: A cellular micro-RNA, let-7i, regulates toll-like receptor 4 expression and contributes to cholangiocyte immune responses against Cryptosporidium parvum infection. J Biol Chem. 2007; 282: 28929–28938. DOI: 10.1074/jbc.M702633200

[85] Ma C, Li Y, Zeng J: Mycobacterium bovis BCG triggered MyD88 induces miR-124 feedback negatively regulates immune response in alveolar epithelial cells. PLoS One. 2014; 9: e92419. DOI: 10.1371/journal.pone.0092419

[86] Mukherjee A, Di Bisceglie AM, Ray RB: Hepatitis C virus-mediated enhancement of microRNA miR-373 impairs the JAK/STAT signaling pathway. J Virol. 2015; 89: 3356–3365. DOI: 10.1128/JVI.03085-14

[87] Landais I, Pelton C, Streblow D: Human cytomegalovirus miR-UL112-3p targets TLR2 and modulates the TLR2/IRAK1/NFkappaB signaling pathway. PLoS Pathog. 2015; 11: e1004881. DOI: 10.1371/journal.ppat.1004881

[88] Michael SF, Zhu X, He Z: MicroRNA-30e* suppresses dengue virus replication by promoting NF-κB–dependent IFN production. PLoS Neglected Tropical Diseases. 2014; 8: e3088. DOI: 10.1371/journal.pntd.0003088

[89] Xu C, He X, Zheng Z: Downregulation of microRNA miR-526a by enterovirus inhibits RIG-I-dependent innate immune response. J Virol. 2014; 88: 11356–11368. DOI: 10.1128/JVI.01400-14

[90] Kim JK, Yuk JM, Kim SY: MicroRNA-125a inhibits autophagy activation and antimicrobial responses during mycobacterial infection. J Immunol. 2015; 194: 5355–5365. DOI: 10.4049/jimmunol.1402557

[91] Park H, Huang X, Lu C: MicroRNA-146a and microRNA-146b regulate human dendritic cell apoptosis and cytokine production by targeting TRAF6 and IRAK1 proteins. J Biol Chem. 2015; 290: 2831–2841. DOI: 10.1074/jbc.M114.591420

[92] Wang S, Zhang X, Ju Y: MicroRNA-146a feedback suppresses T cell immune function by targeting Stat1 in patients with chronic hepatitis B. J Immunol. 2013; 191: 293–301. DOI: 10.4049/jimmunol.1202100

[93] Taganov KD, Boldin MP, Chang KJ: NF-kappaB-dependent induction of microRNA miR-146, an inhibitor targeted to signaling proteins of innate immune responses. Proc Natl Acad Sci U S A. 2006; 103: 12481–12486. DOI: 10.1073/pnas.0605298103

[94] Chang YL, Ho BC, Sher S: miR-146a and miR-370 coordinate enterovirus 71-induced cell apoptosis through targeting SOS1 and GADD45beta. Cell Microbiol. 2015; 17: 802–818. DOI: 10.1111/cmi.12401

[95] Hou ZH, Han QJ, Zhang C: miR146a impairs the IFN-induced anti-HBV immune response by downregulating STAT1 in hepatocytes. Liver Int. 2014; 34: 58–68. DOI: 10.1111/liv.12244

[96] Hou J, Wang P, Lin L: MicroRNA-146a feedback inhibits RIG-I-dependent Type I IFN production in macrophages by targeting TRAF6, IRAK1, and IRAK2. J Immunol. 2009; 183: 2150–2158. DOI: 10.4049/jimmunol.0900707

[97] Wu S, He L, Li Y: miR-146a facilitates replication of dengue virus by dampening interferon induction by targeting TRAF6. J Infect. 2013; 67: 329–341. DOI: 10.1016/j.jinf.2013.05.003

[98] Ho BC, Yu IS, Lu LF: Inhibition of miR-146a prevents enterovirus-induced death by restoring the production of type I interferon. Nat Commun. 2014; 5: 3344. DOI: 10.1038/ncomms4344

[99] Sun X, Zhang J, Hou Z: miR-146a is directly regulated by STAT3 in human hepatocellular carcinoma cells and involved in anti-tumor immune suppression. Cell Cycle. 2015; 14: 243–252. DOI: 10.4161/15384101.2014.977112

[100] Lind EF, Elford AR, Ohashi PS: Micro-RNA 155 is required for optimal CD8+ T cell responses to acute viral and intracellular bacterial challenges. J Immunol. 2013; 190: 1210–1216. DOI: 10.4049/jimmunol.1202700

[101] Iwai H, Funatogawa K, Matsumura K: MicroRNA-155 knockout mice are susceptible to mycobacterium tuberculosis infection. Tuberculosis (Edinb). 2015; 95: 246–250. DOI: 10.1016/j.tube.2015.03.006

[102] Ruelas DS, Chan JK, Oh E: MicroRNA-155 Reinforces HIV Latency. J Biol Chem. 2015; 290: 13736–13748. DOI: 10.1074/jbc.M115.641837

[103] Cheng YQ, Ren JP, Zhao J: MicroRNA-155 regulates interferon-gamma production in natural killer cells via Tim-3 signalling in chronic hepatitis C virus infection. Immunology. 2015; 145: 485–497. DOI: 10.1111/imm.12463

[104] Hentzschel F, Hammerschmidt-Kamper C, Borner K: AAV8-mediated in vivo overexpression of miR-155 enhances the protective capacity of genetically attenuated malarial parasites. Mol Ther. 2014; 22: 2130–2141. DOI: 10.1038/mt.2014.172

[105] Bauernfeind F, Rieger A, Schildberg FA: NLRP3 inflammasome activity is negatively controlled by miR-223. J Immunol. 2012; 189: 4175–4181. DOI: 10.4049/jimmunol.1201516

[106] Haneklaus M, Gerlic M, Kurowska-Stolarska M: Cutting edge: miR-223 and EBV miR-BART15 regulate the NLRP3 inflammasome and IL-1beta production. J Immunol. 2012; 189: 3795-3799. DOI: 10.4049/jimmunol.1200312

[107] Stern-Ginossar N, Elefant N, Zimmermann A: Host immune system gene targeting by a viral miRNA. Science. 2007; 317: 376–381. DOI: 10.1126/science.1140956

[108] Nachmani D, Stern-Ginossar N, Sarid R: Diverse herpesvirus microRNAs target the stress-induced immune ligand MICB to escape recognition by natural killer cells. Cell Host Microbe. 2009; 5: 376–385. DOI: 10.1016/j.chom.2009.03.003

[109] Bauman Y, Nachmani D, Vitenshtein A: An identical miRNA of the human JC and BK polyoma viruses targets the stress-induced ligand ULBP3 to escape immune elimination. Cell Host Microbe. 2011; 9: 93–102. DOI: 10.1016/j.chom.2011.01.008

[110] Nachmani D, Lankry D, Wolf DG: The human cytomegalovirus microRNA miR-UL112 acts synergistically with a cellular microRNA to escape immune elimination. Nat Immunol. 2010; 11: 806–813. DOI: 10.1038/ni.1916

[111] Jasinski-Bergner S, Stoehr C, Bukur J: Clinical relevance of miR-mediated HLA-G regulation and the associated immune cell infiltration in renal cell carcinoma. Oncoimmunology. 2015; 4: e1008805. DOI: 10.1080/2162402X.2015.1008805

[112] Zhu XM, Han T, Wang XH: Overexpression of miR-152 leads to reduced expression of human leukocyte antigen-G and increased natural killer cell mediated cytolysis in JEG-3 cells. Am J Obstet Gynecol. 2010; 202: 592 e591–597. DOI: 10.1016/j.ajog.2010.03.002

[113] Vinuesa CG, Cook MC, Angelucci C: A RING-type ubiquitin ligase family member required to repress follicular helper T cells and autoimmunity. Nature. 2005; 435: 452–458. DOI: 10.1038/nature03555

[114] Rasmussen TK, Andersen T, Bak RO: Overexpression of microRNA-155 increases IL-21 mediated STAT3 signaling and IL-21 production in systemic lupus erythematosus. Arthritis Res Ther. 2015; 17: 154. DOI: 10.1186/s13075-015-0660-z

[115] Xin Q, Li J, Dang J: miR-155 Deficiency Ameliorates Autoimmune Inflammation of Systemic Lupus Erythematosus by Targeting S1pr1 in Faslpr/lpr Mice. J Immunol. 2015; 194: 5437–5445. DOI: 10.4049/jimmunol.1403028

[116] Kalis M, Bolmeson C, Esguerra JL: Beta-cell specific deletion of Dicer1 leads to defective insulin secretion and diabetes mellitus. PLoS One. 2011; 6: e29166. DOI: 10.1371/journal.pone.0029166

[117] Salama A, Fichou N, Allard M: MicroRNA-29b modulates innate and antigen-specific immune responses in mouse models of autoimmunity. PLoS One. 2014; 9: e106153. DOI: 10.1371/journal.pone.0106153

[118] Yang M, Ye L, Wang B: Decreased miR-146 expression in peripheral blood mononuclear cells is correlated with ongoing islet autoimmunity in type 1 diabetes patients 1miR-146. J Diabetes. 2015; 7: 158–165. DOI: 10.1111/1753-0407.12163

[119] Lu LF, Boldin MP, Chaudhry A: Function of miR-146a in controlling Treg cell-mediated regulation of Th1 responses. Cell. 2010; 142: 914–929. DOI: 10.1016/j.cell.2010.08.012

[120] Banerjee A, Schambach F, DeJong CS: Micro-RNA-155 inhibits IFN-gamma signaling in CD4+ T cells. Eur J Immunol. 2010; 40: 225–231. DOI: 10.1002/eji.200939381

[121] Okoye IS, Czieso S, Ktistaki E: Transcriptomics identified a critical role for Th2 cell-intrinsic miR-155 in mediating allergy and antihelminth immunity. Proc Natl Acad Sci U S A. 2014; 111: E3081–3090. DOI: 10.1073/pnas.1406322111

[122] Zhou Q, Haupt S, Kreuzer JT: Decreased expression of miR-146a and miR-155 contributes to an abnormal Treg phenotype in patients with rheumatoid arthritis. Ann Rheum Dis. 2015; 74: 1265–1274. DOI: 10.1136/annrheumdis-2013-204377

[123] Ivanov II, McKenzie BS, Zhou L: The orphan nuclear receptor RORgammat directs the differentiation program of proinflammatory IL-17+ T helper cells. Cell. 2006; 126: 1121–1133. DOI: 10.1016/j.cell.2006.07.035

[124] Du C, Liu C, Kang J: MicroRNA miR-326 regulates TH-17 differentiation and is associated with the pathogenesis of multiple sclerosis. Nat Immunol. 2009; 10: 1252–1259. DOI: 10.1038/ni.1798

[125] Moore CS, Rao VT, Durafourt BA: miR-155 as a multiple sclerosis-relevant regulator of myeloid cell polarization. Ann Neurol. 2013; 74: 709–720. DOI: 10.1002/ana.23967

4

Utility of Potent Anti-Viral MicroRNAs in Emerging Infectious Diseases

Zhabiz Golkar, Donald G. Pace and Omar Bagasra

Abstract

MicroRNAs (miRNAs) are small, noncoding RNA molecules that have emerged as important posttranscriptional regulators of gene expression. miRNA provides intracellular immune defense when the body is faced with challenges from transgenes, viruses, transposons, and aberrant mRNAs. miRNA molecules trigger gene silencing in eukaryotic cells. To date, more than 3,000 different human miRNAs (*hsa-miRs*) have been identified, and it is generally agreed that cellular gene regulation is significantly impacted by the presence of miRNAs. A single miRNA has the complex capacity to target multiple genes simultaneously. In a viral infection context, miRNAs have been connected with the interplay between host and pathogen, and occupy a major role in the host–parasite interaction and pathogenesis. While numerous viral miRNAs from DNA viruses have been identified, characterization of functional RNA virus-encoded miRNAs and their potential targets is still ongoing. Here, we describe an in silico approach to analyze the most recent Ebola virus (EBOV) genome sequences causing West African epidemics. We identified numerous "candidate" miRNAs that can be utilized to quell the Ebola virus. Future approaches will focus on experimental validation of these miRNAs during quelling the Ebola target transcripts for further elucidating their biological functions in primates and other animal models.

Keywords: Ebola virus, gene alignment, miRNA, prevention, vaccine

1. Introduction

1.1. Inhibition of Ebola virus by anti-Ebola miRNAs In silico

Since the HIV-1 pandemic of the 1980s and more recent outbreaks of bird flu, severe acute respiratory syndrome (SARS), and Middle East respiratory syndrome-Corona Virus (MER-CoV), it has been widely believed that there would be new pandemics of highly pathogenic viruses [1]. Fortunately, until recently, many of the new emerging pathogenic agents, such as Ebola virus (EBOV) and Marburg virus (MARV), have failed to demonstrate the transmissibility or animal reservoirs required to become true pandemic threats [2, 3]. Few, if any, antivirals can claim to be specific enough to halt the epidemic. Recently, a whole EBOV replication-defective vaccine—EBOVdVP30—has been found to be very effective in nonhuman primates, while two others are in Phase II trials [4].

The testing of the recently developed replication-defective recombinant chimpanzee adenovirus type 3–vectored ebolavirus (cAd3-EBO) vaccine is based on a demonstration of efficacy in a nonhuman primate model [5]. However, a curious finding has puzzled the investigators —preexisting neutralizing antibodies against cAd6 and cAd68 in human serum samples were found in ~40% of Ugandans and in 15% of the US and European volunteers. The increased prevalence of neutralizing antibodies against chimpanzee adenoviruses in sub-Saharan Africa may indicate cross-species transmission of these viruses from chimpanzees to humans. The possibility of fairly high levels of neutralizing antibodies against cAd3 may complicate the evaluation of the effectiveness of Ebola vaccines currently underway.

1.2. Virology of Ebola virus

Filoviruses are taxonomically classified within the order *Mononegavirales*, a large group of enveloped viruses whose genomes are composed of a nonsegmented, single-stranded minus [2, 3] RNA molecule. Following their discovery, filoviruses were originally grouped with rhabdoviruses, as the appearance of these virus particles appeared similar [3]. However, subsequent filamentous morphology and extensive genetic, physiochemical, and virologic studies of Marburg virus (MARV) and Ebola virus (EBOV) revealed distinctive characteristics, and these viruses were placed into a separate family, the *Filoviridae* [3]. Further characterization of these agents demonstrated that EBOV and MARV represent divergent lineages of filoviruses, and that their variances were significant enough to warrant the formation of the two genera, MARV and EBOV [4]. Subsequent to the International Committee on Taxonomy of Viruses recommendation, the MARV genus contains a single species, the Lake Victoria Marburg virus, as this strain exhibits only limited genetic variation.

EBOV is the causative agent of Ebola virus disease (EVD) [6]. The mortality rate can vary from 40% to 93% depending on the strains [6]. The viral life cycle begins with host cell entry through a mechanism that is still poorly understood. The incubation period for EVD is 2–21 days, and typical early symptoms include fever, chills, malaise, and myalgia (all of which could be misdiagnosed as malaria, which is highly prevalent in West African nations), followed by the onset of symptoms indicative of multi-organ stress and subsequent failure, sometimes followed by hemorrhagic episodes that can easily be misdiagnosed as Lassa fever.

EBOV is a negative, single-stranded RNA virus with an unusual, variable-length, filamentous, branched morphology whose helical capsid is enclosed inside a membrane. The mechanism of attachment and entry into the cell is still not completely defined (see discussion below). Once inside, the viral RNA polymerase (L protein) begins to copy the negative strand (–ve) RNA to make the positive strand (+ve) transcripts that mimic the structure of mRNA and are translated by host ribosomes. Replication is thought to occur in the cytoplasm. An unusual feature of the transcription and translation of the Ebola genes is the fact that the glycoproteins (GP) are only expressed through transcriptional editing. The genome of the Zaire Ebola virus (EBOV), the most pathogenic among all species of EBOV, is 18,959 nucleotides (nts) in length and contains seven transcriptional units that guide synthesis of at least nine distinct primary translation products: the nucleoprotein (NP), virion protein (VP) 35, VP40, glycoprotein (GP), soluble glycoprotein (sGP), small soluble glycoprotein (ssGP), VP30, VP24, and the large (L) protein. L is the catalytic subunit of the viral polymerase complex (Figure 1). Similar to other nonsegmented negative-sense (NNS) RNA viruses, EBOVs encode a multiprotein complex to carry out replication and transcription. In the case of EBOV, viral RNA synthesis requires the viral NP, VP35, VP30, and L proteins. Transcription of filovirus mRNAs is presumed to occur as in other NNS viruses, where there is a gradient of viral mRNAs with the abundance of each mRNA transcript decreasing as the polymerase transcribes toward the 5′ end of the template [7]. Each EBOV mRNA is presumed to be efficiently modified with a 5′–7′-methylguanosine (m^7G) cap and a 3′p (A) tail [8].

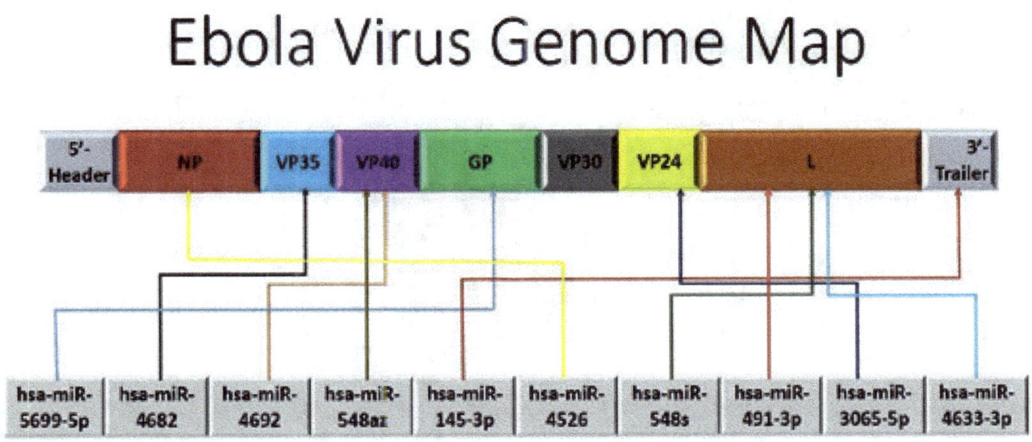

Figure 1. The genome of EBOV, 18 9 kb in length, has the following gene order: 3′ leader nucleoprotein (NP), virion proteins (VP) VP35-VP40, membrane glycoprotein (GP), viral polymerase (VP) VP30-VP24, viral polymerase L protein, and 5′ trailer.

The Ebola virus genus possesses greater diversity, and four viral species have been recognized: Zaire Ebola, Sudan Ebola, Reston Ebola, and Ivory Coast Ebola (EBOV-Z, EBOV-S, EBOV-R, and EBOV-IC, respectively). Each of the EBOV species has a different degree of pathogenicity and mortality rate [9]. Therefore, EBOV-S and EBOV-Z, which are the predominant EBOVs associated with known outbreaks, are more pathogenic than EBOV-R and EBOV-IC [10]. EBOV-IC has only caused a single nonfatal human infection, but EBOV-R has caused fatal infection in nonhuman primates [8]. However, EBOV-S, EBOV-Z, and EBOV-B often cause severe hemorrhagic diseases with markedly high case fatality rates (40–90%) [10]. The EBOV genome is 18.9 kb in length with the following gene order: 3′ leader nucleoprotein (NP), virion protein (VP) 35-VP40, glycoprotein (GP), VP30, VP24, polymerase (L), and 5′ trailer. The GP differences between any two species range from 37% to 41% at the nucleotide level and from

34% to 43% at the amino acid level [40]. However, variations within EBOV-Z species are very low (~2–3%) [11]. Thus, GP nucleotides are usually used in the phylogenetic analysis of EBOV (Figure 2).

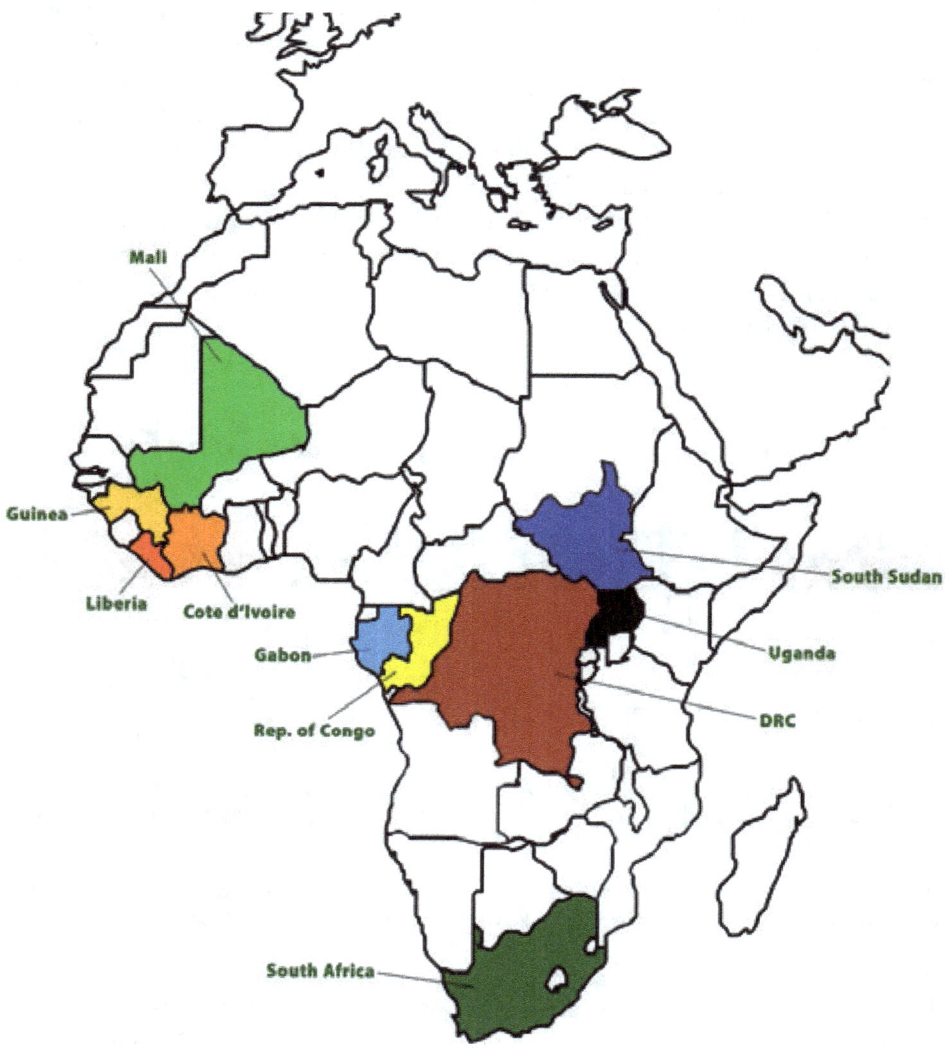

Figure 2. The Ebola Pandemic Map depicts the history of Ebola in Africa. The sporadic cases of Ebola were common in the central African countries such as the DRC (988 cases with 767 fatalities), Uganda (606 cases with 283 fatalities), South Sudan (335 cases with 180 fatalities), Gabon (214 cases with 150 fatalities), the Republic of the Congo (248 cases with 210 fatalities), and South Africa (2 cases with 1 fatality).

Because of their high mortality rate, which can vary from 40% to 93%, and their potential for person-to-person transmission and lack of an approved vaccine or antiviral therapy, MARV and EBOV are classified as biosafety level 4 (BSL-4) viruses by World Health Organization [12, 13]

1.3. History of MARV and EBOV

Viruses are obligate intracellular parasites and essentially rely on host cells for raw materials, replication, transcription, and translations of their genetic codes. Until a few years ago, we assumed that the major intracellular defenses against viral pathogens were interferons [13]. Since the discovery of RNA interference (RNAi) and miRNAs, we know that one of the fundamental functions of miRNAs is to prevent replication of foreign viruses by pre- and posttranscriptions and suppressions of viral expression [12]. Therefore, besides endogenous gene regulation, miRNAs are the primary intracellular immune defense system [13]. Viruses have also evolved to counter the antiviral effects of miRNAs by viral miRNAs (vmiRNAs).

Recently, Li and Chen [14] have conducted molecular epidemiologic analyses of presently extant Ebola viral genomes to ascertain their evolutionary viral history. Of considerable potential importance are interpretations derived from a dataset that is between 1,000 and 2,100 years old and includes four Ebola species (EBOV-Z, EBOV-S, EBOV-TF, EBOV-R) [15]. Logically, one could assume that over the past 2,000 years, humans have evolved countermeasures to the Ebola virus via innate, adaptive, and miRNA-based immunity. The identification in a human database of 71 miRNAs capable of potentially quelling EBOV strongly suggests that *Homo sapiens* already have developed primary intracellular defenses to quell EBOV infection [16]. This raises a question: Why have EBOVs been circulating for about 2,000 years, and yet they seem to have emerged only recently? The earliest known cases of Ebola date to the 1970s. One theory proposes that EBOV-Z experienced a recent genetic bottleneck [17]. Before Ebola viral strains were introduced to primates, they had already been circulating among small mammals, including bats, rodents, marsupials, shrews, and so on [16]. Although these bats and other animals were infected [15, 16], no evidence demonstrated that such infections were fatal to them [18]. This indicates that a natural balance had been achieved between the viruses' pathogenicity and the host's immune system, especially at the intracellular levels where miRNAs provide immunological protection [19]. This homeostasis, this balance, apparently was broken in 1900, when EBOV genetic diversity experienced a dramatic drop [16]. Accordingly, most lineages of the various EBOV species became extinct because of such influences as threatening human activities, climate change, and a steep decline in the number of animals to serve as a reservoir for viral replication. Probably due to altered patterns of positive selection in the glycoprotein (GP), which diversified substantially and was found to be part of fusion and receptor binding within cellular membranes, infection patterns through direct exposure were changing. Therefore, by about 1970, few lineages that possessed broader tropism and enhanced fitness had the capacity to infect primates via direct exposure [16]. Similar examples can be seen in the emergence of HIV-1, which appeared to have surfaced in the 1950s through a zoonotic event that involved common infections among chimpanzees (i.e., SIV) and then accidentally jumped to humans [16–18]. Due to the paucity of significant differences in EBOV genetic diversity since 1970, the decreased number of surviving viruses may have become the only circulating lineages in primates and viral reservoirs. EBOV-Z has the ability to traverse a long distance through bats, which serve as a migratory reservoir. Outbreaks with their epicenter in Congo have been caused by the EBOV-Z species [20–23].

Through analysis of miRNA numbers that demonstrate high homologies in seed sequences and that show high identity to EBOV species, we have deduced that the genetic variations at the GP may serve as a type of Achilles' heel. After all, only one miRNA showed identity to GP, while eight proved capable of blocking polymerase steps. This indicates that minor variations within the GP amino acid sequence could allow for viral entrance into host target cells in humans. The subsequent transcription of negative-stranded RNA viruses into positive RNA strands occurs amid a struggle to overcome the miRNAs with quelling potential that can halt this process. It is possible that at the time of exposure to EBOV, all of the protective miRNAs may not be present in the target cells, or may be present, but not in sufficient quantities to block early EBOV replication [24].

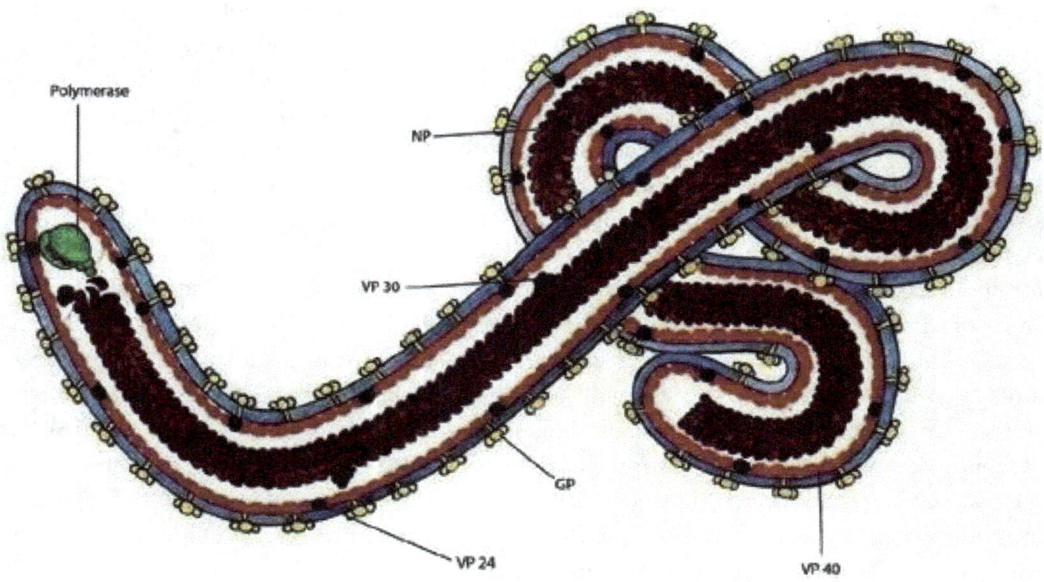

Figure 3. The illustration depicts a simplified structure of Ebola virus. The functions of various viral proteins are described in the text. GP, glycoprotein; NP, nucleoprotein; VP40, matrix protein; VP30, transcription factor; and polymerase enzyme.

Figure 3 shows the VP24, VP30, VP35, VP40, and L nucleoproteins that constitute the nucleocapsid, which is crucial in both the transcription and viral replication processes [25, 26]. The glycoprotein is located in the lipid membrane of the Ebola virus; this is also the place in the host target cells where receptors that facilitate viral entry are embedded [27]. Viral matrix proteins VP40 and VP24 are essential to viral budding, stability, and structure. VP40 is the primary matrix protein, and is the viral protein that is expressed most abundantly. It plays a central role in the process of Ebola budding from the plasma membrane. For example, in mammalian cells, the mere expression of VP40 is sufficient to create virus-like particles (VLPs) with morphological characteristics that are similar to those of the actual Ebola virus [28, 29]. Given VP40's absence, studies have found that the nucleocapsid was not transported effectively into the plasma membrane, and as this membrane is the site of assembly, budding, and incorporation into the virions, considerable attention should be given to the role of this matrix protein [30]. The utilization of miRNAs that specifically target VP40 mRNA degradation is important to our understanding of just how VP40 functions and what potential roles it might play in the regulation of VLP assembly in both in vitro and live cell settings. *hsa-miR-4692* and *hsa-miR-548-az* effectively target VP40; therefore, the overexpression of these particular miRNAs within host cells could totally disrupt the viral life cycle and may have a decisive impact in the categorization of therapeutic targets (data unpublished). The tendency of Ebola VP40 to assemble virus-like particles (VLPs) presents an appealing model for analysis of the Ebola viral assembly at biosafety level 2 made possible by the noninfectious nature of genetically engineered VLPs [31].

VP40's association with the plasma membrane is of fundamental importance [30]; it is here that assembly is initiated as well as oligomerization [31], and nucleoprotein recruitment. Besides membrane association, VP40 also associates or otherwise interacts with host cell factors, including the endosomal sorting complex that supports transport (ESCRT) machinery [27, 29], the vesicle coat II proteins (COPII) [24], as well as the protein actin [25, 30]; these host cell factors, respectively, have been shown to enable VP40 budding, transport, and movement. Moreover, host cell protein kinases could contribute to Ebola infectivity as c-Abl1 can phosphorylate Tyr^{13} in VP40 [32, 33]. Still we have an inadequate understanding of how VP40 actually assembles on the plasma membrane before virion release occurs. Localization of VP40 in the plasma membrane is believed to be important as studies give evidence that hydrophobic residues located within the C-terminal domain, including Leu^{213}, are essential in the localization and budding processes [32]. Detection of VP40 oligomers in VLPs and UV-inactivated virions has occurred [34, 35]; they have been detected mainly in filamentous structures stemming from the plasma membrane [36]. Therefore, VP40 oligomerization apparently occurs on the same plasma membrane in which oligomers selectively have found to reside [37]. In terms of structure, VP40 has predominantly been found to oligomerize into either hexamers or octamers [38, 39]. These share a comparable monomer–monomer (or intradimeric) antiparallel interface. However, the detection of oligomeric structures in live cells suggests that these structures, too, could exert a critical influence on both viral assembly and egress [40]. We discovered that *hsa-miR-4692* and *hsa-miR-548-az* both target VP40 (data unpublished).

The formation of virus-like particles (VLPs) requires VP40 oligomers; these are associated with membranes that are resistant to detergent [41], which underscores the active part that the plasma membrane may play in VP40 oligomerization. Moreover, on the plasma membrane, matrix protein oligomerization may function as a scaffold in host protein recruitment, and also supply the force needed to effect the formation of virus particles and the deformation of membranes. A comprehension of VP40 plasma membrane association thus becomes crucial to our understanding of how the formation of protein buds occurs on the plasma membrane. Gupta K [42] recently investigated the role that the VP40 C-terminal domain plays in membrane association as well as in membrane penetration. These investigators utilized the monolayer penetration methodology to conduct in vitro research into the molecular basis of the penetration of the VP40 membrane. To study VP40 assembly and its associated egress in cells, they employed a multipronged methodology that blended cellular imaging, number and brightness (N&B) analysis, analysis of the egress of virus-like particles, site-directed mutagenesis, and total internal reflection (TIRF) microscopy. N&B analysis permitted them to ascertain the average number of molecules and also the brightness within each pixel within a fluorescence microscopy image. This permitted them to detect the oligomeric status of proteins that are labeled fluorescently. They concluded that within the VP40 C-terminal domain, a hydrophobic interface actually penetrates the plasma membrane, which plays a key role in the oligomerization of VP40. The knocking out of plasma membrane penetration by hydrophobic mutants also substantially reduces the egress of VLPs [38, 39]. Therefore, degradation of VP40 mRNA by a two-pronged attack from *hsa-miR-4692* and *hsa-miR-548-az* can stop Ebola.

A distinguishing characteristic of filovirus genomes is their 3′- and 5′-UTRs that are long related to other RNA viruses of the nonsegmented negative-strand (NNS) variety [40]. Of particular note, Kochetov AV [41] concentrated on the 5′-UTRs in the mRNA of seven EBOV viruses, due to the critical importance of the 5′-UTRs in translation initiation. In four of these seven mRNAs, small alternate upstream open reading frames (uORFs) were identified, but their significance is yet to be fully characterized. In cellular mRNAs, uORFs are known to be a common feature; they are critical in modulating translation of primary ORFs (pORFs), which was accomplish by reducing the efficiency and quantity of the scanning ribosomes associated with the reinitiation that occurs at the start codon of pORFs [42]. At a uAUG, rather than a pAUG, translation initiation frequency is affected by a variety of factors, including the strength of the Kozak consensus sequence that surrounds the uAUG. Moreover, between the pAUG and the upstream open reading frame (uORF) is an intercistronic space that, combined with the phosphorylation status of and the eIF-2α [43, 44], controls whether translation takes place at the principal protein initiation site (pAUG) or at the termination codon (uAUG).

When eIF-2α~P is absent, cap-dependent translation has been found to be efficient, which permits higher ribosome initiation rates at the uORF [45]. When eIF2α~P is enhanced, impairment of translation initiation occurs, which causes a ribosome to continue scanning beyond the uAUG; in this case, initiation occurs at the pAUG. In short, when cell stress occurs, eIF2α~P facilitates translation initiation of select mRNAs that possess uORFs at the primary open ready frame (pORF) [46].

They characterized how the EBOV 5′-UTRs modulate translation. Mutating any of the four uAUGs present in the EBOV genome enhances translation at the corresponding pORF. The most dramatic effect was with the L gene where the L uAUG can potently suppress pORF translation; however, in response to eIF2α~P, the L uAUG maintains L translation. Modulating viral polymerase levels is biologically significant as ablating the L uORF in a recombinant EBOV reduces viral titers 10- to 100-fold in cell culture, severely impairs viral RNA synthesis, and functions to maintain virus titers in cells treated with stress-inducing agents. These data suggest that a uORF in the EBOV L mRNA regulates polymerase expression in response to the status of the cellular innate immune response and is required for optimal virus replication.

It would be relatively easy to incorporate a combination of relevant miRNAs in a miRNA-expression vector to test the utility of these miRNAs in genetically engineered VLP cell models in vitro that can be performed in a BSL-2 facility, and then to extend these studies in animal models utilizing safe vectors in a BSL-4 environment.

Currently, there are several genetically engineered vaccines containing genes for surface proteins (GP) that are in clinical trial. The first among these is a vaccine that Ebola GP genes stitched into a weakened chimpanzee adenovirus that serves as a vector. The second vaccine contains the Ebola surface protein gene inside a weakened version of vesicular stomatitis virus (VSV), which commonly infects farm animals. The potential dangers of employing of VSV are obvious: it can save men but potentially harm livestock in West Africa. The chimpanzee adenovirus will be a zoonotic event itself, and its potential danger cannot be underestimated [47, 48].

The third vaccine uses a vector known as MVA, a modified version of the smallpox vaccine virus, and involves protection from an Ebola virus "challenge" 10 months after the last vaccination.

We noted that none of these three approaches mentioned a simple and well-tested method of human and animal vaccination. What happened to the simple, whole formalin-killed or UV-killed, less pathogenic EBOV vaccines that have been tried in so many viral vaccinations [49, 50]?

With viruses like the major Ebola strands, where the mortality rate is over 50%, it will be difficult to find a reasonable and ethical way to carry out an unbiased clinical trial. However, if one can prepare a "dead Ebola virus" with antigenicity intact, it would be easy to immunize "high risk groups" without utilizing unusual vectors as exemplified by "harmless" chimpanzee adenovirus, VSV or MVA (modified smallpox virus), each with unknown long-term risk factors and accompanied by immediate concerns of viral vector-induced antigenic competition that may potentially quell proper immune responses to the Ebola antigens [51]. We believe that a dead vaccine may induce the protective miRNAs and quell the pandemic. Increasingly, miRNA-induced intracellular immunity is being better understood, and several clinical trials are under way to treat viral diseases and cancers [52–55]. The cost of each of these vaccines would run into millions of dollars and would be prohibitively expensive to any of the individuals who are predicted to be infected with the virus in West African nations. In contrast to the proposed recombinant vaccines, each of the more traditional "killed vaccines" has been very inexpensive to produce and has benefited billions of humans [56].

2. Conclusions

The current ongoing Ebola outbreaks in West Africa that began almost three years ago in March 2013 have already claimed 11,000 lives and over 27,000 cases. The rapid spread of the infection demands the need for rapid prevention methods. Currently, there are several vaccines that are in different phases of clinical trials. In this report, we highlight an alternative to the standard vaccine for Ebola prevention. We show that a preventive method based on miRNAs could be utilized and tested in nonhuman primates. Some of the lessons that we have learned from the recent West Africa Ebola outbreaks is to test the vaccine and other preventive methods that are currently available against Ebola before the major outbreaks occur. Therefore, we recommend that vaccines and preventive methods must be developed to the point that the measures correlate for human protection (Phase I level), so when the outbreaks occur, the vaccine and other measures can be rolled out quickly to prevent the spread of the disease.

Acknowledgements

We would like to thank Dr. Donald Gene Pace for his editorial assistance.

Author details

Zhabiz Golkar[1], Donald G. Pace[2] and Omar Bagasra[3*]

*Address all correspondence to: obagasra@claflin.edu

1 Department of Biology, School of Health and Natural Science, Voorhees College, Denmark, SC, USA

2 School of Humanities & Social Science, Claflin University, Orangeburg, SC, USA

3 School of Natural Science, Claflin University, Orangeburg, SC, USA

References

[1] Na W, Park N, Yeom M, Song D. Ebola outbreak in Western Africa 2014: what is going on with Ebola virus? ClinExp Vaccine Res. 2015; 4:1:17-22. DOI:10.7774/cevr.2015.4.1.17

[2] Zhou Y, Simmons G. Development of novel entry inhibitors targeting emerging viruses Expert Rev Anti Infect Ther. 2012; 10: 1129–1138 t. DOI:10.1586/eri.12.104

[3] Misasi J, Chandran K, Yang JY. Filoviruses require endosomal cysteine proteases for entry but exhibit distinct protease preferences. J. Virol. 2012; 86:6:3284–3292. DOI:10.1128/JVI.06346-11

[4] Sarwar UN, Costner P, Enama ME, Berkowitz N, Hu Z, Hendel CS, Sitar S, Plummer S, Mulangu S, Bailer RT, Koup RA, Mascola JR, Nabel GJ, Sullivan NJ, Graham BS, Ledgerwood JE. Safety and immunogenicity of DNA vaccines encoding Ebola virus and Marburg virus wild-type glycoproteins in a phase I clinical trial. J Infect Dis. 2015; 211:4:549–557. DOI:10.1093/infdis/jiu511

[5] Zhang Q, Seto DChimpanzee Adenovirus Vector Ebola Vaccine--Preliminary Report. N Engl J Med. 2015 Aug 20; 373(8):775–6. DOI:10.1056/NEJMc1505499#SA1

[6] Gao J, Yin L. Drug development for controlling Ebola epidemic – a race against time.Drug DiscovTher. 2014; 85:229–31.

[7] Drake JW, Holland JJ. "Mutation rates among RNA viruses". Proc. Natl. Acad. Sci. 1999; 96:24:13910–13913. DOI:10.1073/pnas.96.24.13910

[8] Adu-Gyamfi E, Soni SP, Xue Y, Digman MA, Gratton E, Stahelin RV. The Ebola virus matrix protein penetrates into the plasma membrane: a key step in viral protein 40 (VP40) oligomerization and viral egress. J Biol Chem. 2013; 288:8:5779–5789. DOI: 10.1074/jbc.M112.443960

[9] Shabman RS, Hoenen T, Groseth A, Jabado O, Binning JM. An Upstream Open Reading Frame Modulates Ebola Virus Polymerase Translation and Virus Replication. 2013. PLoSPathog 9(1): e1003147. DOI:10.1371/journal.ppat.1003147

[10] Harty RN. No exit: Targeting the budding process to inhibit filovirus replication. Antiviral 2009; 81:189–197. DOI:10.1016/j.antiviral. 2008.12.003.

[11] Feldmann HME, Randolf A, Will C, Kiley MP, Sanchez A. Marburg virus, a Filovirus: messenger RNAs, gene order, and regulatory elements of the replication cycle. 1992; 24:1–19.

[12] Adu-Gyamfi E, Soni SP, Xue Y, Digman MA, Gratton E, Stahelin RV. The Ebola virus matrix protein penetrates into the plasma membrane: a key step in viral protein 40 (VP40) oligomerization and viral egress. J Biol Chem. 2013; 288:8:5779–5789. DOI: 10.1074/jbc.M112.443960

[13] Sanchez AKM. Identification and analysis of Ebola virus messenger RNA. Virology. 1987; 157:414–420.

[14] Weik M, Modrof J, Klenk HD, Becker S, Muhlberger E. Ebola Virus VP30-Mediated Transcription Is Regulated by RNA Secondary Structure Formation. J Virol. 2012; 76:8532–8539. DOI:10.1128/JVI.76.17.8532-8539.2002

[15] Bryan R. Cullen. The role of RNAi and microRNAs in animal virus replication and antiviral immunity. Genes & Dev. 2009; 23:1151–1164. DOI:10.1101/gad.1793309.

[16] Haasnoot J, Vries WD, Geutjes EJ, Prins M, Haan PD, Berkhout B.The Ebola virus VP35 protein is a suppressor of RNA silencing. PLoSPathog. 2007; 3:e86, DOI: 10.1371/journal.ppat.0030086

[17] Li YH, Chen SP. Evolutionary history of Ebola virus. Epidemiol Infect. 2014;142(6): 1138–1145. DOI: 10.1017/S0950268813002215.

[18] Biek R. Recent common ancestry of Ebola Zaire virus found in a bat reservoir. PLoS Pathogens. 2006; 2:e90. DOI: 10.1371/journal.ppat.0020090.

[19] Ramanan P, Shabman RS, Brown CS, Amarasinghe GK, Basler CF, Leung DW. Filoviral immune evasion mechanisms. Viruses. 2011; 3:9:1634-1649. DOI:10.3390/v3091634

[20] Taylor DJ, Leach RW, Bruenn J. Filoviruses are ancient and integrated into mammalian genomes. BMC evolutionary biology. 2010; 22:10:193. DOI: 10.1186/1471-2148-10-193

[21] Hunt CL, Kondratowicz AS, Bowman J, Sinn PL, McCray PB Jr, Quinn K, Weller ML, Chiorini JA, Maury W. Tyrosine kinase receptor Axl enhances entry of Zaire ebolavirus without direct interactions with the viral glycoprotein.Virology. 2011; 5:415:2: 83-94. DOI:10.1016/j.virol.2011.04.002

[22] Soni SP, Adu-Gyamfi E, Yong SS, Jee CS, Stahelin RV. The Ebola Virus Matrix Protein Deeply Penetrates the Plasma Membrane: An Important Step in Viral Egress. Biophysical Journal. 2013; 104:9:1940-1949. DOI:10.1016/j.bpj.2013.03.021

[23] Warfield KL, Warren TK, Lovejoy C, Hassinger JN, Ruthel G, Blouch RE, Moulton HM, Weller DD, Iversen PL, Bavari S. Chemical modifications of antisense morpholino oligomers enhance their efficacy against Ebola virus infection. Antimicrob Agents Chemother. 2009; 53:5:2089–2099. DOI:10.1128/AAC.00936-08

[24] Reynard O, Nemirov K, Volchkov VE. Conserved proline-rich region of Ebola virus matrix protein VP40 is essential for plasma membrane targeting and virus-like particle release. J. Infect. Dis. 2011; 204:3: 884–891. DOI:10.1093/infdis/jir305

[25] Makino A, Yamayoshi S, Kawaoka Y. Identification of amino acids in Marburg virus VP40 that are important for virus-like particle budding. J. Infect. Dis. 2011; 204: 3:871–877. DOI:10.1093/infdis/jir309.

[26] Harty RN, Brown ME, Hayes FP. A PPxY motif within the VP40 protein of Ebola virus interacts physically and functionally with a ubiquitin ligase: implications for filovirus budding. Proc. Natl. Acad. Sci. 2000; 97:13871–13876.

[27] Licata JM, Simpson-H M, Harty RN. Overlapping motifs (PTAP and PPEY) within the Ebola virus VP40 protein function independently as late budding domains: involvement of host proteins TSG101 and VPS-4.J. Virol. 2003; 77:1812–1819.

[28] Hoenen T, Volchkov V, Weissenhorn W. VP40 octamers are essential for Ebola virus replication. J. Virol. 2005; 79:1898–1905. DOI: 10.1128/JVI.00737-10

[29] Dessen A, Volchkov V, Weissenhorn W. Crystal structure of the matrix protein VP40 from Ebola virus. EMBO J. 2000; 19:4228–4236. DOI:10.1093/emboj/19.16.4228

[30] Adu-Gyamfi E, Soni SP, Stahelin RV. The Ebola virus matrix protein penetrates into the plasma membrane: a key step in viral protein 40 (VP40) oligomerization and viral egress. J. Biol. Chem. 2013; 288:5779–5789. DOI:10.3390/v6103837

[31] Adu-Gyamfi E, Digman MA, Stahelin RV. Investigation of Ebola VP40 assembly and oligomerization in live cells using number and brightness analysis. Biophys. J. 2012; 102:2517–2525. DOI:10.1016/j.bpj.2012.04.022

[32] Licata JM, Simpson-HM, Wright N T, Han Z, Paragas J, Harty RN. Overlapping motifs (PTAP and PPEY) within the Ebola virus VP40 protein function independently as

late budding domains: involvement of host proteins TSG101 and VPS-4. J. Virol. 2003; 77: 1812–1819.

[33] Neumann G, Ebihara H, Takada A, Noda T, Kobasa D, Jasenosky LD, Watanabe S, Kim J H, FeldmannH, Kawaoka Y. Ebola virus VP40 late domains are not essential for viral replication in cell culture. J. Virol. 2005; 79:10300–10307. DOI: 10.1128/JVI.79.16.10300-10307.2005

[34] Yamayoshi S, Noda T, Ebihara H, Goto H, Morikawa Y, Lukashevich IS, Neumann G, Feldmann H, Kawaoka Y. Ebola virus matrix protein VP40 uses the COPII transport system for its intracellular transport. Cell Host Microbe. 2008; 3:168–177. DOI: 10.1016/j.chom.2008.02.001

[35] García M, Cooper A, Shi W, Bornmann W, Carrion R, Kalman D, Nabel GJ. Produtive replication of Ebola virus is regulated by the c-Abl1 tyrosine kinase. Sci. Transl. Med. 2012; 4: 123ra24. DOI: 10.1126/scitranslmed.3003500

[36] McCarthy SE, Johnson RF, Zhang YA, Sunyer JO, Harty RN. Role for amino acids 212KLR214 of Ebola virus VP40 in assembly and budding. J. Virol. 2007; 81:11452–11460. DOI:10.1128/JVI.00853-07

[37] Hoenen T, Volchkov V, Kolesnikova L, Mittler E, Timmins J, Ottmann M, Reynard O, Becker S, Weissenhorn W. VP40 octamers are essential for Ebola virus replication. J. Virol. 2005; 79: 1898–1905. DOI:10.1128/JVI.79.3.1898-1905.2005

[38] Morris DR, Geballe AP. Upstream Open Reading Frames as Regulators of mRNA Translation. Molecular and Cellular Biology. 2000; 20: 8635–8642. DOI: 10.1128/MCB.20.23.8635-8642.2000

[39] Kozak M. Initiation of translation in prokaryotes and eukaryotes. Gene. 1999; 234:187–208.

[40] Meijer HA, Thomas AAM. Control of eukaryotic protein synthesis by upstream open reading frames in the 5′-untranslated region of an mRNA. BiochemJ. 2002; 367:1–11. DOI:10.1042/BJ20011706

[41] Kochetov AV, Ahmad S, Ivanisenko V, Volkova OA, Kolchanov NA, et al. uORFs, reinitiation and alternative translation start sites in human mRNAs. FEBS Letters 2008; 582:1293–1297. DOI:10.1016/j.febslet.2008.03.014

[42] Gupta KA. Regulation and Deregulation of mRNA translation during myeloid maturation. Experimental hematology. 2011; 39(2):133–141. DOI:10.1016/j.exphem.2010.10.011

[43] Wek RC, Jiang HY, Anthony TG. Coping with stress: eIF2 kinases and translational control. BiochemSoc Trans. 2006; 34: 7–11.

[44] Bukreyev AA, DiNapoli JM, Yang L, Murphy BR, Collins PL. Mucosal parainfluenza virus-vectored vaccine against Ebola virus replicates in the respiratory tract of vec-

tor-immune monkeys and is immunogenic. Virology. 2010; 399:2:290-298. DOI: 10.1016/j.virol.2010.01.015

[45] Passi D, Sharma S, Dutta SR, Dudeja P, Sharma V.Ebola Virus Disease (The Killer Virus): Another Threat to Humans and Bioterrorism: Brief Review and Recent Updates. J ClinDiagn Res. 2015; 9:6:LE01–8. DOI:10.7860/JCDR/2015/13062.6100

[46] Isere EE, Fatiregun AA, Ajayi IO.An overview of disease surveillance and notification system in Nigeria and the roles of clinicians in disease outbreak prevention and control. Niger Med J. 2015; 56:3:161–8. DOI: 10.4103/0300-1652.160347

[47] Sesmero E, Thorpe IF.Using the Hepatitis C Virus RNA-Dependent RNA Polymerase as a Model to Understand Viral Polymerase Structure, Function and Dynamics.Viruses. 2015 ; 7:7:3974–94. DOI: 10.3390/v7072808.

[48] Alexander KA, Sanderson CE, Marathe M, Lewis BL, Rivers CM, Shaman J, Drake JM, Lofgren E, DatoVM,Eisenberg MC, Eubank S.What factors might have led to the emergence of Ebola in West Africa?PLoSNegl Trop Dis. 2015; 9:6:e0003652. DOI: 10.1371/journal.pntd.0003652

[49] Falasca L, Agrati C, Petrosillo N, Di Caro A, Capobianchi MR, Ippolito G, Piacentini M.Molecular mechanisms of Ebola virus pathogenesis: focus on cell death.Cell Death Differ. 2015; 22:8:1250–9. DOI:10.1038/cdd.2015.67

[50] Rewar S, Mirdha D. Transmission of ebola virus disease: an overview. Ann Glob Health. 2014; 80:6:444–51. DOI: 10.1016/j.aogh.2015.02.005

[51] Cenciarelli O, Pietropaoli S, Malizia A, Carestia M, D'Amico F, Sassolini A, Di Giovanni D, Rea S, GabbariniV,Tamburrini A, Palombi L, Bellecci C, Gaudio P. Ebola virus disease 2013-2014 outbreak in west Africa: an analysis of the epidemic spread and response. Int J Microbiol. 2015; 2015:769121. DOI:10.1155/2015/769121

[52] Roca A, Afolabi MO, Saidu Y, Kampmann B.Ebola: a holistic approach is required to achieve effective management and control. J Allergy ClinImmunol. 2015; 135:4:856-67. DOI: 10.1016/j.jaci.2015.02.015

[53] Ibrahim F, Thio TH, Faisal T, Neuman M. The application of biomedical engineering techniques to the diagnosis and management of tropical diseases: a review. Sensors (Basel). 2015; 15:3:6947–95. DOI:10.3390/s150306947

[54] Shurtleff AC, Whitehouse CA, Ward MD, Cazares LH, Bavari S. Pre-symptomatic diagnosis and treatment of filovirus diseases. Front Microbiol. 2015; 20:6:108. DOI: 10.3389/fmicb.2015.00108

[55] Litterman N, Lipinski C, Ekins S. Small molecules with antiviral activity against the Ebola virus.F1000Res. 2015; 9:4:38. DOI:10.12688/f1000research.6120.1

[56] Bociaga-Jasik M, Piatek A, Garlicki A. Ebola virus disease – pathogenesis, clinical presentation and management. Folia Med Cracov. 2014; 54 :3:49–55.

5

RNA Interference as a Tool to Reduce the Risk of Rejection in Cell-Based Therapies

Constanca Figueiredo and Rainer Blasczyk

Abstract

Remarkable progress in the experimental and clinical applications of cell-based therapies has identified stem cells and their derived products as potential candidates for regenerative therapies for many disorders. The use of autologous stem cells as source for regenerative therapeutic products is strongly limited by their low availability. Therefore, the future applications of *in vitro* pharmed therapeutic cell products will most likely occur in an allogeneic manner. However, the high variability of the human leukocyte antigen (HLA) represents a major obstacle to the application of off-the-shelf products. We have developed a strategy to decrease the immunogenicity of *in vitro* generated cell products by silencing HLA expression using RNAi. HLA expression was permanently silenced in CD34+ hematopoietic stem and progenitor cells and induced the pluripotent stem cells to generate HLA-universal cells sources, which were then used for the differentiation of low immunogenic cell products. In this chapter, we will provide an overview about an RNAi-based strategy to reduce the immunogenicity of cell-based therapies, and in particular in the generation of HLA-universal platelets and tissues.

Keywords: HLA, immunogenicity, transplant rejection, blood pharming

1. Introduction

The high variability of the human leukocyte antigen (HLA) constitutes a major hurdle in allogeneic transplantation and to the application of off-the-shelf cell products in regenerative medicine. Recently, remarkable progresses in the field of stem cell biology, cell pharming, and tissue engineering have made feasible the differentiation of cells and tissues that might serve as a bridging strategy or even an alternative to the very scarce donated tissues and organs. However, HLA incompatibility may pose a threat to the applicability of such *in vitro* generated cell products by increasing the risk of immune rejection after the transplantation.[1] To overcome this major hurdle in the fields of transplantation, cell and tissue engineering, we have developed an RNA interference (RNAi)-based approach to reduce the immunogenicity of cells and tissues, allowing their application in an universal manner. A lentiviral vector encoding for specific short hairpins RNA (shRNA), targeting HLA transcripts were used to achieve a permanent silencing of HLA expression. As HLA residual expression is crucial to prevent the natural killer (NK) cell activity, RNAi appears as a superior tool in comparison to gene editing technologies that cause a complete gene deletion such as the transcription activator-like effector nuclease (TALEN) or clustered regularly interspaced short palindromic repeats (CRISPR)/Cas9 systems.[2-4] By decreasing the immunogenicity of cells and tissues, the need for immunosuppressive regimens might be reduced after HLA-mismatched transplantation. Furthermore, as HLA plays a pivotal role in the recognition of virus-infected cells and cancer cells, the combination of conditional promoter systems allows the re-expression of HLA and constitutes a safety mechanism. The generation of low immunogenic cells and tissues would bring enormous benefits to the patients and open novel horizons in the field of transplantation and regenerative medicine.

2. The HLA system

Evolution conferred highly refined mechanisms to all animals from sponges to mammals to distinguish self from non-self, and thereby allowing an immune response against potential pathogens. In humans, a tight interplay between adaptive and innate immune systems allows their defense against virtually all pathogens and cancer cells.[5, 6] Nevertheless, those sophisticated surveillance mechanisms pose a major hurdle to allogeneic transplantation. The alloimmune responses are mainly based on the recognition of mismatched major histocompatibility complex (MHC) antigens by antibodies and T-cells. In humans, the MHC is known as HLA and it comprises a group of linked genes. MHC class I and II regulate the immune response through the presentation of peptides to T-cells. Allogeneic MHC in the graft's antigen-presenting cells (APCs) is recognized after transplantation through a direct pathway. Afterwards, own patient APCs process and present the allogeneic antigens to T-cells by an indirect alloantigen recognition pathway.[7, 8] HLA loci are encoded on the short arm of human chromosome 6. Based on their structure, HLA molecules are grouped into class I and class II (Figure 1). HLA class I classical genes comprise the A, B, and C loci, and are expressed in the majority of cells. HLA class II genes include DR, DQ, and DP and are constitutively expressed only in professional APCs.[9] The non-self recognition mediated by the engagement of the T-cell receptor with the donor HLA is the basis for the allogeneic immune response.

2.1. HLA incompatibility increases the risk of rejection

Despite the progresses in the field of transplantation, graft rejection remains the major concern regarding the application of off-the-shelf products. HLA comprises the most polymorphic loci of the entire human genome. The probability to find a complete HLA-matched donor for a specific patient is very low and, therefore, in most of the cases, patients will be treated with partially HLA-mismatched tissues and organs. In addition, even in fully HLA donor/recipient

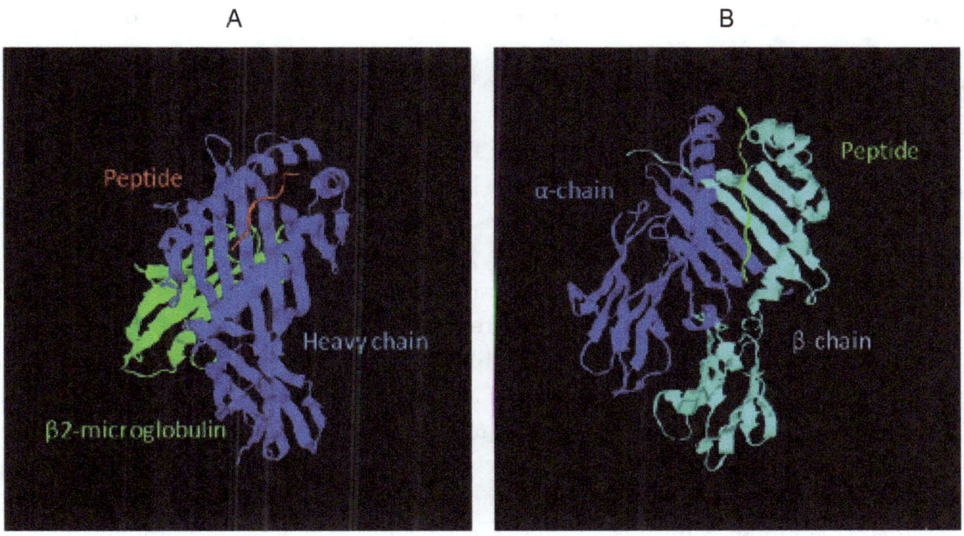

Figure 1. Structure representation of (A) HLA class I (HLA-B) and (B) HLA class II (HLA-DQ) molecules. The structures were designed using the software http://www.mh-hannover.de/institute/transfusion/histocheck/.

pairs, disparities at the minor histocompatibility antigens (mHAg) derived from other polymorphic proteins and presented at the HLA complexes are capable of triggering antigen-specific immune responses that cause graft rejection. Improved use of post-transplant immunosuppression to prevent acute and chronic rejection allowed allogeneic transplantation as a widespread, successful therapy.[10-13] However, graft rejection remains a major concern in the field of transplantation. The registry of the International Society for Heart and Lung Transplantation (ISHLT) reported that within the first year after lung transplantation, up to 55% patients need to be treated for acute rejection and only 50% are alive after five years.[14] Also, the number of HLA mismatches between a donor/recipient pair is associated with stronger immunosuppressive regimens. In particular, the number of HLA-DR mismatches and the number of HLA-A and -B mismatches as well as rejection treatment showed significant associations with the dose of maintenance steroids. Although immunosuppression allows the acceptance of the allogeneic graft, it has severe side effects that may contribute to death even with a functioning graft.[15] The occurrence of post-transplant complications related to the immunosuppressive therapy such as cancer, opportunistic infection, toxicity, and hip fractures have indicated the necessity to develop alternative strategies to allow the therapeutical use of off-the-shelf HLA and mHAg-mismatched cell-based products.[16] Furthermore, due to the shortage of organs and tissues for transplantation, there is a high demand regarding the development of *in vitro* pharmed cell products, and engineered tissues or organs. Progresses in the fields of stem cell biology and tissue engineering have demonstrated the feasibility to generate *in vitro* potential alternative cell-based products that might serve as an alternative or overcome the need for using donated tissues. Nevertheless, the future use of such products will occur in an allogeneic manner, and therefore, it will be required that those products will be able to escape an allogeneic immune response.

2.2. RNAi-mediated HLA targeting as a strategy to decrease the cell immunogenicity

Rejection of allogeneic grafts is based on the recognition of the HLA complexes by the specific pre-formed complement-binding anti-HLA antibodies or by the engagement of the T-cell receptor, which leads to T-cell activation and the initiation of the immune response.[17, 18] RNA interference is an invaluable technique in cell biology and regenerative strategies to silence the target gene expression. Our studies have focused on the downregulation of HLA class I and class II expression on the graft cells. So far, several strategies have been developed to induce the acceptance of the allogeneic graft. Similar to the immunosuppression, those strategies involve the modulation of immune responses and aim the induction of tolerance to the graft. In our studies, we genetically modify the graft to silence its HLA expression to prevent the recognition of the allogeneic graft as non-self by the recipient's immune system. In this approach, we do not induce tolerance toward the allogeneic graft, but we generate a condition of immunological blindness in which the recipient's immune system is not able to recognize the allogeneic cells (due to the missing HLA) but is fully capable of defending the patient against common clinical conditions associated with the use of immunosuppressive drugs such as opportunistic infections and leukemia. To prevent the recognition of the grafted cells as off the shelf, we have downregulated the expression of HLA class I and class II antigens using RNAi. We have constructed lentiviral vectors encoding for short-hairpin RNA sequences targeting β2-microglobulin (shβ2m) or the alpha-chain of HLA-DR (shDRA) to silence the expression of HLA class I and class II antigens, respectively. Our studies demonstrated the feasibility to stably downregulate HLA class I and II expression in several cell lines (e.g., B-LCL, MonoMac-6, HeLa) as well as in primary cells (e.g., endothelial cells, CD34+ progenitor, induced pluripotent stem cells). Cell transduction for the delivery of shRNAs targeting specific HLA transcripts resulted in a decrease by up to 90% of β2m or HLA-DRA transcript levels and HLA class I expression. *In vitro* assays have shown that HLA class I-silenced cells were protected against the antibody-mediated complement-dependent cytotoxicity. Furthermore, in T-cell cytotoxicity assays, significantly lower cell lysis rates were observed when HLA-silenced cells were used as targets in comparison to fully HLA-expressing cells. In addition, HLA-silenced cells demonstrated to induce significantly lower T-cell proliferation, pro-inflammatory cytokine secretion, and degranulation. The residual HLA class I expression showed to be sufficient to prevent NK cell cytotoxicity. Altogether, HLA-silenced cells showed a protective effect against the humoral and cellular allogeneic immune response.[2, 3, 19]

2.3. MHC-silenced cells survive after fully HLA-incompatible transplantation

Despite the widespread use of immunosuppressive regimens to prevent graft rejection, their therapeutic window is very narrow. Immunosuppressive drugs frequently cause adverse effects including thrombocytopenia, leukopenia, hypercholesterolemia, stomatitis, nephro-toxicity, and diarrhea, and they lead to an increased risk for infections and cancer.[20, 21] Silencing HLA expression using RNAi may represent an alternative to immunosuppression; hence it has the potential to offer many benefits for the patients. In addition, silencing HLA expression may allow the future application of HLA-mismatched off-the-shelf products in a universal manner independently of the genetic background of the donor and recipient. In an allogeneic transplantation rat model, we have confirmed the improved capacity of MHC-silenced cells to survive in allogeneic environment upon transplantation and even in the absence of immunosuppression. A lentiviral vector encoding for a shRNA sequence targeting rat MHC class I (RT1-A) and the sequence for firefly luciferase as a reporter gene was used to silence MHC class I Lewis rat-derived fibroblasts. In contrast to nonmodified fibroblasts, MHC class I-silenced fibroblasts were able to survive after subcutaneous transplantation in a complete MHC-mismatched setting. MHC class I-silenced fibroblasts were able to engraft and were detectable during the entire monitoring period (8 weeks). Nonmodified cells were rejected in all animals.[22] This study showed the superior performance of MHC-silenced cells after MHC-incompatible transplantation.

2.4. Generation of HLA-silenced platelets

Since the 1950s, blood transfusion therapy has become routine clinical practice; however, the concept of blood pharming – ex vivo production of mature blood cells – is quite new. In humans, platelet production is sustained by a well-regulated process known as thrombopoiesis. In the bone marrow, CD34+ progenitor cells differentiate into polyploid megakaryocytes (the precursor of platelets). Megakaryocytes lack the expression of CD34, but express several glycoproteins essential for the platelet function.[23, 24] In general, platelet numbers in blood range from 150×10^9 to 400×10^9 per liter, and an estimated 1×10^{11} platelets are produced each day in the adult human. Thrombocytopenia and severe thrombocytopenia characterized as platelet counts less than 50×10^9 and 10×10^9 per liter, respectively, increase the risk of spontaneous bleeding and represent a threat for the patient's life.[25] Platelet transfusion has been widely used to prevent and treat life-threatening thrombocytopenia; however, preparation of a unit of concentrated platelets for transfusion requires at least 4–6 units of whole blood, thereby significantly increasing the risk of blood-borne infections and adverse immunologic reactions. Furthermore, platelet transfusion refractoriness – lack of adequate post-transfusion platelet counts – remains a major complication often observed in patients receiving multiple transfusions. This condition is frequently caused by the development of antibodies specific to HLA. Currently, platelet transfusion relies on volunteer blood donation; however, the demand for blood products in particular of platelets often exceeds their availability.[25]

The potential of multipotent progenitor and stem cells in regenerative medicine has been recognized.[26, 27] Platelet transfusion refractoriness due to the presence of anti-HLA antibodies constitutes a life-threatening risk for many patients suffering from hematological disorders, and hence require multiple platelet transfusions. Thus, it would be highly desirable to produce HLA-deficient platelets to facilitate the management of severe alloimmunized thrombocytopenic patients. In our studies, we have combined the concept of blood pharming with RNAi as a strategy to downregulate HLA gene expression. The ultimate goal of this approach is the large-scale production of platelets *in vitro* that may be used as an alternative to the conventional donated blood platelets. In addition, we aim for the production of genetically modified platelets with the capacity to survive even under platelet transfusion refractoriness.

In our studies, CD34+ hematopoietic progenitor cells and induced pluripotent stem cells (iPSCs) were used to produce HLA-silenced platelets *in vitro*. CD34+ cells or iPSCs were transduced with a lentiviral vector encoding for the shRNA sequence targeting β2m which induces HLA class I silencing. We have demonstrated the feasibility to generate HLA-universal CD34+ cells and iPSCs which might be used for the differentiation of HLA-silenced cell-products. In our studies, we have differentiated HLA-silenced megakaryocytes and platelets from both cell sources. In our previous studies, we have demonstrated the possibility to generate HLA-silenced platelets with comparable function to blood-derived platelets. However, in contrast to blood-derived platelets, *in vitro* generated HLA-silenced platelets were able to escape antibody-mediated complement-dependent cytotoxicity as well as cellular-dependent cytotoxicity. Also, in a platelet transfusion refractoriness mouse model, HLA-silenced platelets showed the capacity to survive and were even detectable 10 days after transfusion.[28] The limited availability of CD34+ cells derived from G-CSF mobilized donors is a major obstacle to the large-scale production of *in vitro* pharmed platelets. The breakthrough Nobel Prize–winning research by Yamanaka and colleagues to induce pluripotency in somatic cells has reshaped the field of stem cell research. Human iPSCs can be used for studying embryogenesis, disease modeling, drug testing, and regenerative medicine.[29] In contrast to CD34+ cells, iPSCs represent an unlimited cell source for the *in vitro* production of a variety of cell-based products including platelets. Therefore, we have recently established an efficient protocol for the differentiation of megakaryocytes and platelets from iPSCs (Figure 2). First, we have generated an HLA-universal iPSC line. Then, the lentiviral vector containing the shRNA targeting β2-microglobulin was used to silence HLA expression on iPSCs. A significant and durable reduction of HLA expression was observed even after passaging. Nevertheless, the HLA-silenced iPSC line showed comparable expression of pluripotency markers (such as SSEA-4 and Tra-1-60) as the original HLA class I-expressing iPSC line (Figure 3). The data indicate that silencing HLA expression does not affect the pluripotency potential of iPSCs.

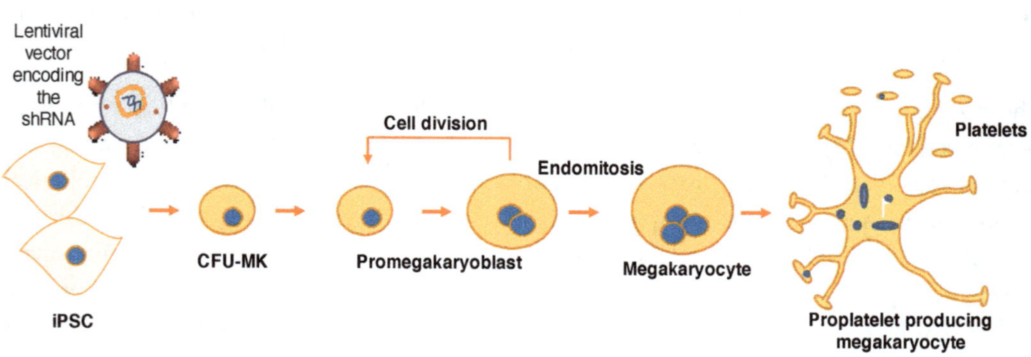

Figure 2. Schematic representation of the differentiation of HLA-silenced platelets from iPSCs. A lentiviral vector encoding for an HLA-specific shRNA is used to transduce the iPSCs. Afterward, HLA-silenced iPSCs will be differentiated using a cytokine cocktail containing thrombopoietin (TPO) until the release of platelets.

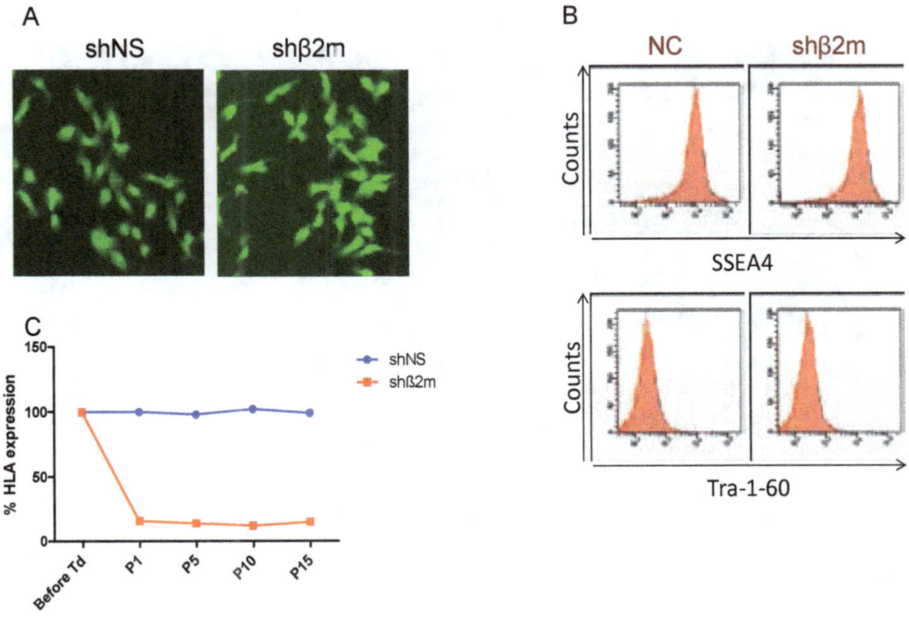

Figure 3. Generation of an HLA-universal iPSC line. (A) iPSCs were adapted to monolayer culture conditions and transduced with a lentiviral vector encoding for a nonspecific shRNA (shNS) or a β2-microglobulin-specific shRNA to silence the expression of HLA class I; (B) expression of SSEA4 and Tra-1-60 on nonmodified and shβ2m-expressing iPSCs; (C) expression of HLA class I of a HLA-silenced shNS-expressing iPSC lines. Cells were stained with an HLA class I antibody (W6/32) and the expression of HLA was measured by flow cytometry after different number of passages. Mean fluorescence intensities (MFI) detected on HLA-silenced iPSCs were normalized to the MFI measured on shNS-expressing iPSCs at the same passage.

In addition, the future application of iPSCs will occur most likely in an allogeneic manner to facilitate their availability during the time of need and standardization of the protocols. Hence, the use of HLA-silenced iPSCs may facilitate the application of HLA-mismatched iPSC-derived cell products. For megakaryocyte differentiation, HLA-silenced iPSCs were cultured in monolayer in the presence of vascular endothelial growth factor (VEGF) and BMP-4 for mesoderm induction and afterward in the presence of TPO. During ontogeny, definitive hematopoietic cells are generated de novo from a specialized subset of endothelium, known as hemogenic endothelium. Endothelial-to-hematopoietic transition during embryogenesis provides the first long-term hematopoietic stem and progenitor cells in the embryo.[30] In our differentiation cultures of iPSCs into megakaryocytes, structures resembling the hemogenic endothelium were observed (Figure 4). In suspension, megakaryocytes could be detected by an increase in DNA content higher than 4n and the expression of typical megakaryocytic markers such as CD41 and CD42a. In addition, the megakaryocytes showed the capability to build pro-platelets. Moreover, the shRNA-mediated silencing effect was maintained during the entire differentiation. Importantly, iPSC-derived megakaryocytes and pro-platelets showed a significant reduction of β2-microglobulin and HLA class I antigens in comparison to those differentiated from iPSC expressing a nonspecific shRNA (control) (Figure 5). Differentiation rates of iPSC into megakaryocytes by up to 82% were observed (Figure 6).

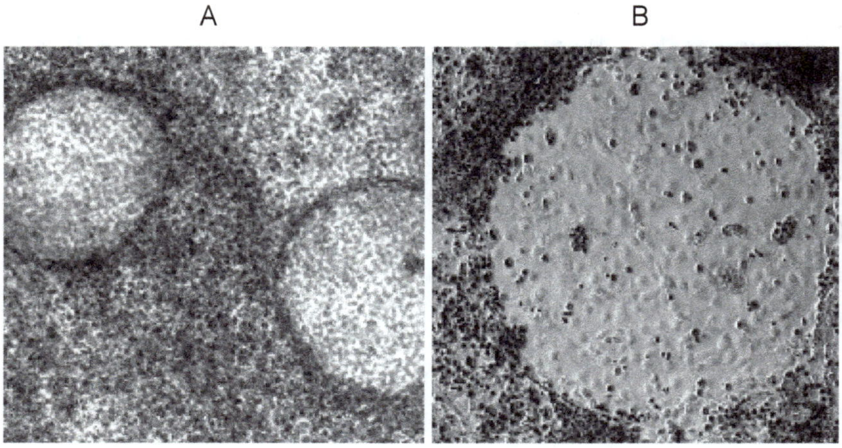

Figure 4. Formation of hemogenic-like endothelium during the differentiation of iPSCs into megakaryocytes. The photos display an island of hemogenic-like endothelium at a magnification of (A) 10x; (B) 20x.

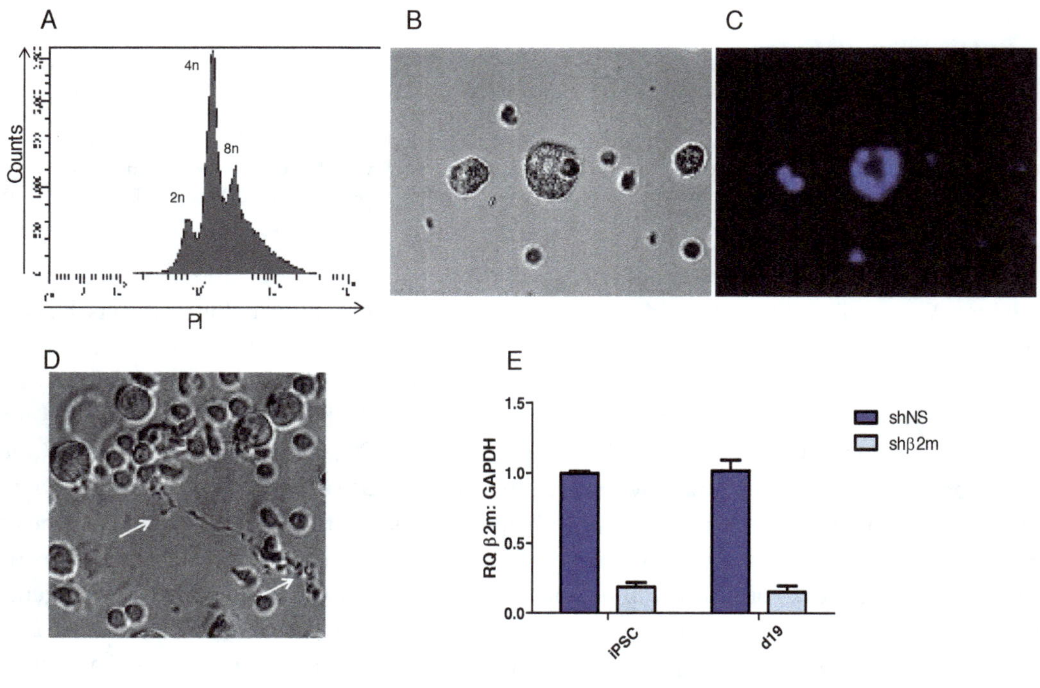

Figure 5. Differentiation of HLA-universal megakaryocytes from HLA-silenced iPSC. (A) The histogram represents the flow cytometric analysis of HLA-silenced iPSC-derived megakaryocytes after staining with propidium iodide; (B) light microscopic and (C) fluorescence microscopic analysis of an iPSC-derived megakaryocyte after staining with 4′,6-Diamidin-2-phenylindol (DAPI, blue); (D) light microscopic analysis of pro-platelets indicated with white arrows; (E) real-time PCR analysis of β2-microglobulin levels in megakaryocytes derived from iPSCs transduced with a lentiviral vector encoding the shRNA targeting β2-microglobulin (shβ2m) or a nonspecific shRNA (shNS) as a control.

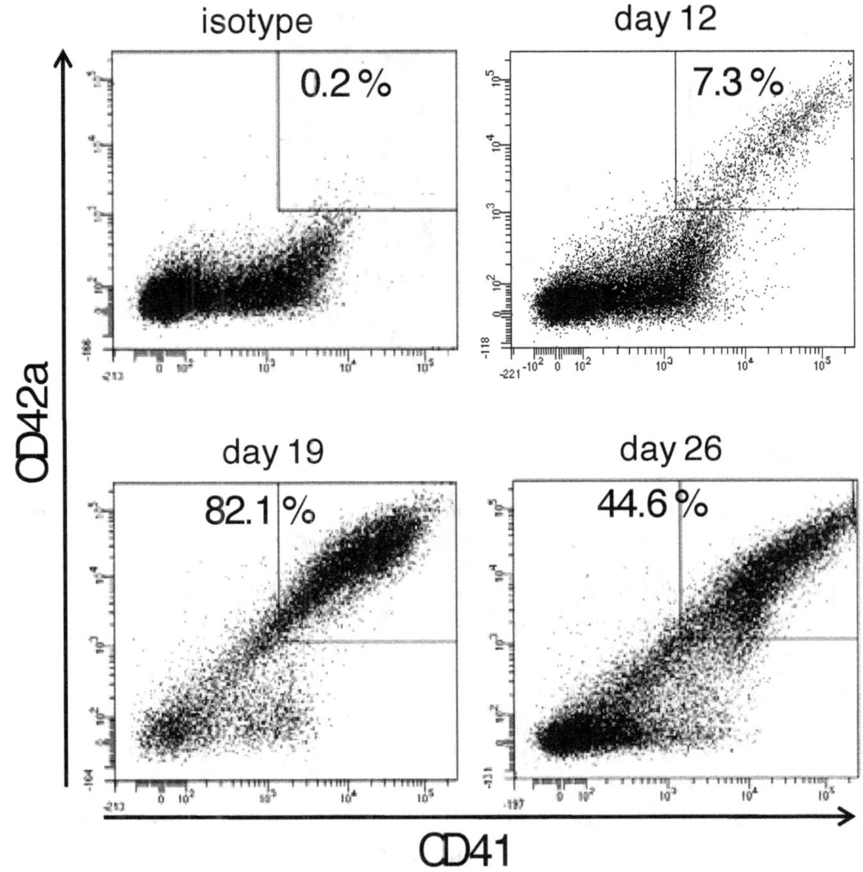

Figure 6. Phenotypic analysis of HLA-universal megakaryocytes derived from iPSCs. The expression of the megakaryocyte markers CD41 and CD42a was measured by flow cytometry in the cells harvested from the iPSC differentiation cultures at different time points. The gates in the dotplots indicate megakaryocytes characterized by the double expression of CD41 and CD42a.

The complement-dependent cytotoxic (CDC) crossmatch is an informative assay that detects alloantibodies in pre- and post-transplant patients, which may guide the most appropriate clinical management of transplant patients.[31] The capacity of *in vitro* generated HLA-silenced megakaryocytes and platelets to escape antibody-mediated complement-dependent cytotoxicity was evaluated in CDC tests. HLA-silenced megakaryocytes incubated with specific HLA antibodies and complement showed comparable cell lyses rates to the megakaryocytes incubated with nonspecific HLA antibodies. In contrast, significantly higher cell lysis rates were observed when HLA-expressing megakaryocytes were incubated with specific anti-HLA antibodies (Figure 7). These data suggest that HLA-universal iPSC-derived megakaryocytes are protected from anti-HLA antibody-mediated complement-dependent cytotoxicity and have the potential to survive under refractoriness conditions.

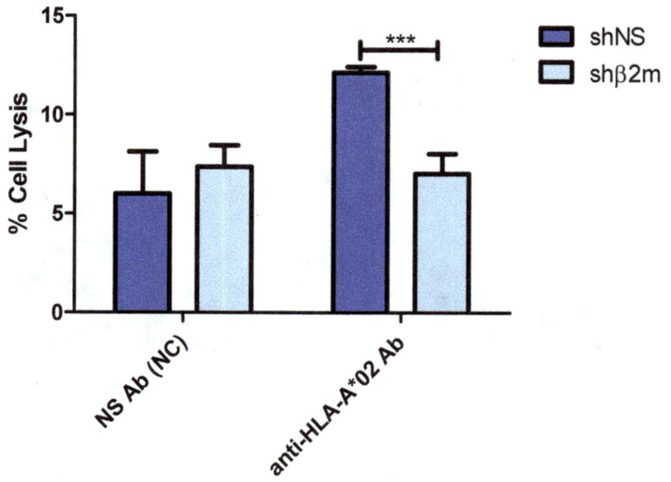

Figure 7. HLA-silenced megakaryocytes are protected from antibody-mediated complement-dependent cytotoxicity. HLA-expressing (shNS) or HLA-silenced (shβ2m) iPSC-derived megakaryocytes were incubated with a nonspecific antibody (NC) or an HLA-specific antibody and complement. Cell lysis was detected by flow cytometric analysis upon staining with propidium iodide. The bar graph represents means and standard deviations of three independent experiments. Statistical significance was calculated using Student's *t*-test (*$p < 0.05$, **$p < 0.01$; ***$p < 0.001$).

2.5. Generation of HLA-silenced tissues

Due to the high variability of the HLA loci and the shortage of organs and tissues for transplantation, it is very difficult to find a complete HLA-matched graft for a given recipient. The number of HLA mismatches between the graft and the recipient are associated with a higher risk for graft rejection and even morbidity and mortality due to immunosuppression-related side effects. Thus, it would be desirable to engineer the grafts in order to decrease their immunogenicity by silencing HLA expression. Worldwide, the demand for organs and tissues for transplantation is very high and it is not possible to satisfy all needs. This discrepancy is even accentuated in the Middle East and countries in the East such as India and China. According to the World Health Organization (WHO), there are over 10 million people in the world who are blind in one or both eyes due to corneal injury or disease and up to 45 million people could benefit from corneal transplants. However, according to data from eye banks and health agencies, less than 150,000 corneal transplants are done annually worldwide due to the shortage of human cadaver corneas. Furthermore, during the first five years after penetrating keratoplasty, rejection is responsible for 28–35% of total corneal graft loss. High risk-corneal recipients even showed increased rejection rates (30–56%).[32, 33]

The cornea presents a simple anatomical structure, in which the endothelium is easily accessible to the shRNA-encoding viral vector containing supernatant (Figure 8). The integrity of the endothelial cell layer is crucial for the transparency of the cornea and it is the major target for rejection. Therefore, silencing HLA expression on the corneal endothelium may improve cornea survival in high-risk patients after allogeneic keratoplasty.

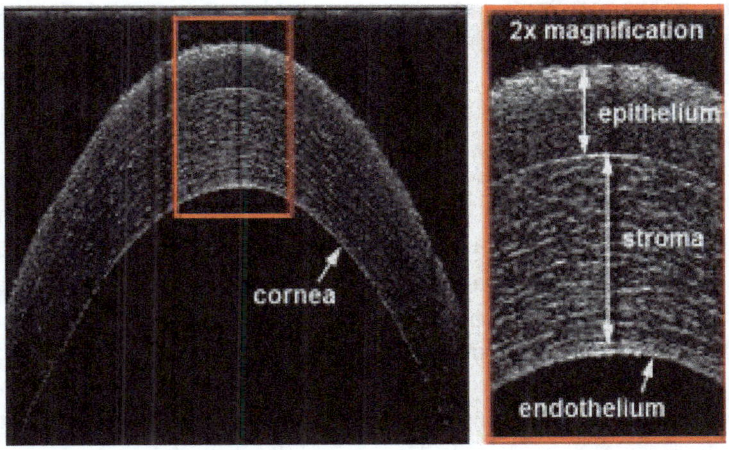

Figure 8. Anatomy of the cornea. Optical coherence tomography of a mouse cornea showing the three main layers.

We have silenced HLA expression in human and mice corneas. The tissue was transduced for 8 h with the lentiviral vector encoding for the MHC-specific shRNAs as described above. We were able to silence the MHC expression on the cornea endothelium, which is the major target during graft rejection. In this study, we demonstrated the feasibility to generate HLA universal tissues in their original 3D structure (Figure 9). Silencing HLA expression on tissues is expected to significantly improve graft survival rates in high-risk keratoplasty patients.

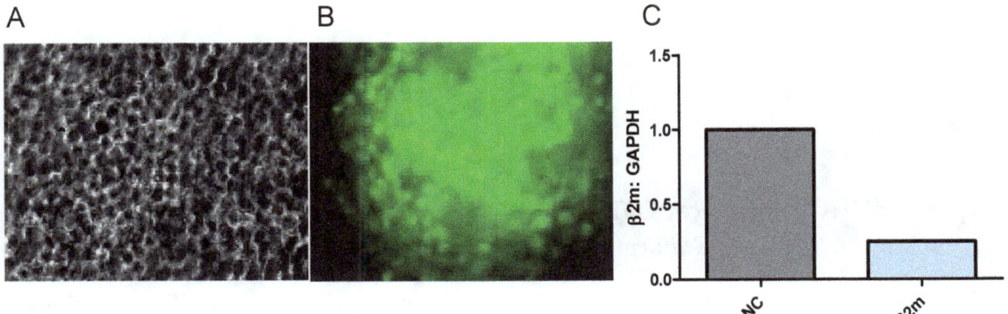

Figure 9. Generation of MHC-silenced corneas. A mouse cornea was explanted and transduced with a lentiviral vector encoding the shβ2m to cause a downregulation of MHC class I antigens and the expression of green fluorescence protein (GFP) sequences. (A) Light microscopic and (B) fluorescence microscopic analyses of a transduced mouse cornea.

2.6. Conclusion

Recently, gene regulation or editing strategies have emerged as powerful tools to improve the design and efficacy of personalized cell-based therapies. In the field of histocompatibility and transplantation, RNAi seems to be a favorite approach to reduce the immunogenicity of allogeneic and *in vitro* generated cells and tissues. The lentiviral vector-mediated delivery of shRNAs targeting HLA transcripts prevents the activation of cellular and humoral allogeneic immune responses that cause the rejection of the foreign cells. However, this RNAi-based strategy permits the residual expression of HLA class I antigens which are crucial to inhibit NK cell cytotoxicity. With the establishment of iPSCs, the concept of cell pharming came one step closer to reality as iPSCs may serve as unlimited cell sources for different cell products such as platelets. The combination of RNAi-mediated HLA silencing and the capacity to generate platelets *in vitro* may represent a novel therapeutic approach for the management of alloimmunized thrombocytopenic patients with an increased risk to develop refractoriness to platelet transfusion. Furthermore, our results also indicate the feasibility to reduce MHC expression in the 3D original structure of tissues. Abrogating the histocompatibility barrier between donors and recipients may improve therapeutic efficacy, reduce the adverse events associated with strong immunosuppressive regimens, and improve transplant patient life's quality. In conclusion, RNAi-mediated silencing of HLA expression may open new avenues in tissue engineering and transplantation.

Author details

Constanca Figueiredo* and Rainer Blasczyk

*Address all correspondence to: figueiredo.constanca@mh-hannover.de

Institute for Transfusion Medicine, Hannover Medical School, Hannover, Germany

References

[1] Barry J, Hyllner J, Stacey G, Taylor CJ, Turner M. Setting up a Haplobank: issues and solutions. *Curr Stem Cell Rep*. 2015;1(2):110–117.

[2] Figueiredo C, Seltsam A, Blasczyk R. Class-, gene-, and group-specific HLA silencing by lentiviral shRNA delivery. *J Mol Med (Berl)*. 2006;84(5):425–437.

[3] Jaimes Y, Seltsam A, Eiz-Vesper B, Blasczyk R, Figueiredo C. Regulation of HLA class II expression prevents allogeneic T-cell responses. *Tissue Antigens*. 2011;77(1): 36–44.

[4] Wiegmann B, Figueiredo C, Gras C, et al. Prevention of rejection of allogeneic endothelial cells in a biohybrid lung by silencing HLA-class I expression. *Biomaterials*. 2014;35(28):8123–8133.

[5] Hirano M, Das S, Guo P, Cooper MD. The evolution of adaptive immunity in vertebrates. *Adv Immunol*. 2011;109:125–157.

[6] Buchmann K. Evolution of innate immunity: clues from Invertebrates via fish to mammals. *Front Immunol*. 2014;5:459.

[7] Ali JM, Bolton EM, Bradley JA, Pettigrew GJ. Allorecognition pathways in transplant rejection and tolerance. *Transplantation*. 2013;96(8):681–688.

[8] Sagoo P, Lombardi G, Lechler RI. Relevance of regulatory T cell promotion of donor-specific tolerance in solid organ transplantation. *Front Immunol*. 2012;3:184.

[9] Shiina T, Hosomichi K, Inoko H, Kulski JK. The HLA genomic loci map: expression, interaction, diversity, and disease. *J Hum Genet*. 2009;54(1):15–39.

[10] Almoguera B, Shaked A, Keating BJ. Transplantation genetics: current status and prospects. *Am J Transplant*. 2014;14(4):764–778.

[11] de Rham C, Villard J. Potential and limitation of HLA-based banking of human pluripotent stem cells for cell therapy. *J Immunol Res*. 2014;2014:518135.

[12] Hess SM, Young EF, Miller KR, et al. Deletion of naive T cells recognizing the minor histocompatibility antigen HY with toxin-coupled peptide-MHC class I tetramers inhibits cognate CTL responses and alters immunodominance. *Transpl Immunol*. 2013;29(14):138–145.

[13] Kwun J, Malarkannan S, Burlingham WJ, Knechtle SJ. Primary vascularization of the graft determines the immunodominance of murine minor H antigens during organ transplantation. *J Immunol*. 2011;187(8):3997–4006.

[14] Trulock EP, Christie JD, Edwards LB, et al. Registry of the International Society for Heart and Lung Transplantation: twenty-fourth official adult lung and heart-lung transplantation report-2007. *J Heart Lung Transplant*. 2007;26(8):782–795.

[15] Opelz G, Dohler B. Association between steroid dosage and death with a functioning graft after kidney transplantation. *Am J Transplant*. 2013;13(8):2096–2105.

[16] Robson R, Cecka JM, Opelz G, Budde M, Sacks S. Prospective registry-based observational cohort study of the long-term risk of malignancies in renal transplant patients treated with mycophenolate mofetil. *Am J Transplant*. 2005;5(12):2954–2960.

[17] Wood S, Feng J, Chung J, et al. Transient blockade of delta-like Notch ligands prevents allograft rejection mediated by cellular and humoral mechanisms in a mouse model of heart transplantation. *J Immunol*. 2015;194(6):2899–2908.

[18] Wedel J, Bruneau S, Kochupurakkal N, Boneschansker L, Briscoe DM. Chronic allograft rejection: a fresh look. *Curr Opin Organ Transplant*. 2015;20(1):13–20.

[19] Figueiredo C, Horn PA, Blasczyk R, Seltsam A. Regulating MHC expression for cellular therapeutics. *Transfusion*. 2007;47(1):18–27.

[20] Moes DJ, Guchelaar HJ, de Fijter JW. Sirolimus and everolimus in kidney transplantation. *Drug Discov Today*. 2015;20(10):1243-9

[21] Khan S, Khan S, Baboota S, Ali J. Immunosuppressive drug therapy - biopharmaceutical challenges and remedies. *Expert Opin Drug Deliv.* 2015;12(8):1333–1349.

[22] Figueiredo C, Wedekind D, Muller T, et al. MHC universal cells survive in an allogeneic environment after incompatible transplantation. *Biomed Res Int.* 2013;2013:796046.

[23] Thon JN, Italiano JE. Platelet formation. *Semin Hematol.* 2010;47(3):220–226.

[24] Patel-Hett S, Wang H, Begonja AJ, et al. The spectrin-based membrane skeleton stabilizes mouse megakaryocyte membrane systems and is essential for proplatelet and platelet formation. *Blood.* 2011;118(6):1641–1652.

[25] Stanworth SJ, Navarrete C, Estcourt L, Marsh J. Platelet refractoriness - practical approaches and ongoing dilemmas in patient management. *Br J Haematol.* 2015;171(3): 297-305

[26] Crane AM, Kramer P, Bui JH, et al. Targeted correction and restored function of the CFTR gene in cystic fibrosis induced pluripotent stem cells. *Stem Cell Reports.* 2015;4(4):569–577.

[27] Tong Z, Solanki A, Hamilos A, et al. Application of biomaterials to advance induced pluripotent stem cell research and therapy. *EMBO J.* 2015;34(8):987–1008.

[28] Gras C, Schulze K, Goudeva L, Guzman CA, Blasczyk R, Figueiredo C. HLA-universal platelet transfusions prevent platelet refractoriness in a mouse model. *Hum Gene Ther.* 2013;24(12):1018–1028.

[29] Takahashi K, Yamanaka S. Induction of pluripotent stem cells from mouse embryonic and adult fibroblast cultures by defined factors. *Cell.* 2006;126(4):663–676.

[30] Zape JP, Zovein AC. Hemogenic endothelium: origins, regulation, and implications for vascular biology. *Semin Cell Dev Biol.* 2011;22(9):1036–1047.

[31] Lawrence C, Willicombe M, Brookes PA, et al. Preformed complement-activating low-level donor-specific antibody predicts early antibody-mediated rejection in renal allografts. *Transplantation.* 2013;95(2):341–346.

[32] Stuart PM, Yin X, Plambeck S, Pan F, Ferguson TA. The role of Fas ligand as an effector molecule in corneal graft rejection. *Eur J Immunol.* 2005;35(9):2591–2597.

[33] Yin XT, Zobell S, Jarosz JG, Stuart PM. Anti-IL-17 therapy restricts and reverses late-term corneal allorejection. *J Immunol.* 2015;194(8):4029–4038.

6

RNAi — Implications in Entomological Research and Pest Control

Nidhi Thakur, Jaspreet Kaur Mundey and Santosh Kumar Upadhyay

Abstract

RNA interference (RNAi) has progressed swiftly in the past decade to become a convenient and dominant genetic tool that has immense utility in diverse fields. The entomological research, ranging from functional genomics to agriculture, has gained enormous momentum due to this technology. RNAi tool helped to discover the functions of new genes and study the complicated genetic networks, thus providing an evolutionary insight into various processes. RNAi is also becoming a method of choice for controlling insect pest populations. It is envisaged as tailor-made insecticide, which is highly species specific. However, the efficiency of this mechanism is limited by various factors such as the stability of the trigger molecule, the candidate gene selection, delivery system adopted and, most importantly, the choice of the target species. Apart from the successful implication in diverse areas, there are certain drawbacks of this technology such as 'off-target' effects, lack of sensitivity of various species, etc. Further research would relieve these limitations and support the manifestation of this genetic tool with much more reliability.

Keywords: RNAi, insects, pest management, efficiency of RNAi

1. Introduction

RNA interference (RNAi) is a highly conserved, sequence-specific mechanism of gene silencing which is triggered by the presence of double-stranded RNA (dsRNA). Since its discovery in 1998, RNAi has attained the status of a powerful genetic tool [1]. This reverse genetics technique is now immensely used in biomedical research, functional genetics and many other areas of biological research. Broadly, all the reactions that take place for RNA silencing are initiated when a long dsRNA is processed into small dsRNAs of about 21 to 24 bp by the RNaseIII enzyme, called Dicer. These small dsRNAs are called small interfering RNA (siRNA), which when unwound using ATP-dependent activity are incorporated into the multi-subunit RNA-induced silencing complex (RISC). Here, the siRNA guides the RISC complex to degrade cellular RNA molecules that are complementary to its sequence [2]. Earlier this process was described in the experimental RNAi studies, and now it is the most accepted tool for gene knockdown studies.

The advent of RNAi also revolutionised the entomological research, as novel gene functions were efficiently discovered. In 1998, Kennerdell and Carthew were the first to use RNAi *in vivo* to study the genes *Frizzled* and *Frizzled-2* in *Drosophila melanogaster* [3]. The tremendous success of RNAi in model organisms has prompted its use for research in other insect species as well. In genomics and post-genomics era with the availability of a large amount of sequence information, RNAi further provides an opportunity to investigate the vital functions and crucial interactions that are of importance in both biomedical research and agriculture [4–6]. RNAi studies on insects of economic importance would provide new insights into unravelling the molecular interactions between various disease vectors and ultimately helping in the discovery of novel vaccine and drug targets. Disease vectors such as mosquito, ticks, mites, lice and others were studied extensively using RNAi [7]. These insects cause many serious diseases in humans and animals.

Among other applications, this genetic tool is also gaining popularity as a promising technology in controlling a wide array of agricultural pests. There is a substantial amount of literature available which documents the success of RNAi as a feasible and sustainable strategy in managing the agricultural pests [8–11]. The core RNAi machinery being present in all the insects makes it possible to silence a wide variety of target genes to produce diverse physiological, developmental and reproductive restrains. The sequence specificity of endogenous RNAi pathway allows the targeted suppression of genes essential for insect survival and thus offers the development of a specific, logical and sustainable strategy to combat against insect pests.

Agricultural pests are notorious and they cannot be efficiently managed by employing a single control agent or technique. Most commonly, the integrated pest management (IPM) strategies are utilised for combating the diversity of insect pests in the agro-ecosystem [12]. Along with mechanical, cultural, biological and chemical methods, the transgenic technology should also be embraced in the IPM regime. In this regard, RNAi can play an important role along with the available insecticidal molecules. Among various transgenic approaches to manage insect pests, *Bacillus thuringiensis* (Bt) toxin has shown spectacular success [13]; however, many important insect pests (primarily sap-sucking pests) are not amenable to Bt protection [14]. RNAi can be harnessed to defend crops against insect pests. Successful application of RNAi technology in agricultural pest management requires (i) suitable candidate gene where its silencing can cause mortality of the insect and (ii) an effective method of dsRNA delivery. Nevertheless, prior to field application, many aspects of this multi-faceted technology including safety and possible risks to environment need to be evaluated in detail.

In this chapter, we discussed the potential of this technology in gene silencing experiments to study the gene function as well as on opportunity to combat against agricultural pests and other disease vectors. Further, the factors responsible for a successful RNAi experiment, the link with immune response and viral infections have been discussed, highlighting the possible shortcomings of this strategy.

2. RNAi in insects

RNAi offers species-specific molecules that can be flexibly manipulated and used in understanding various complicated biochemical pathways. The research application of RNAi in entomology has elucidated the functions of several genes. Decrease in the mRNA levels of a candidate gene due to introduction of a complementary dsRNA fragment, and the study of the corresponding phenotype, illuminates a gene function. RNAi has been used to study various mechanisms related to insect development (embryonic and post-embryonic), reproduction, behaviour and other complicated biosynthetic pathways [15].

Various insect orders have demonstrated amenability to RNAi-mediated silencing. Species of orders Coleoptera, Lepidoptera, Diptera, Hemiptera, Orthoptera, Blattodea and Hymenoptera have been studied for various aspects using RNAi technique [15]. The silencing efficiency ranges from 0% to 100% in different insects. A large majority of the target genes were gut-specific genes; however, genes from salivary glands, brain and antennae have also been targeted [16]. RNAi-based studies can be carried out by either *in vivo* or *in vitro* studies. The former method is much easier and involves incubating the cells with the dsRNA added to the medium. However, the *in vivo* approach is more useful in the field of functional genomics, especially in case of non-model organisms. Here, the dsRNA dosage and developmental stage of insect can be specified. In addition, RNAi can be very helpful in identifying the mutant genes that are fatal to the organism,. The significance and compilation of various categories of RNAi experiments in entomology are summarised in Table 1 [17–45].

Experiments	Insect	Gene and function
RNAi in developmental biology		
Parental RNAi	*Tribolium castaneum*	Zygotic genes [16]
Parental RNAi is an important method for analysing early embryogenesis. It is crucial for many insects whose eggs are not accessible or do not survive after microinjection.	*Oncopeltus fasciatus*	Determination of the role of the gap genes, *hunchback* and *Krüppel* [17,18]
	Gryllus bimaculatus	Antenna and appendages [19], *hedgehog*, *wingless* and *dpp* in the initiation of proximodistal axis formation during the regeneration of insect legs [20]
	Nasonia vitripennis	Various genes in demonstration of parental RNAi [21]
	Tetranychus urticae	*Distal-less* was used, resulting in phenotypes with canonical limb truncation as well as the fusion of leg segments [22]
Embryonic RNAi	*T. castaneum*	Role of *wingless* (*wg*) in leg development [23]

Experiments	Insect	Gene and function
	N. vitripennis	Role of *bicoid* gene in the structural pattern of the anterior body region. Also in the absence of *bicoid* gene, *orthodenticle, hunchback* and *giant* genes are responsible for proper head and thorax formation [24]
	Oplegnathus. fasciatus	*Hox* genes and genes involved in segmentation and segment specification [25]
Larval/nymphal/pupal RNAi	*T. castaneum* (larval RNAi)	To study the molecular basis of adult morphological diversity in various organs [26]
	T. castaneum (larval RNAi)	*Ubx/Utx* during hindwing/elytron development [27]
	T. castaneum (larval RNAi)	*Laccase* 2 [28]
	Bombyx mori (pupal RNAi)	Fatty acid transport protein (Bm'FATP) [29]
	Schistocerca Americana (Nymphal RNAi)	The eye colour gene of first-instar nymphs triggered a suppression of ommochrome formation in the eye [30]
	S. Americana	Importance of early retinal genes *eyes absent (eya)* or *sine oculis (so)* in eye development [31]
	Blattella germanica (nymphal RNAi)	RXR/USP, along with EcR, of the heterodimeric nuclear receptor of 20-hydroxyecdysone (20E) [32]
	G. bimaculatus	Mechanisms of leg regeneration [33]
	G. bimaculatus	*period* (*per*)gene for circadian-dependent locomotor activity rhythm [34]
	G. bimaculatus	Genes responsible for certain human disorders: *fragile X mental retardation 1* (*fmr1*) and *Dopamine receptor* (*DopR*) [35]
Regeneration-dependent RNAi	*G. bimaculatus*	Insect leg regeneration [36]
	G. bimaculatus	Orthologs of *Drosophila hedgehog* (*Gb'hh*), *wingless* (*Gb'wg*) and *decapentaplegic* (*Gb'dpp*) are expressed during leg regeneration and play essential roles in the establishment of the proximal–distal axis [37]
RNAi in behavioural biology	*Rhodnius prolixus*	Nitrophorin 2 a decrease of anticoagulant activity and less efficient feeding behaviour [38]
	Anopheles gambiae	Apyrase AgApy in the salivary glands shows important role in host probing behaviour [39]
	D. melanogaster	3-Hydroxy-3-methylglutaryl CoA reductase has been identified for the control of

Experiments	Insect	Gene and function
		sexual dimorphism of locomotor activity in [40]]
	B. germanica	Neuropeptide pigment dispersing factor in the regulation of locomotor circadian rhythms [41]
Mechanism of insecticidal action	Mosquitoes	NADPH cytochrome P450 reductase led to increased sensitivity of mosquitoes to pyrethroids [42]
	Spodoptera litura and *Helicoverpa armigera*	Aminopeptidase M led to decreased sensitivity to BT toxin [43]
Understanding the biosynthetic pathway	*T. castaneum*	Chitin synthases *CHS1* and *CHS2* are crucialexoskeleton and the midgut peritrophic matrix [28]
	Bombyx mori	*Bombykol* is the main component of sexual pheromone, as well as pheromone-binding proteins and the receptor of the pheromone biosynthesis activator neuropeptide [44]
	Epiphyas postvittana	Silencing of pheromone-binding protein of the antennae [45]

Table 1. RNAi in the study of gene function in insects.

Apart from deciphering the function of genes involved in various metabolic pathways, RNAi also finds relevance in other aspects of insect science. It is quite beneficial in maintaining the beneficial insects and saving them from various parasites and pathogens. Certainly, this is useful in case of those parasites and pathogens, which have operative RNAi machinery. A successful study in this regard shows the control of honey bee parasite *Nosema ceranae*. When the gene related to energy metabolism was silenced, it was observed that the honey bee population had reduced infestation of *Nosema*, and lower mortality [46]. In another study, multiple genes of an ectoparasite of honey bee *Varroa destructor* were targeted [47]. It poses a great threat to the health of bees, and its control is of utmost importance for the rearing industry. It is a blood-sucking parasite, so the bees were fed on a meal containing dsRNA against the genes of *Varroa*. The RNAi-mediated control decreased the mite population by 50%, causing no evident damage to the bees. RNAi has also been useful in elucidating the importance of various immunological pathways in *D. melanogaster* [48]. Host–parasite relationships such as that of *Anopheles–Plasmodium* have also been studied by using RNAi. Early research was conducted on *defensin* and it was shown to be important for protecting mosquitoes against infections of Gram-positive bacteria [49]. Later, the same group demonstrated how the development of Plasmodium is affected by *Anopheles gambiae* immune genes [50]. Similarly, in *Manduca sexta* haemocytes, knockdown of haemolin (a bacterial recognition protein) decreased the ability of insects to clear *Escherichia coli* from the haemolymph. This eventually reduced their ability to engulf bacteria and highlighted the role of haemolin in the *M. sexta* immune response [51].

3. RNAi in pest control

Plants are damaged by a plethora of insect pests. The losses due to these pests and expenditure on the chemical pesticides amount to billions of dollars. In an attempt to reduce these losses, many reports have been published which demonstrate the successful application of RNAi technique in crop protection. Huvenne and Smagghe [52] have summarised the reports on insects in which RNAi has been applied through feeding, and they discussed several factors that influence the success of RNAi on target insects, such as the concentration of dsRNA, the nucleotide sequence, the length of the dsRNA fragment and the life stage of the target insects. The downregulation of expression of critical genes, caused by dsRNA/siRNA, eventually leads to death/growth retardation of the insect and forms the basis of pest control. In this view, the efficient delivery and uptake of the dsRNA trigger is of prime importance. In contrast to the study of gene function, pest control strategies cannot depend on injection of the molecule. The deployment of pest controlling siRNA/miRNA molecules would involve oral exposure, either as transgenic plants or as sprays. Most of the nutrients from gut lumen are absorbed in the midgut tissue of the insect; therefore, this tissue is an attractive target for RNAi. After ingestion, the dsRNA enters into the gut lumen of the insect. Insect gut is divided into foregut, midgut and hindgut. While both foregut and hindgut are covered with chitin, it is only the midgut that has exposed cell surfaces. It is the site of nutrient exchange between the haemolymph and the gut contents. Therefore, midgut epithelium is an attractive target as it is the primary tissue exposed to dsRNA in the gut lumen. The stability of dsRNA molecule and the efficiency of the silencing process (discussed in section 5) is determined by the gut pH and nucleases.

A breakthrough research in RNAi-mediated pest control was published in 2007 on the western corn rootworm, *Diabrotica virgifera virgifera* (WCRW) [53], and cotton bollworm *Helicoverpa armigera* (CBW) [54]. In the former study, a candidate gene was screened based on the complete cDNA library. Out of a total of 290 dsRNAs, *Vacoular ATPase (V-ATPase)* subunit A was finally selected for the development of transgenic corn plants. The larvae reared on transformed plants caused much less damage to the roots and also showed the reduced expression of the target gene. The other study of Mao et al. [9] targeted the pesticide detoxifying gene *Cytochrome P450 (CYP6AE14)*, which provides gossypol tolerance to the insect. Transgenic plants expressing dsRNA corresponding to *CYP6AE14* levels of this transcript in insect body was decreased and the larval growth was retarded. Following these two studies, many research groups started to consider RNAi as a feasible technique which could be employed in the transgenic approaches to manage insects. As we know from the various studies conducted, the Bt (*Bacillus thuringiensis*) toxins are effective on lepidopteran and coleopteran pests but fail to work against hemipteran pests like aphids, whiteflies, phyllids, etc. [55–58].

RNAi-engineered plants can be more useful in case of these phloem-feeding hemipteran pests, which are notorious not only because of feeding damages but also because of their ability to transmit plant viruses [59]. The midgut genes of *Nilaparvata lugens* were downregulated by feeding on transgenic rice expressing dsRNA against three separate genes, but no lethal phenotype was detected in this case [60]. Pitino et al. [61] demonstrated RNAi in aphid *Myzus persicae* directed towards the receptor of activated kinase (*Rack-1*) gene by transgenic expression in *Arabidopsis thaliana*. Another important pest, the whitefly, is also now amenable to RNAi [62]. Its control was demonstrated both by feeding on artificial diet and by feeding on transgenic tobacco plants expressing dsRNA of *V-ATPase A* gene [11, 63]. RNAi experiments conducted on agricultural pests as well as on insect vectors of several human diseases are summarised in Table 2 [53–118].

Insect pests	**Mode of delivery**	**Gene target**
		Order Coleopteran
Diabrotica virgifera virgifera	Artificial diet and transgenic plant	*a*-Tubulin, vacuolar ATPase subunit A [53]
Phyllotreta striolata	Plant tissue	Arginine kinase [64]
Leptinotarsa decemlineata	Artificial diet	Vacuolar ATPase subunit A and E [53]
Diabrotica undecimpunctata howardi	Artificial diet	Vacuolar ATPase subunit A and E, *a*-tubulin [53]
Monochamus alternates	Injection	*Laccase* gene [65]
		Order Diptera
Aedes aegypti	Blood meal Artificial diet Feeding	Inverted repeat (IR) RNA derived from the premembrane protein coding region of the DENV-2 RNA genome [66] V-ATPase A [67] ATP-dependent efflux pump [68]
Anopheles gambiae	Feeding	Chitin synthase [69]
Glossina morsitans morsitans	Feeding	Midgut protein Tsetse EP; transferrin [70]
Bactrocera dorsalis	Feeding and injection	Rpl19; V-ATPase D subunit; fatty acid elongase Noa; small GTPase Rab11 [71]
		Order Hemiptera
Acyrthosiphon pisum	Injection Feeding	Calreticulin, cathepsin-L [72] C002 [73] Hunchback [74] V-ATPase [75] aquaporin [76]
Cimex lectularius	Injection	Cpr gene[77]
Diaphorina citri	Topical In planta (virus induced)	Abnormal wing disc [78] Abnormal wing disc [79]
Laodelphax striatellus	Feeding	Disembodied [80]
Rhodnius prolixus	Injection	Nitrophorins1–4 [81] *a*-Glucosidase [82] Gap gene giant [83] Phospholipase A2 [84]

Insect pests	Mode of delivery	Gene target
Sitobion avenae	Feeding In planta	Catalase [85] CbE E4 [86]
Lygus lineolaris	Injection Injection	Inhibitor of apoptosis gene (IAP) [87] Polygalacturonase (PG) [88]
Oncopeltus fasciatus	Injection	Hunchback [89]
Riptortus pedestris	Injection Injection and feeding	Circadian clock gene, mammalian-type cryptochrome; Bla [90] Gland nitrophorin 2 (*NP2*) [91]
Nilaparvata lugens	Feeding and transgenic Feeding Feeding and injection	Hexose transporter; carboxypeptidase; trypsin-like serine protease [92] ATP synthase subunit [93] Trehalose phosphate synthase [94] Cathepsin B-like protease; nicotinic acetylcholine receptors [95]
Myzus persicae	Transgenic plant	*MpC002* and *Rack-1* [96]
Bemisia tabaci	Injection Artificial diet Transgenic plant	Snap, Chickadee, CG5885, GATAd [62] Actin; ADP/ATP translocase; α-tubulin; ribosomal protein L9; V-ATPase [63] V-ATPase subunit A [11]
Bactericerca cockerelli	Injection/feeding	Actin, V-ATPase [97]
	Order Hymenoptera	
Athalia rosae	Injection	*Ar white gene*
	Order Isoptera	
Reticulitermes flavipes	Feeding	Endogenous digestive cellulase enzyme, hexamerin storage protein [98]
	Order Lepidoptera	
Ostrinia furnacalis	Spraying	LIM protein 1; myosin 3 light chain; chymotrypsin-like serine protease; chymotrypsin-like protease C1; chymortypsin-like serine protease C3; hydroxybutyrate dehydrogenase; Kazal-type serine proteinase inhibitor 1; fatty acid binding protein 1; unknown; caboxypeptidse 4 [99]
Ostrinia nubilalis	Spraying	Chitinase (*OnCht*); chitin synthase (*OnCHS2*) [100]
Epiphyas postvittana	Feeding	Carboxylesterase gene (*EposCXE1*); pheromone binding protein [101]

Insect pests	Mode of delivery	Gene target
Helicoverpa armigera	Feeding Transgenic plant Transgenic plant Feeding and transgenic plant	Acetylcholinesterase (*AChE*) [102] Cytochrome P450; gluthatione-S-transferase[9, 103] Ecdysone receptor EcR [104] HaHR3 moulting factor [105]
Hyalophora cecropia	Injection	*Haemolin* [106]
Manduca sexta	Injection	*Cadherin* [107]
Spodoptera litura	Injection	Vitellogenin receptor [108]
Spodoptera exigua	Feeding	Chitin synthase gene A [109]
Spodoptera littoralis	Injection	β-Actin gene [110]
Spodoptera frugiperda	Allatostatin C; allototropin 2; cytochrome	Feeding [111]
Plutella xylostella	Feeding	Rieske iron–sulphur protein (RISP) [112]
	Order Orthtoptera	
Gryllus bimaculatus	Injection Injection Injection Injection Injection	Delta; Notch [113] Insulin receptor; insulin receptor substrate; phosphatase and tensin homolog; target of rapamycin; PRS6-p70-protein kinase; forkhead box O; epidermal growth factor receptor [114] Nitric oxide synthase gene *NOS* [115] Circadian clock gene *per* [116] Sulfakinins [117]
Schistocerca americana		Eye colour gene vermilion [118]

Table 2. Different insect pests targeted by RNAi.

The choice of a suitable target gene is central to pest control strategy. The gene selection approaches can be based on choosing the gene with known function such as detoxification enzymes, cell synthesis, nutrition, metabolism and cytoskeleton structure. These types of genes can be selected as insect pest control targets. For this, expressed sequence tag (EST) library of European corn borer (*Ostrinia nubilalis*) was screened to find out that a *chitinase* gene (*OnCht*) and a *chitin synthase* gene (*OnCHS2*), which are very important in regulating the growth and development of this insect [119]. Likewise, the EST library of *Bemisia tabaci* was also used to screen out few important genes for RNAi-mediated control [63]. The cDNA library screening approach was also used. Mao et al. [9] constructed a cDNA library from RNAs expressed in the midgut of fifth-instar larvae exposed to gossypol. Several cDNA libraries of WCR (*D. virgifera virgifera*) were prepared and considered upon the underlying principle that genes encoding proteins with essential functions would be the best RNAi targets for causing lethality [8].

As an extension of the cDNA library screening approach, the next-generation sequencing (NGS) technologies have led to novel opportunities for expression profiling in organisms lacking any genome or transcriptome sequence information. It enables the direct sequencing of cDNA generated from mRNA (RNA-seq) [120, 121]. Hence, it provides the *de novo* generation of the transcriptome for a non-model organism, including various pests. Wang et al. [99] adopted Illumina's RNA-seq and digital gene expression tag profile (DGE-tag) to screen optimal RNAi targets from Asian corn borer (ACB; *Ostrinia furnacalis*). The same technique has been used for the grain aphid, *Sitobion avenae* and *Spodoptera litura* [122, 123]. It seems likely that the combination of DGE-tag with RNA-seq is a rapid, high-throughput, cost-effective and easy way to select for candidate target genes for RNAi, which may not be only limited to the midgut tissue but can also be selected from the whole insect.

The convenience of RNAi to target specific pests while not harming other species is a perfect method of pest management. However, target gene selection and efficient delivery methods are the two major cornerstones of pest management by RNAi. The candidate gene for RNAi can be tailored to be species specific or they can also have a broad spectrum. Specificity can be achieved by designing dsRNAs that target the more variable regions of genes, such as untranslated regions (UTRs). It was first demonstrated in *Drosophila* where UTR of the *gamma-tubulin* gene was targeted and even closely related species could be targeted selectively [75]. However, it can also be possible to target multiple organisms with a single gene. One such example is of *V-ATPase* gene, which is an effective target in *B. tabaci*, *D. virgifera* and *B. dorsalis* [8, 63, 124]; all of these insects belong to different orders. In this case, either a conserved region can be selected which could affect closely related species or a mixture of dsRNA fragments from different genes belonging to different species can be selected.

Delivery methods that ensure continuous supply of dsRNA/siRNA will be applicable in the fields. A more reliable and verified method would be transgenic plants as the dsRNA can be applied as bait, sprays, or supplied through irrigation systems [125, 126]. The application approach by spray could be quite practical like the spray of chemical pesticides. Gan et al. [127] have also demonstrated the control of viral infection using dsRNA spraying. Similar results were obtained with Asian corn borer, *Ostrinia furnacalis*. This study showed that larval lethality or developmental disorders can be achieved by gene-specific RNAi, and spraying can be an efficient method for continuous supply of dsRNA [99]. The coating of dsRNA molecule with liposomes is used for delivering siRNA to mammalian cells, specific tissues and some insects [128, 75]. This coating prevents the degradation of the molecule and enhances its uptake ability; spraying may also be explored for such particles. Zhang et al. [129] used the chitosan nanoparticle based RNAi technology to suppress the expression of two chitin synthase genes (*AgCHS1* and *AgCHS2*) in African malaria mosquito (*A. gambiae*) larvae. Bacterial expression or chemical synthesis allows large-scale production of dsRNA at efficient costs [75, 130, 131].

4. RNAi: Link with immunity and viral infections

The RNAi mechanisms evolved primarily as a defence mechanism against viruses and transposons [132]. Research has established that RNAi pathway also contributes to the innate immunity of the insects against the viruses having either dsRNA genome or such replicative intermediates. It was demonstrated that the *Drosophila* S2 cells utilise the endocytosis-mediated pathway involving the pattern recognition scavenger receptors for the uptake of dsRNA from the surroundings. These receptors are key players in the innate immune responses of the cell [133, 134]. Saleh et al. [135] demonstrated the strong link of dsRNA uptake pathway and the activation of the immune response in the infected cells. The normal cells used dsRNA uptake pathway to internalise viral dsRNA and subsequently showed manifestation of antiviral response in these cells. On the contrary, the mutant cells (defective genes used for dsRNA uptake) did not show activation of any antiviral response. Mutants in the core siRNA components Dicer-2, AGO-2 and R2D2 are more susceptible to viral infections [140].

Further, it was also reported that receptors such as Sr-CI and Eater, which contribute to majority of dsRNA uptake in the *Drosophila* S2 cells, were significantly down-regulated after pathogenic virus treatments, and significant changes in phagocytic activity were observed. The role of RNAi in antiviral defence has also been firmly established in mosquitoes [136]. Viruses can also affect the availability of RNAi machinery for other candidate dsRNA molecules. They can saturate the RNAi machinery and affect the efficiency of RNAi mechanism. Many viruses are known to produce viral suppressors of RNA silencing (VSRs), which bind to the key elements of the RNAi pathway rendering it unavailable. Many of the viral proteins (viz. B2 protein from Flockhouse virus, 1A proteins from *Drosophila* C virus and cricket paralysis virus) are known to interfere in the siRNA pathway of RNA-mediated silencing [137–140]. These viral proteins may affect the biogenesis of the trigger molecule by binding to important enzymes such as dicer, which generate the siRNA from long dsRNA or affect the target cleavage by binding to RISC. The viral proteins may also sequester the dsRNA signal molecule or form complexes with the replicative intermediates of the siRNA pathway.

Viruses also produce large amount of RNAs and small RNAs that accumulate in the infected cells. It has also been hypothesised that the occurrence of alternative and effective antiviral pathway may become important in controlling the viral infections and may supersede the RNAi pathway. Few of these possible pathways have been worked upon. Goic et al. [141] have reported the potential interaction of nucleic acid-based acquired immunity with the core RNAi machinery in the study of persistent infection of S2 cells by Flock House Virus (FHV). The insects also protect themselves from foreign nucleic acids by becoming refractory to RNAi. In the oriental fruit fly, *Bactrocera dorsalis*, orally administered dsRNA-targeting endogenous genes, resistance to RNAi was seen due to a blockade in the dsRNA uptake pathway. A very interesting hypothesis is presented by Swevers et al. [142] about the possible impact of persistent viral infection in the insects. In their work, the authors have analysed various factors that determine the response to exogenous dsRNA in the background of viral infection.

5. Efficiency of RNAi

Though RNAi is a conserved mechanism in eukaryotes, its efficiency is governed by various factors. The response of different insect species towards this mechanism of gene silencing is imperative for successful implementation in the study of gene function and more importantly in the pest management programs. Also, the efficacy is governed by many factors which are not intrinsic to the organism such as the delivery, dosage and choice of the candidate gene. Comprehending these factors will provide a better insight into designing the experiments for successful application of RNAi. The available reports indicate that the lower *Insecta* species such as that of *Blatella* show a much robust and persistent RNAi response, while higher *Insecta* species belonging to the orders Lepidoptera and Diptera are non-compliant [15]. The sensitivity could vary within and among the orders. For instance, many Lepidopteran insects are resistant to RNAi. Terenius et al. [143] have reviewed various factors that may be contributing to the poor responsiveness of these insects. The efficiency can vary with insect species, target gene, developmental stage of the organism, expression of RNAi machinery, method of delivery, stability of dsRNA, etc. A few factors that may be crucial in determining the efficiency of RNAi are discussed below.

5.1. The RNAi machinery

RNAi evolved in organisms as a defence mechanism against viral infections at the cellular level [144, 145]. The differences in the expression of core RNAi machinery can be a prime reason affecting the adequacy of RNAi mechanism. The systemic RNA-interference-deficient 1 (sid-1) protein forms a gated channel which is selective for dsRNA molecule. Its role is well established in the systemic spread of the RNAi signal in the model organism *Caenorhabditis elegans* [146]. The presence of *SID-1*gene orthologs in insects varies with the insect orders [52]. The dipterans lack this gene completely. The mosquito *Culex quinquefasciatus* also lacks sid-1 ortholog but shows the systemic spread of the dsRNA trigger [147]. On the one hand, honey bee (*Apis mellifera*) showed an increase in the expression of *SID-1* during the RNAi experiments, indicating its role in the uptake pathway [148]. On the other hand, in *Tribolium castaneum*, the silencing of all three orthologs of *SID-1* casted no influence on the efficiency of RNAi [149].

In *Bombyx mori*, three orthologs are present but no significant success has been found in this lepidopteran, while mosquitoes show systemic RNAi despite the absence of *sid-1* in several species [149–152]. R2D2, a cofactor of dicer-2 enzyme which cleaves long dsRNA into siRNA for loading into the RISC, is absent in *B. mori* making the insect very insensitive to RNAi. Another important enzyme RNA-dependent RNA polymerase (RdRP), which amplifies the primary siRNA signal in *C. elegans*, is entirely not reported in the insects [149]. *T. castaneum* showed a robust systemic RNAi, but a wide survey of RNAi related genes did not show any traces of RdRP [149]. However, RdRP-like activity was substituted in *Drosophila* cell lines by certain other enzymatic pathways. In many cases, the absence of certain well-known genes of the RNAi pathway is directly responsible for the poor response of the organism while in several other examples, the absence is compensated by other genes/pathways which play key roles of their counterparts.

5.2. The RNAi molecule

The exogenous dsRNA molecule is the trigger for initiating the RNAi pathway. These molecules are delivered in the form of dsRNA, siRNA or hairpin RNA. Apart from sequence specificity, other parameters are also crucial in determining the efficiency of RNAi experiments. The study on the administration of dsRNA (feeding by means of artificial diet, natural diet, droplet method, blood meal, transgenic plants, etc.) in insects has used varied length of dsRNA molecule. The nucleotide length used in these reports ranges from 134 to 1842 bp, while most of the studies used 300–500 bp as the optimal length [153]. However, silencing effects have also been observed in the case of single siRNA synthesised chemically (administration in *H. armigera*) or a cocktail of siRNA (obtained by using dicer enzyme to chop the dsRNA molecule) [154]. In the cell line experiments done on the *Drosophila* S2 cell line, 211 bp was found to be the optimum length of dsRNA that could be absorbed by the cells [135]. Not only the length but also the specificity of the RNAi molecule is a concern. It can be understood by the reports on *Drosophila* that feeding specific sequence of *V-ATPase* dsRNA caused no silencing in non-target species [75], which implies the specificity of the process. On the contrary, various other studies report non-specific silencing. Off-target effects were reported in *Rhodnius prolixus* [81] and Colorado potato beetle (*Leptinotarsa decemlineata*) [8]. Single mismatches are known to impair the RNAi effect in the mammalian cell lines [155]. Further studies will clarify whether single mismatches show similar impact in insects as well. In case of pest management programs, long dsRNAs (>200 bp) are generally used which generate many probable siRNA maximising the RNAi response [153]. The dosage of the dsRNA molecule also plays an important role in determining the efficiency of the process. Higher doses are required in case of feeding experiments as compared to injection. The silencing effect in *R. prolixus* was enhanced by multiple doses [38]. Therefore, it follows that doses and types of administration (oral or injectable) also need to be optimised according to the life stage of the organism and the target tissue.

5.3. Delivery of the molecule/uptake of silencing signal

One of the most decisive factors for inducing RNAi is the efficient delivery of the dsRNA molecule. The common methods of delivery are by microinjection, soaking, oral delivery and transgenic technique [156]. Microinjection-based delivery is the most commonly used technique in studying gene functions. It has proven to work well for *Tribolium, Drosophila* and many other lepidopteran insects. Although it works well for larger insects, success with smaller insects is limited due to the invasive nature of this technique. The survival of aphids after microinjection procedure is highly dependent on the injected volume [157].

Further, factors such as needle choice, optimal volume and place of injection are very crucial considerations and tend to vary with organisms and laboratories. Feeding-based experiments involve either *in vitro* synthesised or bacterially expressed dsRNA molecules. The success of oral delivery methods indicates the possible employment of RNAi technique for target pest control. However, the stability of the molecule will always be a concern in the gut lumen. Artificial diet mixed with dsRNA could not induce RNAi in *Drosophila* spp. Ingested dsRNA against a gut-specific *aminopeptidase N* gene also failed to develop RNAi response in *Spodoptera litura* [43]. Therefore, it can be suggested that oral delivery is not equally suitable for all species. Another convenient method of delivery is soaking. Nevertheless, this method is more applicable for cell line experiments rather than whole insects.

After the delivery of the molecules, the next step is the uptake of the molecules by insects. Huvenne and Smagghe [52] have elaborately reviewed the basic mechanisms involved in the uptake of dsRNA in the insects. The spreading of the RNAi signal, i.e., systemic RNAi, is an important determinant of the efficiency of RNAi. In cases of functional genetics, cell autonomous RNAi has been successfully employed to study the function of genes; however, for implementation in the pest control programs, non-cell autonomous RNAi is important. The systemic spread of the silencing signal is absent in the most studied model insect *Drosophila*. In contrast, the most studied insect *Tribolium* shows a powerful systemic silencing effect [149].

5.4. Potency of the silencing signal

The manifestation of the RNAi effect also depends on the stability and persistence of the dsRNA molecule. In *Acyrthosiphon pisum*, the silencing effect on the aquaporin gene began to reduce after five days [157]. The early stability of dsRNA molecule may be disrupted by the non-specific nucleases as reported in many of the lepidopteran insects [143]. These are extracellular enzymes different from dicer and digest the trigger molecule, thereby preventing the RNAi cascade. In certain cases, the activity of dsRNA degrading enzymes have been studied and their levels were measured in different stages, which was found related to the developmental stage. The dsRNase activity is also found in the digestive juices of *Bombyx mori*, saliva of *Linus lineolaris* and in haemolymph of *Manduca sexta* [87, 158, 159]. The existence/stability/mode of action of these enzymes are not sufficiently studied and future research in this direction needs to be carried out to comprehend the stability of dsRNA molecule in the *in vivo* studies. The choice of gene can also decrease the strength of the silencing signal. Ideally, the protein whose function is to be silenced should have a short half-life, whilst the mRNA turnover number should be high. The stability of protein explained the weak RNAi response in both *D. melanogaster* and *T. casteneum* [160]. However, such studies have not been conducted for the majority of the genes and therefore it can be concluded that expression of RNAi is limited by many uncovered phenomena.

6. Conclusions

The advent of RNA interference has been a crucial phase of the modern day science. The wide array of applications in the entomological research has led to many momentous findings. The functionality of many genes has been understood by this technique. Its implication in functional genomics is not only restricted to the study of a given set of genes but is also used to unveil the interaction of different genes in a particular metabolic pathway. The rapid pace of RNAi-based research suggests that it would soon facilitate better understanding of evolution, circadian rhythms, behavioural pattern, reproductive biology and interaction between host and parasites/pathogens. However, successful manifestation of RNAi is dependent on several factors. The insect species might lack the basic RNAi machinery [161] or may rapidly degrade alien dsRNA. Such factors could be intrinsic to the concerned tissue or gene. The gene might have high transcription rate and could evade the effect of RNAi or the target mRNA may be too transient.

As happens with every phenomenon, this mechanism can also undergo selection pressure. Viruliferous insects that also have RNAi suppressors would be able to thrive on RNAi-protected crops. Furthermore, single nucleotide polymorphisms (SNPs) that result in lower effectiveness of the RNAi could potentially be selected for and lead to the evolution of resistance [153]. Genetic variations among insect species are already a challenge for RNAi. Therefore, parallel research must be carried out to develop strategies, which would minimise the resistance development and selective pressures.

RNAi has proved its utility as a futuristic tool of insect pest management. However, there are several issues that need to be addressed before the implementation of this technology in fields. The knowledge gaps underlying large-scale implications of pesticidal RNAi-based crops on the environment should be identified and bridged. The off-target gene silencing is a serious concern where unintended organisms are adversely affected [162]. The non-target effects can be categorised as off-target gene silencing, silencing the target gene in non-target organisms, immune stimulation and saturation of the RNAi machinery [163]. A balanced approach should be taken with maximum effects on the target pests with minimal effects on non-target organisms.

Acknowledgements

SKU is thankful to the Department of Science and Technology, India, for DST-INSPIRE faculty fellowship and Panjab University for facility.

Author details

Nidhi Thakur[1,2], Jaspreet Kaur Mundey[3] and Santosh Kumar Upadhyay[3*]

*Address all correspondence to: skupadhyay@pu.ac.in

1 Plant Molecular Biology Lab, CSIR-National Botanical Research Institute, Lucknow, India

2 Academy of Scientific and Innovative Research, Anusandhan Bhawan, New Delhi, India

3 Department of Botany, Panjab University, Chandigarh, India

References

[1] Fire A, Xu S, Montgomery MK, Kostas SA, Driver SE, Mello CC. Potent and specific genetic interference by double-stranded RNA in Caenorhabditis elegans. *Nature* 1998:391, 806–811. DOI:10.1038/35888.

[2] Meister G, Tuschl T. Mechanisms of gene silencing by double-stranded RNA. *Nature* 2004:431(7006), 343–349. DOI:10.1038/nature02873.

[3] Kennerdell JR, Carthew RW. Use of dsRNA-mediated genetic interference to demonstrate that frizzled and frizzled 2 act in the wingless pathway. *Cell* 1998:95(7), 1017–1026. DOI: http://dx.doi.org/10.1016/S0092-8674(00)81725-0.

[4] Angaji SA, Hedayati SS, Poor RH, Madani S, Poor SS, Panahi S. Application of RNA interference in treating human diseases. *Journal of Genetics* 2010:89(4), 527–537.

[5] Ambesajir A, Kaushik A, Kaushik J, Petros S. RNA interference: A futuristic tool and its therapeutic applications. *Saudi Journal of Biological Sciences* 2012:19, 395–403. DOI: 10.1016/j.sjbs.2012.08.001.

[6] Younis A, Siddique MI, Kim C, Lim K. RNA interference (RNAi) induced gene silencing: A promising approach of hi-tech plant breeding. *International Journal of Biological Science* 2014:10(10), 1150–1158. DOI: 10.7150/ijbs.10452.

[7] Gu L, Knipple DC. Recent advances in RNA interference research in insects: Implications for future insect pest management strategies. *Crop Protection* 2013:45, 36–40. DOI:10.1016/j.cropro.2012.10.004.

[8] Baum JA, Bogaert T, Clinton W, Heck GR, Feldmann P, Ilagan O et al. Control of coleopteran insect pests through RNA interference. *Nature Biotechnology* 2007:25(11), 1322–1326. DOI: 10.1038/nbt1359.

[9] Mao YB, Cai WJ, Wang JW, Hong GJ, Tao XY, Wang LJ, Huang YP, Chen XY. Silencing a cotton bollworm P450 monooxygenase gene by plant-mediated RNAi impairs larval tolerance of gossypol. *Nature Biotechnology* 2007:25(11), 1307–1313. DOI: 10.1038/nbt1352.

[10] Chen J, Zhang D, Yao Q, Zhang J, Dong X, Tian H et al. Feeding-based RNA interference of a trehalose phosphate synthase gene in the brown planthopper, *Nilaparvata lugens*. *Insect Molecular Biology* 2010:19(6), 777–786. DOI:10.1111/j.1365-2583.2010.01038.x.

[11] Thakur N, Upadhyay SK, Verma PC, Chandrashekar K, Tuli R, Singh PK. Enhanced whitefly resistance in transgenic tobacco plants expressing double stranded RNA of v-ATPase a gene. *PLoS One* 2014:9(3), e87235. DOI: 10.1371/journal.pone.0087235.

[12] Saini RK, Yadav GS, Kumari B. Novel approaches in pest and pesticide management in agro-ecosystem. http://hau.ernet.in/coa/pdf/ento4789.pdf

[13] Sanahuja G, Banakar R, Twyman RM, Capell T, Christou P. *Bacillus thuringiensis*: A century of research, development and commercial applications. *Journal of Plant Biotechnology* 2011:9, 283–300. DOI: 10.1111/j.1467-7652.2011.00595.x.

[14] Bergé JB, Ricroch AE. Emergence of minor pests becoming major pests in GE cotton in China: What are the reasons? What are the alternatives practices to this change of status? *GM Crops* 2010:1, 214–219. DOI: 10.4161/gmcr.1.4.13421.

[15] Bellés X. Beyond drosophila: RNAi in vivo and functional genomics in insects. *Annual Review of Entomology* 2010:55, 111–128. DOI: 10.1146/annurev-ento-112408-085301.

[16] Bucher G, Scholten J, Klingler M. Parental RNAi in *Tribolium* (Coleoptera). *Current Biology* 2002:12, R85–R86. DOI: http://dx.doi.org/10.1016/S0960-9822(02)00666-8.

[17] Liu PZ, Kaufman TC. Hunchback is required for suppression of abdominal identity, and for proper germband growth and segmentation in the intermediate germband insect Oncopeltus fasciatus. *Development* 2004a:131, 1515–1527. DOI: 10.1242/dev.01046.

[18] Liu PZ, Kaufman TC. Kruppel is a gap gene in the intermediate germband insect Oncopeltus fasciatus and is required for development of both blastoderm and germband-derived segments. *Development* 2004b:131, 4567–4579. DOI: 10.1242/dev.01311.

[19] Ronco M, Uda T, Mito T, Minelli A, Noji S, Klingler M. Antenna and all gnathal appendages are similarly transformed by homothorax knock-down in the cricket *Gryllusbimaculatus. Developmental Biology* 2008:313, 80–92. DOI:10.1016/j.ydbio.2007.09.059.

[20] Mito T, Inoue Y, Kimura S, Miyawaki K, Niwa N, Shinmyo Y et al. Involvement of *hedgehog, wingless*, and *dpp* in the initiation of proximodistal axis formation during the regeneration of insect legs, a verification of the modified boundary model. *Mechanisms of Development* 2002:114, 27–35. DOI:10.1016/S0925-4773(02)00052-7.

[21] Lynch JA, Desplan C. A method for parental RNA interference in the wasp Nasonia vitripennis. *Nature Protocols* 2006:1, 486–494. DOI:10.1038/nprot.2006.70.

[22] Khila A, Grbic M. Gene silencing in the spider mite Tetranychus urticae: dsRNA and siRNA parental silencing of the Distal-less gene. *Development Genes and Evolution* 2007:217, 241–251.

[23] Grossmann D, Scholten J, Prpic NM. Separable functions of wingless in distal and ventral patterning of the *Tribolium* leg. *Development Genes and Evolution* 2009:219, 469–479. DOI: 10.1007/s00427-009-0310-z.

[24] Brent AE, Yucel G, Small S, Desplan C. Permissive and instructive anterior patterning rely on mRNA localization in the wasp embryo. *Science* 2007:315, 1841–1843. DOI: 10.1126/science.1137528.

[25] Hughes CL, Kaufman TC. RNAi analysis of deformed, proboscipedia and sex combs reduced in the milkweed bug oncopeltus fasciatus: Novel roles for Hox genes in the hemipteran head. *Development* 2000:127, 3683–3694.

[26] Tomoyasu Y, Denell RE. Larval RNAi in *Tribolium* (Coleoptera) for analyzing adult development. *Development Genes and Evolution* 2004:214, 575–578. DOI: 10.1007/s00427-004-0434-0.

[27] Tomoyasu Y, Wheeler SR, Denell RE. *Ultrabithorax* is required for membranous wing identity in the beetle *Tribolium castaneum*. *Nature* 2005:433, 643–647. DOI:10.1038/nature03272.

[28] Arakane Y, Muthukrishnan S, Beeman RW, Kanost MR, Kramer KJ. Laccase 2 is the phenoloxidase gene required for beetle cuticle tanning. *Proceedings of the National Academy of Sciences of the United States of America* 2005:102, 11337–11342. DOI: 10.1073/pnas.0504982102.

[29] Ohnishi A, Hashimoto K, Imai K, Matsumoto S. Functional characterization of the *Bombyx mori* fatty acid transport protein (*Bm*FATP) within the silkmoth pheromone gland. *The Journal of Biological Chemistry* 2009:284, 5128–5136. DOI: 10.1074/jbc.M806072200.

[30] Dong Y, Friedrich M. Nymphal RNAi: Systemic RNAi mediated gene knockdown in juvenile grasshopper. *BMC Biotechnology* 2005:5, 25. DOI: 10.1186/1472-6750-5-25.

[31] Dong Y, Friedrich M. Enforcing biphasic eye development in a directly developing insect by transient knockdown of single eye selector genes. *Journal of Experimental Zoology Part B: Molecular and Developmental Evolution* 2010:314, 104–114. DOI: 10.1002/jez.b.21313.

[32] Martin D, Maestro O, Cruz J, Mane-Padros D, Belles X. RNAi studies reveal a conserved role for RXR in molting in the cockroach *Blattella germanica*. *Journal of Insect Physiology* 2006:52, 410–416. DOI:10.1016/j.jinsphys.2005.12.002.

[33] Nakamura T, Mito T, Tanaka Y, Bando T, Ohuchi H, Noji S. Involvement of canonical Wnt/Wingless signalling in the determination of the positional values within the leg segment of the cricket *Gryllus bimaculatus*. *Development, Growth & Differentiation* 2007:49, 79–88. DOI: 10.1111/j.1440-169X.2007.00915.x.

[34] Moriyama Y, Sakamoto T, Karpova SG, Matsumoto A, Noji S, Tomioka K. RNA interference of the clock gene period disrupts circadian rhythms in the cricket Gryllus bimaculatus. *Journal of Biological Rhythms* 2008:23, 308–318. DOI: 10.1177/0748730408320486.

[35] Hamada A, Miyawaki K, Honda-sumi E, Tomioka K, Mito T, Ohuchi H et al. Loss-offunction analyses of the fragile X-related and dopamine receptor genes by RNA interference in the cricket Gryllus bimaculatus. *Developmental Dynamics* 2009:238, 2025–2033. DOI: 10.1002/dvdy.22029.

[36] Nakamura T, Mito T, Bando T, Ohuchi H, Noji S. Dissecting insect leg regeneration through RNA interference. *Cellular and Molecular Life Sciences* 2008:65, 64–72. DOI: 10.1016/j.mod.2011.07.001.

[37] Mito T, Inoue Y, Kimura S, Miyawaki K, Niwa N, Shinmyo Y et al. Involvement of *hedgehog*, *wingless*, and *dpp* in the initiation of proximodistal axis formation during

the regeneration of insect legs, a verification of the modified boundary model. *Mechanisms of Development* 2002:114, 27–35. DOI:10.1016/S0925-4773(02)00052-7.

[38] Araujo RN, Santos A, Pinto FS, Gontijo NF, Lehane MJ, Pereira MH. RNA interference of the salivary gland Nitrophorin 2 in the triatomine bug Rhodnius prolixus (Hemiptera: Reduviidae) by dsRNA ingestion or injection. *Insect Biochemistry and Molecular Biology* 2006:36, 683–693. DOI:10.1016/j.ibmb.2006.05.012.

[39] Boisson B, Jacques JC, Choumet V, Martin E, Xu J, Vernick K, et al. Gene silencing in mosquito salivary glands by RNAi. *FEBS Letters* 2006:580, 1988–1992. DOI: http://dx.doi.org/10.1016/j.febslet.2006.02.069.

[40] Belgacem YH, Martin JR. Hmgcr in the corpus allatum controls sexual dimorphism of locomotor activity and body size via the insulin pathway in Drosophila. *PLoS One* 2007:2, e187. DOI: 10.1371/journal.pone.0000187.

[41] Lee CM, Su MT, Lee HJ. Pigment dispersing factor: An output regulator of the circadian clock in the German cockroach. *Journal of Biological Rhythms* 2009:24, 35–43. DOI: 10.1177/0748730408327909.

[42] Lycett GJ, McLaughlin LA, Ranson H, Hemingway J, Kafatos FC, Loukeris TG et al. Anopheles gambiae P450 reductase is highly expressed in oenocytes and in vivo knockdown increases permethrin susceptibility. *Insect Molecular Biology* 2006:15, 321–27. DOI: 10.1111/j.1365-2583.2006.00647.x.

[43] Sivakumar S, Rajagopal R, Venkatesh GR, Srivastava A, Bhatnagar RK. Knockdown of aminopeptidase-N from Helicoverpa armigera larvae and in transfected Sf21 cells by RNA interference reveals its functional interaction with Bacillus thuringiensis insecticidal protein Cry1Ac. *Journal Biological Chemistry* 2007:282, 7312–7319. DOI: 10.1074/jbc.M607442200.

[44] Ohnishi A, Hull JJ, Matsumoto S. Targeted disruption of genes in the Bombyx mori sex pheromone biosynthetic pathway. *Proceedings of National Academy of Science of the United States of America* 2006:103, 4398–4403. DOI: 10.1073/pnas.0511270103.

[45] Turner CT, Davy MW, MacDiarmid RM, Plummer KM, Birch NP, Newcomb RD. 2006. RNA interference in the light brown apple moth, Epiphyas postvittana (Walker) induced by double-stranded RNA feeding. *Insect Molecular Biology* 2006:15, 383–391. DOI: 10.1111/j.1365-2583.2006.00656.x.

[46] Paldi N, Glick E, Oliva M, Zilberberg Y, Aubin L, Pettis J et al. Effective gene silencing in a microsporidian parasite associated with honeybee (Apis mellifera) colony declines. *Applied and Environmental Microbiology* 2010:76, 5960–5964. DOI:10.1128/AEM.01067-10.

[47] Garbian Y, Maori E, Kalev H, Shafir S, Sela I. Bidirectional transfer of RNAi between honey bee and Varroa destructor: Varroa gene silencing reduces Varroa population. *PLoS Pathogens* 2012:8, e1003035. DOI: 10.1371/journal.ppat.1003035.

[48] Goto A, Blandin S, Royet J, Reichhart JM, Levashina EA. Silencing of Toll pathway components by direct injection of double-stranded RNA into Drosophila adult flies. *Nucleic Acids Research* 2003:31, 6619–6623. DOI: 10.1093/nar/gkg852.

[49] Blandin S, Moita LF, Kocher T, Wilm M, Kafatos FC, Levashina EA. Reverse genetics in the mosquito Anopheles gambiae: Targeted disruption of the defensin gene. *EMBO Reports* 2002:3, 852–856. DOI: 10.1093/embo-reports/kvf180.

[50] Osta MA, Christophides GK, Kafatos FC. Effects of mosquito genes on Plasmodium development. *Science* 2004:303, 2030–2032. DOI:10.1126/science.1091789.

[51] Eleftherianos I, Gokcen F, Felfoldi G, Millichap PJ, Trenczek TE, ffrench-Constant RH et al. The immunoglobulin family protein hemolin mediates cellular immune responses to bacteria in the insect Manduca sexta. *Cell Microbiology* 2007:9, 1137–1147. DOI: 10.1111/j.1462-5822.2006.00855.x.

[52] Huvenne H, Smagghe, G. Mechanisms of dsRNA uptake in insects and potential of RNAi for pest control: A review. *Journal of Insect Physiology* 2010:56, 227–235. DOI: 10.1016/j.jinsphys.2009.10.004.

[53] Baum JA, Bogaert T, Clinton W, Heck GR, Feldmann P, Ilagan O et al. Control of coleopteran insect pests through RNA interference. *Nature Biotechnology* 2007:25, 1322–1326. DOI:10.1038/nbt1359.

[54] Mao YB, Cai WJ, Wang JW, Hong GJ, Tao XY, Wang LJ et al. Silencing a cotton bollworm P450 monooxygenase gene by plant-mediated RNAi impairs larval tolerance of gossypol. *Nature Biotechnology* 2007:25(11), 1307–1313. DOI: 10.1038/nbt1352.

[55] Li J, Chen Q, Lin Y, Jiang T, Wu G, Hua H. RNA interference in Nilaparvata lugens (Homoptera: Delphacidae) based on dsRNA ingestion. *Pest Management Science* 2011:67, 852–859. DOI: 10.1002/ps.2124.

[56] Elaine BA, Miguel SS, Christopher RM. Mechanisms of hopperburn: An overview of insect taxonomy, behavior, and physiology. *Annual Review of Entomology* 2005:50, 125–151. DOI: 10.1146/annurev.ento.49.061802.123310.

[57] Liu S, Ding Z, Zhang C, Yang B, Liu Z. Gene knockdown by intro-thoracic injection of double-stranded RNA in the brown planthopper, Nilaparvata lugens. *Insect Biochemistry and Molecular Biology* 2010:40, 666–671. DOI:10.1016/j.ibmb.2010.06.007.

[58] Gatehouse JA, Price DRG. Protection of crops against insect pests using RNA interference. *Insect Biotechnology* 2011:2, 145–168. DOI: 10.1007/978-90-481-9641-8_8.

[59] Navas-Castillo J, Fiallo-Olivé E, Sánchez-Campos S. Emerging virus diseases transmitted by whiteflies. *Annual Review of Phytopathology* 2011:49, 219–248. DOI: 10.1146/annurev-phyto-072910-095235.

[60] Zha W, Peng X, Chen R, Du B, Zhu L, He G. Knockdown of midgut genes by dsRNA-transgenic plant-mediated RNA interference in the hemipteran insect Nilaparvata lugens. *PLoS One* 2011:6, e20504. DOI: 10.1371/journal.pone.0020504.

[61] Pitino M, Coleman AD, Maffei ME, Ridout CJ, Hogenhout SA. Silencing of aphid genes by dsRNA feeding from plants. *PLoS One* 2011:6, e25709. DOI: 10.1371/journal.pone.0025709.

[62] Ghanim M, Kontsedalov S, Czosnek H. Tissue-specific gene silencing by RNA interference in the whitefly Bemisia tabaci (Gennadius). *Insect Biochemistry and Molecular Biology* 2007:37, 732–738. DOI:10.1016/j.ibmb.2007.04.006.

[63] Upadhyay SK, Chandrashekar K, Thakur N, Verma PC, Borgio JF, Singh PK et al. RNA interference for the control of whiteflies (Bemisia tabaci) by oral route. *Journal of Biosciences* 2011:36, 153–161. DOI: 10.1007/s12038-011-9009-1.

[64] Zhao YY, Yang G, Wang-Pruski G, You MS. Phyllotreta striolata Coleoptera: Chrysomelidae): Arginine kinase cloning and RNAi-based pest control. *European Journal of Entomology* 2008:105, 815–822. DOI: 10.14411/eje.2008.108.

[65] Niu BL, Shen WF, Liu Y, Weng HB, He LH, Mu JJ et al. Cloning and RNAi-mediated functional characterization of MaLac2 of the pine sawyer, Monochamus alternatus. *Insect Molecular Biology* 2008:17, 303–312. DOI: 10.1111/j.1365-2583.2008.00803.x.

[66] Franz AW, Sanchez-Vargas I, Adelman ZN, Blair CD, Beaty BJ, James AA et al. Engineering RNA interference-based resistance to dengue virus type 2 in genetically modified Aedes aegypti. *Proceedings of the National Academy of Sciences of the United States of America* 2006:103(11), 4198–4203. DOI: 10.1073/pnas.0600479103.

[67] Coy MR, Sanscrainte ND, Chalaire KC, Inberg A, Maayan I, Glick E et al. Gene silencing in adult Aedes aegypti mosquitoes through oral delivery of double-stranded RNA. *Journal of Applied Entomology* 2012:136(10), 741–748. DOI: 10.1111/j.1439-0418.2012.01713.x.

[68] Figueira-Mansur J, Ferreira-Pereira A, Mansur JF, Franco TA, Alvarenga ESL, Sorgine MHF et al. Silencing of P-glycoprotein increases mortality in temephos-treated Aedes aegypti larvae. *Insect Molecular Biology* 2013:22(6), 648–658. DOI: 10.1111/imb.12052.

[69] Zhang X, Zhang J, Zhu KY. Chitosan/double-stranded RNA nanoparticle-mediated RNA interference to silence chitin synthase genes through larval feeding in the African malaria mosquito (Anopheles gambiae). *Insect Molecular Biology* 2010:19(5), 683–693. DOI: 10.1111/j.1365-2583.2010.01029.x.

[70] Walshe DP, Lehane SM, Lehane MJ, Haines LR. Prolonged gene knockdown in the tsetse fly Glossina by feeding double stranded RNA. *Insect Molecular Biology* 2009:(1), 11–19. DOI: 10.1371/journal.pone.0017788.

[71] Li X, Zhang M, Zhang H. RNA interference of four genes in adult Bactrocera dorsalis by feeding their dsRNAs. *PLoS One* 2011:6(3), e17788. DOI: 10.1371/journal.pone.0017788.

[72] Jaubert-Possamai S, Le Trionnaire G, Bonhomme J, Christophides GK, Rispe C, Tagu D. Gene knockdown by RNAi in the pea aphid Acyrthosiphon pisum. *BMC Biotechnology* 2007:7, 63. DOI:10.1186/1472-6750-7-63.

[73] Mutti NS, Park Y, Reese JC, Reeck GR. RNAi knockdown of a salivary transcript leading to lethality in the pea aphid, Acyrthosiphon pisum. *Journal of Insect Science* 2006:6, 1–7. DOI: 10.1673/031.006.3801.

[74] Mao J, Zeng F. Feeding-based RNA interference of a gap gene is lethal to the pea aphid, Acyrthosiphon pisum. *Plos One* 2012:7, e48718. DOI: 10.1371/journal.pone.0048718.

[75] Whyard S, Singh AD, Wong S. Ingested double-stranded RNAs can act as species-specific insecticides. *Insect Biochemistry and Molecular Biology* 2009:39, 824–832. DOI: 10.1016/j.ibmb.2009.09.007.

[76] Shakesby A, Wallace I, Isaacs H, Pritchard J, Roberts D, Douglas A. A water-specific aquaporin involved in aphid osmoregulation. *Insect Biochemistry and Molecular Biology* 2009:39, 1–10. DOI: 10.1016/j.ibmb.2008.08.008.

[77] Zhu F, Sams S, Moural T, Haynes KF, Potter MF, Palli SR. RNA interference of NADPH-cytochrome P450 reductase results in reduced insecticide resistance in the bed bug, Cimex lectularius. *PLos One* 2012:7, e31037. DOI: 10.1371/journal.pone.0031037.

[78] El-Shesheny I, Hajeri S, El-Hawary I, Gowda S, Killiny N. Silencing abnormal wing disc gene of the Asian citrus psyllid, Diaphorina citri disrupts adult wing development and increases nymph mortality. *PLos One* 2013:8, e65392. DOI: 10.1371/journal.pone.0065392.

[79] Hajeri S, Killiny N, El-Mohtar C, Dawson WO, Gowda S. Citrus tristeza virus-based RNAi in citrus plants induces gene silencing in Diaphorina citri, a phloem-sap sucking insect vector of citrus greening disease (Huanglongbing). *Journal of Biotechnology* 2014:176, 42–49. DOI: 10.1016/j.jbiotec.2014.02.010.

[80] Wan P-J, Jia S, Li N, Fan J-M, Li G-Q. RNA interference depletion of the halloween gene disembodied implies its potential application for management of planthopper Sogatella furcifera and Laodelphax striatellus. *PLos One* 2014:9, e86675. DOI: 10.1371/journal.pone.0086675.

[81] Araujo RN, Soares AC, Paim RM, Gontijo NF, Gontijo AF, Lehane MJ et al. The role of salivary nitrophorins in the ingestion of blood by the triatomine bug Rhodnius prolixus (Reduviidae: Triatominae). *Insect Biochemistry and Molecular Biology* 2009:39, 83–89. DOI: 10.1016/j.ibmb.2008.10.002.

[82] Mury FB, da Silva JR, Ferreira LS, dos Santos Ferreira B, de Souza-Filho GA, de Souza-Neto JA et al. Alpha-glucosidase promotes hemozoin formation in a blood-suck-

ing bug: An evolutionary history. *PLoS One* 2009:4, e6966. DOI: 10.1371/journal.pone.0006966.

[83] Paim RM, Araujo RN, Lehane MJ, Gontijo NF, Pereira MH. Longterm effects and parental RNAi in the blood feeder Rhodnius prolixus (Hemiptera; Reduviidae). *Insect Biochemistry and Molecular Biology* 2013:43, 1015–1020. DOI: 10.1016/j.ibmb.2013.08.008.

[84] Defferrari M, Lee D, Fernandes C, Orchard I, Carlini C. A phospholipase A2 gene is linked to Jack bean urease toxicity in the Chagas' disease vector Rhodnius prolixus. *Biochimica et Biophysica Acta* 2014:1840, 396–405. DOI: 10.1016/j.bbagen.2013.09.016.

[85] Deng F, Zhao Z. Influence of catalase gene silencing on the survivability of Sitobion avenae. *Archives of Insect Biochemistry and Physiology* 2014:86, 46–57. DOI: 10.1002/arch.21161.

[86] Xu L, Duan X, Lv Y, Zhang X, Nie Z, Xie C, Ni Z, Liang R. Silencing of an aphid carboxylesterase gene by use of plant-mediated RNAi impairs Sitobion avenae tolerance of Phoxim insecticides. *Transgenic Research* 2014:23, 389–396. DOI: 10.1007/s11248-013-9765-9.

[87] Walker WB, Allen ML. Expression and RNA interference of salivary polygalacturonase genes in the tarnished plant bug, Lygus lineolaris. *Journal of Insect Science* 2010:10, 173. DOI: 10.1673/031.010.14133.

[88] Walker WB, Allen ML. RNA interference-mediated knockdown of IAP in Lygus lineolaris induces mortality in adult and preadult life stages. *Entomologia Experimentalis et Applicata* 2011:138, 83–92. DOI: 10.1111/j.1570-7458.2010.01078.x.

[89] Liu PZ, Kaufman TC. Hunchback is required for suppression of abdominal identity, and for proper germband growth and segmentation in the intermediate germ band insect Oncopeltus fasciatus. *Development* 2004:131, 1515–1527. DOI: 10.1242/dev.01046.

[90] Ikeno T, Numata H, Goto SG. Circadian clock genes period and cycle regulate photoperiodic diapause in the bean bug Riptortus pedestris males. *Journal of Insect Physiology* 2011a:57, 935–938. DOI: 10.1016/j.jinsphys.2011.04.006.

[91] Araujo RN, Santos A, Pinto FS, Gontijo NF, Lehane MJ, Pereira MH. RNA interference of the salivary gland nitrophorin 2 in the triatomine bug Rhodnius prolixus (Hemiptera: Reduviidae) by dsRNA ingestion or injection. *Insect Biochemistry and Molecular Biology* 2006:36, 683–693. DOI:10.1016/j.ibmb.2006.05.012.

[92] Zha W, Peng X, Chen R, Du B, Zhu L, He G. Knockdown of midgut genes by dsRNA-transgenic plant-mediated RNA interference in the hemipteran insect Nilaparvata lugens. *PLoS One* 2011:6(5), e20504. DOI: 10.1371/journal.pone.0020504.

[93] Li J, Chen Q, Lin Y, Jiang T, Wu G, Hua H. RNA interference in Nilaparvata lugens (Homoptera: Delphacidae) based on dsRNA ingestion. *Pest Management Science* 2011:67(7), 852–859. DOI: 10.1002/ps.2124.

[94] Chen J, Zhang D, Yao Q, Zhang J, Dong X, Tian H et al. Feeding-based RNA interference of a trehalose phosphate synthase gene in the brown planthopper, Nilaparvata lugens. *Insect Molecular Biology* 2010:19(6), 777–786. DOI: 10.1111/j.1365-2583.2010.01038.x.

[95] Zhang Y, Wang X, Yang B, Hu Y, Huang L, Bass C et al. Reduction in mRNA and protein expression of a nicotinic acetylcholine receptor $\alpha 8$ subunit is associated with resistance to imidacloprid in the brown planthopper, Nilaparvata lugens. *Journal of Neurochemistry*. 2015. DOI: 10.1111/jnc.13281.

[96] Pitino M, Coleman AD, Maffei ME, Ridout CJ, Hogenhout SA. Silencing of aphid genes by dsRNA feeding from plants. *PLoS One* 2011:6, e25709. DOI: 10.1371/journal.pone.0025709.

[97] Wuriyanghan H, Rosa C, Falk BW. Oral delivery of doublestranded RNAs and siRNAs induces RNAi effects in the potato/tomato psyllid, Bactericerca cockerelli. *PLoS One* 2011:6, e27736. DOI: 10.1371/journal.pone.0027736.

[98] Zhou XG, Wheeler MM, Oi FM, Scharf ME. RNA interference in the termite Reticulitermes flavipes through ingestion of double-stranded RNA. *Insect Biochemistry and Molecular Biology* 2008:38, 805–815. DOI: 10.1016/j.ibmb.2008.05.005.

[99] Wang YB, Zhang H, Li HC and Miao XX. Second generation sequencing supply an effectiveway to screen RNAi targets in large scale for potential application in pest insect control. *PLoS One* 2011:6(4), e18644. DOI: 10.1371/journal.pone.0018644.

[100] Khajuria C, Buschman LL, Chen MS, Muthukrishnan S, Zhu KY. A gut-specific chitinase gene essential for regulation of chitin content of peritrophic matrix and growth of *Ostrinia nubilalis* larvae. *Insect Biochemistry and Molecular Biology* 2010:40, 621–629. DOI: 10.1016/j.ibmb.2010.06.003.

[101] Turner CT, Davy MW, Macdiarmid RM, Plummer KM, Birch NP, Newcomb RD. RNA interference in the light brown apple moth, *Epiphyas postvittana* (Walker) induced by double-stranded RNA feeding. *Insect Molecular Biology* 2006:15, 383–391. DOI: 10.1111/j.1365-2583.2006.00656.x.

[102] Kumar M, Gupta GP, Rajam MV. Silencing of acetylcholinesterase gene of Helicoverpa armigera by siRNA affects larval growth and its life cycle. *Journal of Insect Physiology* 2009:55, 273–278. DOI: 10.1016/j.jinsphys.2008.12.005.

[103] Mao YB, Tao XY, Xue XY, Wang LJ, Chen XY. Cotton plants expressing *CYP6AE14* double-stranded RNA show enhanced resistance to bollworms. *Transgenic Research* 2011:20, 665–673. DOI: 10.1007/s11248-010-9450-1.

[104] He HJ, Wang Q, Zheng WW, Wang JX, Song QS, Zhao XF. Function of nuclear transport factor 2 and Ran in the 20E signal transduction pathway in the cotton bollworm, Helicoverpa armigera. *BMC Cell Biology* 2010:11, 1. DOI:10.1186/1471-2121-11-1.

[105] Xiong Y, Zeng H, Zhang Y, Xu D, Qiu D. Silencing the HaHR3 gene by transgenic plant-mediated RNAi to disrupt Helicoverpa armigera development. *International Journal of Biological Sciences* 2013:9(4), 370–381. DOI: 10.7150/ijbs.5929.

[106] Bettencourt R, Terenius O, Faye I. *Hemolin* gene silencing by ds-RNA injected into Cecropia pupae is lethal to next generation embryos. *Insect Molecular Biology* 2002:11, 267–271. DOI: 10.1046/j.1365-2583.2002.00334.x.

[107] Porta H, Jimenez G, Cordoba E, Leon P, Soberon M, Bravo A. Tobacco plants expressing the Cry1AbMod toxin suppress tolerance to Cry1Ab toxin of Manduca sexta cadherin-silenced larvae. *Insect Biochemistry and Molecular Biology* 2011:41, 513–519. DOI: 10.1016/j.ibmb.2011.04.013.

[108] Shu YH, Wang JW, Lu K, Zhou JL, Zhou Q, Zhang GR. The first vitellogenin receptor from a Lepidopteran insect: Molecular characterization, expression patterns and RNA interference analysis. *Insect Molecular Biology* 2011:20, 61–73. DOI: 10.1111/j.1365-2583.2010.01054.x.

[109] Tian H, Peng H, Yao Q, Chen H, Xie Q, Tang B et al. Developmental control of a lepidopteran pest *Spodoptera exigua* by ingestion of bacteria expressing dsRNA of a non-midgut gene. *PLoS One* 2009:4(7), e6225. DOI: 10.1371/journal.pone.0006225.

[110] Gvakharia BO, Bebas P, Cymborowski B, Giebultowicz JM. Disruption of sperm release from insect testes by cytochalasin and beta-actin mRNA mediated interference. *Cellular and Molecular Life Sciences* 2003:60, 1744–1751. DOI: 10.1007/s00018-003-3139-z.

[111] Griebler M, Westerlund SA, Hoffmann KH, Meyering-Vos M. RNA interference with the allatoregulating neuropeptide genes from the fall armyworm *Spodoptera frugiperda* and its effects on the JH titer in the hemolymph. *Journal of Insect Physiology* 2008:54, 997–1007. DOI: 10.1016/j.jinsphys.2008.04.019.

[112] Gong LA, Yang XQ, Zhang BL, Zhong GH, Hu MY. Silencing of Rieske iron-sulfur protein using chemically synthesised siRNA as a potential biopesticide against *Plutella xylostella. Pest Management Science* 2011:67, 514–520. DOI: 10.1002/ps.2086.

[113] Mito T, Nakamura T, Bando T, Ohuchi H, Noji S. The advent of RNA interference in entomology. *Entomological Science* 2011:14, 1–8. DOI: 10.1111/j.1479-8298.2010.00408.x.

[114] Dabour N, Bando T, Nakamura T, Miyawaki K, Mito T, Ohuchi H, Noji S. Cricket body size is altered by systemic RNAi against insulin signaling components and epidermal growth factor receptor. *Development Growth & Differentiation* 2011:53, 857–869. DOI: 10.1111/j.1440-169X.2011.01291.x.

[115] Takahashi T, Hamada A, Miyawaki K, Matsumoto Y, Mito T, Noji S et al. Systemic RNA interference for the study of learning and memory in an insect. *Journal of Neuroscience Methods* 2009:179, 9–15. DOI:10.1016/j.jneumeth.2009.01.002.

[116] Moriyama Y, Sakamoto T, Karpova SG, Matsumoto A, Noji S, Tomioka K. RNA interference of the clock gene period disrupts circadian rhythms in the cricket Gryllus bimaculatus. *Journal of Biological Rhythms* 2008:23, 308–318. DOI: 10.1177/0748730408320486.

[117] Meyering-Vos M, Muller A. RNA interference suggests sulfakinins as satiety effectors in the cricket *Gryllus bimaculatus*. *Journal of Insect Physiology* 2007:53, 840–848. DOI:10.1016/j.jinsphys.2007.04.003.

[118] Dong Y, Friedrich M. Nymphal RNAi: Systemic RNAi mediated gene knockdown in juvenile grasshopper. *BMC Biotechnology* 2005:5, 25. DOI:10.1186/1472-6750-5-25.

[119] Khajuria C, Buschman LL, Chen MS, Muthukrishnan S, Zhu KY. A gut-specific chitinase gene essential for regulation of chitin content of peritrophic matrix and growth of Ostrinia nubilalis larvae. *Insect Biochemistry and Molecular Biology* 2010:40, 621–629. DOI: 10.1016/j.ibmb.2010.06.003.

[120] Wang Z, Gerstein M, Snyder M. RNA-Seq: A revolutionary tool for transcriptomics. *Nature Reviews Genetics* 2009:10, 57–63. DOI:10.1038/nrg2484.

[121] Haas BJ, Zody MC. Advancing RNA-Seq analysis. *Nature Biotechnology* 2010:28, 421–423. DOI: 10.1038/nbt0510-421.

[122] Zhang M, Zhou Y, Jones HD, Gao Q, Wang D, Ma Y, et al. Identifying potential RNAi targets in grain aphid (*Sitobion aveane* F.) based on transcriptome profiling of its alimentary canal after feeding on wheat plants. *BMC Genomics* 2013:14, 560. DOI: 10.1186/1471-2164-14-560.

[123] Li H, Jiang W, Zhang Z, Xing Y, Li F. Transcriptome analysis and screening for potential target genes for RNAi-mediated pest control of the beet armyworm, *Spodoptera exigua*. *PLoS One*. 2013:8(6), e65931. DOI:10.1371/journal.pone.0065931.

[124] Li X, Zhang M, Zhang H. RNA interference of four genes in adult Bactrocera dorsalis by feeding their dsRNAs. *PLoS One* 2011:6, e17788. DOI:10.1371/journal.pone.0017788.

[125] Hunter W, Ellis J, Vanengelsdorp D, Hayes J, Westervelt D, Glick E et al. Large-scale field application of RNAi technology reducing Israeli acute paralysis virus disease in honey bees (Apis mellifera, Hymenoptera: Apidae). *PLoS Pathogens* 2010:6, e1001160. DOI: 10.1371/journal.ppat.1001160.

[126] Hunter WB, Glick E, Paldi N, Bextine BR. Advances in RNA interference: dsRNA treatment in trees and grapevines for insect pest population suppression. *Southwestern Entomologist* 2012:37, 85–87. DOI: http://dx.doi.org/10.3958/059.037.0110.

[127] Gan D, Zhang J, Jiang H, Jiang T, Zhu S, Cheng B. Bacterially expressed dsRNA protects maize against SCMV infection. *Plant Cell Reports* 2010:29, 1261–1268. DOI: 10.1007/s00299-010-0911-z.

[128] Kurreck J. RNA interference: From basic research to therapeutic applications. *Angewandte Chemie (International Edition in English)* 2009:48, 1378–1398. DOI: 10.1002/anie.200802092.

[129] Zhang X, Zhang J, Zhu KY Chitosan/double-stranded RNA nanoparticle-mediated RNA interference to silence chitin synthase genes through larval feeding in the African malaria mosquito (Anopheles gambiae). *Insect Molecular Biology* 2010:19(5), 683–693. DOI: 10.1111/j.1365-2583.2010.01029.x.

[130] Gong LA, Yang XQ, Zhang BL, Zhong GH, Hu MY. Silencing of Rieske iron-sulfur protein using chemically synthesised siRNA as a potential biopesticide against *Plutella xylostella. Pest Management Science* 2011:67, 514–520. DOI: 10.1002/ps.2086.

[131] Zhu F, Xu JJ, Palli R, Ferguson J, Palli SR. Ingested RNA interference for managing the populations of the Colorado potato beetle, *Leptinotarsa decemlineata. Pest Management Science* 2011:67, 175–182. DOI: 10.1002/ps.2048.

[132] Obbard DJ, Gordon KH, Buck AH, Jiggins FM. The evolution of RNAi as a defence against viruses and transposable elements. *Philosophical Transactions of the Royal Society B: Biological Sciences* 2009:364(1513), 99–115. DOI: 10.1098/rstb.2008.0168.

[133] Saleh MC, Tassetto M, van Rij RP, Goic B, Gausson V, Berry B, Jacquier C, Antoniewski C, Andino R. Antiviral immunity in Drosophila requires systemic RNA interference spread. *Nature* 2009:458, 346–351. DOI: 10.1038/nature07712.

[134] Ulvila J, Parikka M, Kleino A, Sormunen R, Ezekowitz RA, Kocks C, Ramet M. Double-stranded RNA is internalized by scavenger receptor-mediated endocytosis in Drosophila S2 cells. *Journal of Biological Chemistry* 2006:281, 14370–14375. DOI: 10.1074/jbc.M513868200.

[135] Saleh MC, van Rij RP, Hekele A, Gillis A, Foley E, O'Farrell PH et al. The endocytic pathway mediates cell entry of dsRNA to induce RNAi silencing. *Nature Cell Biology* 2006:8, 793–802. DOI: 10.1038/ncb1439.

[136] Campbell CL, Keene KM, Brackney DE, Olson KE, Blair CD, Wilusz J et al. Aedes aegypti uses RNA interference in defense against Sindbis virus infection. *BMC Microbiology* 2008:8(1), 47. DOI: 10 1186/1471-2180-8-47.

[137] Aliyari R, Wu Q, Li WH, Wang XH, Li F, Green LD, et al. Mechanism of induction and suppression of antiviral immunity directed by virus-derived small RNA sin Drosophila. *Cell Host & Microbe* 2008:4, 387–397. DOI:10.1016/j.chom.2008.09.001.

[138] Li H, Li WX, Ding SW. Induction and suppression of RNA silencing by an animal virus. *Science* 2002:296, 1319–1321. DOI:10.1126/science.1070948.

[139] Nayak A, Berry B, Tassetto M, Kunitomi M, Acevedo A, Deng C, et al. Cricket paralysis virus antagonizes Argonaute2 to modulate antiviral defensein Drosophila. *Nature Structural and Molecular Biology* 2010:17, 547–554. DOI:10.1038/nsmb.1810.

[140] Wang XH, Aliyari R, Li WX, Li HW, Kim K, Carthew R, et al. RNA interference directs innate immunity against viruses in adult Drosophila. *Science* 2006:312, 452–454. DOI:10.1126/science.1125694.

[141] Goic B, Vodovar N, Mondotte JA, Monot C, Frangeul L, Blanc H, et al. RNA-mediated interference and reverse transcription control the persistence of RNA viruses in the insect model Drosophila. *Nature Immunology* 2013:14, 396–403. DOI:10.1038/ni.2542.

[142] Swevers L, Broeck JV, Smagghe G. The possible impact of persistent virus infection on the function of the RNAi machinery in insects: A hypothesis. *Frontiers in Physiology* 2013:4, 319. DOI: 10.3389/fphys.2013.00319.

[143] Terenius O, Papanicolaou A, Garbutt JS, Eleftherianos I, Huvenne H, Kanginakudru S, et al. RNA interference in Lepidoptera: An overview of successful and unsuccessful studies and implications for experimental design. *Journal of Insect Physiology* 2011:57, 231–245. DOI:10.1016/j.jinsphys.2010.11.006.

[144] Blair CD. Mosquito RNAi is the major innate immune pathway controlling arbovirus infection and transmission. *Future Microbiology* 2011:6, 267–277. DOI: 10.2217/fmb.11.11.

[145] Schnettler E, Sterken MG, Leung JY, Metz SW, Geertsema C, Goldbach RW et al. Noncoding flavivirus RNA displays RNA interference suppressor activity in insect and mammalian cells. *Journal of Virology* 2012:86, 13486–13500. DOI: 10.1128/JVI.01104-12.

[146] Winston WM, Molodowitch C, Hunter CP. Systemic RNAi in C. elegans requires the putative transmembrane protein SID-1. *Science* 2002:295, 2456–2459. DOI:10.1126/science.1068836.

[147] Barnard AC, Nijhof AM, Fick W, Stutzer C, Maritz-Olivier C. RNAi in arthropods: Insight into the machinery and applications for understanding the pathogen-vector interface. *Genes* 2012:3(4), 702–741. DOI:10.3390/genes3040702.

[148] Aronstein K, Pankiw T, Saldivar E. SID-1 is implicated in systemic gene silencing in the honey bee. *Journal of Apicultural Research* 2006:45, 20–24. DOI:10.3896/IBRA.1.45.1.05.

[149] Tomoyasu Y, Miller SC, Tomita S, Schoppmeier M, Grossmann D, Bucher G. Exploring systemic RNA interference in insects: A genome-wide survey for RNAi genes in Tribolium. *Genome Biology* 2008:9(1), R10. DOI: 10.1186/gb-2008-9-1-r10.

[150] Boisson B, Jacques JC, Choumet V, Martin E, Xu JN, Vernick K et al. Gene silencing in mosquito salivary glands by RNAi. *FEBS Letters* 2006:580, 1988–1992. DOI: http://dx.doi.org/10.1016/j.febslet.2006.02.069.

[151] Volz J, Muller HM, Zdanowicz A, Kafatos FC, Osta MA. A genetic module regulates the melanization response of Anopheles to Plasmodium. *Cellular Microbiology* 2006:8, 1392–1405. DOI: 10.1111/j.1462-5822.2006.00718.x.

[152] Zhu JS, Chen L, Raikhel AS. Posttranscriptional control of the competence factor beta FTZ-F1 by juvenile hormone in the mosquito Aedes aegypti. *Proceedings of the National Academy of Sciences of the United States of America* 2003:100, 13338–13343. DOI: 10.1073/pnas.2234416100.

[153] Scott JG, Michel K, Bartholomay LC, Siegfried BD, Hunter WB, Smagghe G et al. Towards the elements of successful insect RNAi. *Journal of Insect Physiology* 2013:59(12), 1212–1221. DOI: 10.1016/j.jinsphys.2013.08.014.

[154] Kumar M, Gupta GP, Rajam MV. Silencing of acetylcholinesterase gene of Helicoverpa armigera by siRNA affects larval growth and its life cycle. *Journal of Insect Physiology* 2009:55, 273–278. DOI: 10.1016/j.jinsphys.2008.12.005.

[155] Wu H, Ma H, Ye C, Ramirez D, Chen S, Montoya J et al. Improved siRNA/shRNA functionality by mismatched duplex. *PLoS One* 2011:6(12), e28580. DOI: 10.1371/journal.pone.0028580.

[156] Yu N, Christiaens O, Liu J, Niu J, Cappelle K, Caccia S et al. Delivery of dsRNA for RNAi in insects: An overview and future directions. *Insect Science* 2013:20(1), 4–14. DOI: 10.1111/j.1744-7917.2012.01534.x.

[157] Shakesby AJ, Wallace IS, Isaacs HV, Pritchard J, Roberts DM, Douglas AE. A water-specific aquaporin involved in aphid osmoregulation. *Insect Biochemistry and Molecular Biology* 2009:39, 1–10. DOI: 10.1016/j.ibmb.2008.08.008.

[158] Arimatsu Y, Kotani E, Sugimura Y, Furusawa T. Molecular characterization of a cDNA encoding extracellular dsRNase and its expression in the silkworm, *Bombyx mori. Insect Biochemistry and Molecular Biology* 2007:37, 176–183. DOI:10.1016/j.ibmb.2006.11.004.

[159] Garbutt JS, Belles X, Richards EH, Reynolds SE. Persistence of double stranded RNA in insect hemolymph as a potential determiner of RNA interference success: Evidence from Manduca sexta and Blattella germanica. *Journal of Insect Physiology* 2013:59, 171–178. DOI: 10.1016/j.jinsphys.2012.05.013.

[160] Rinkevich FD, Scott JG. Limitations of RNAi of a6 nicotinic acetylcholine receptor subunits for assessing the in vivo sensitivity to spinosad. *Insect Science* 2013:20, 101–108. DOI: 10.1111/j.1744-7917.2012.01523.x.

[161] Upadhyay SK, Dixit S, Sharma S, Singh H, Kumar J, Verma PC, Chandrashekar K. siRNA machinery in whitefly (*Bemisia tabaci*). Plos ONE 2013: 8(12), e83692. DOI: 10.1371/journal.pone.0083692.

[162] Lundgren JG, Duan JJ. RNAi-based insecticidal crops: Potential effects on non-target5 species. Bioscience 2013:63(8), 657–665. DOI: http://dx.doi.org/10.1525/bio.2013.63.8.8.

[163] Jackson AL, Linsley PS. Noise amidst the silence: Off-target effects of siRNAs? Trends in Genetics 2004:20(11), 521–524. DOI: http://dx.doi.org/10.1016/j.tig.2004.08.006.

7

Management of Insect Pest by RNAi — A New Tool for Crop Protection

Thais Barros Rodrigues and Antonio Figueira

Abstract

The fast-growing human population requires the development of new agricultural technologies to meet consumers' demand, while minimizing environmental impacts. Insect pests are one of the main causes for losses in agriculture production, and current control technologies based on pesticide application or the use of transgenic crops expressing *Bacillus thuringiensis* toxin proteins are facing efficacy challenges. Novel approaches to control pests are urgently necessary. RNA interference (RNAi) is a gene silencing mechanism triggered by providing double-stranded RNA (dsRNA), that when ingested into insects can lead to death or affect the viability of the target pest. Transgenic plants expressing dsRNA version of insect specific target genes are the new generation of resistant plants. However, the RNAi mechanism is not conserved among insect orders, and its elucidation is the key to develop commercial RNAi crops. In this chapter, we review the core RNAi pathway in insects and the dsRNA uptake, amplification, and spread of systemic silencing signals in some key insect species. We also highlight some of the experimental steps before developing an insect-pest-resistant "RNAi plant". Lastly, we review some of the most recent development studies to control agricultural insect pests by RNAi transgenic plants.

Keywords: Biotechnology, dsRNA, Entomology, Gene silencing, Insect control, RNA interference

1. Introduction

Agriculture has to continually adapt to rising environmental concerns in conjunction with meeting the increasing consumers' demand. The fast-growing human population creates the need for the sustainable intensification of agriculture throughout the world which can be acomplished by adopting mechanization and new technologies to close yield gaps while minimizing environmental impacts. In the past few decades, insect pest control has been mainly conducted by the application of chemical pesticides because of the low cost and efficacy; but their indiscriminate use has caused escalating problems with the evolution of insect resistance to the pesticides together with secondary pest outbreaks. The development of new biotechnological approaches, with the introduction of transgenic crops expressing *Bacillus thuringiensis* (Bt) Cry toxin proteins, also known as insect-resistant transgenic Bt-plants, decreased pesticide utilization in certain key crops, such as cotton and maize, and brought economical and environmental benefits [1-3]. But once again, insect resistance has arisen, now against the Bt toxins, and outbreaks of nontarget pests have emerged [1, 4], which makes necessary the development of novel approaches to control selected agriculture pests.

RNA interference (RNAi) is a gene silencing mechanism at the cellular level triggered by double-stranded RNA (dsRNA) and is likely to be the new approach underlying the next generation of insect-resistant transgenic plants. In some studies, successful delivery of dsRNA molecules to insects by ingestion resulted in the expected essential gene target silencing [5, 6], which led to death or affected the viability of the target insect, resulting in control of the pest.

In general, long dsRNAs are processed by species-specific RNase-III-like enzymes, resulting in smaller double-stranded molecules. These shorter RNAs are loaded into RNA complexes as a guide for finding target mRNAs that are either cleaved or blocked for translation in posttranscriptional silencing, or inducing histone modifications when involved in transcriptional silencing response [7, 8]. However, the RNAi systemic spreading mechanism is not conserved across organisms, and its elucidation is an essential step in developing an efficient method to control agricultural pests by RNAi technology.

In this chapter, we review how the RNAi mechanism occurs in insects, highlighting the core RNAi pathway and components, and new developments regarding dsRNA uptake, amplification, and the spread of systemic silencing signals in some key insect species. We also discuss the critical experimental steps before developing an "RNAi plant" protected against a specific insect pest, with consideration to application. Lastly, we review some of the most recent published studies to control agriculturally important insect pests based on RNAi transgenic plants.

2. RNAi mechanism

RNAi is an important and natural antiviral defense mechanism, protecting organisms from RNA viruses, or even avoiding the random integration of transposons [9]. Over time, with the discovery of some aspects of the mechanism, RNAi has become a widely used tool to knock down and analyze the function of genes. Most of the RNAi pathways have dsRNA as the precursor triggering molecule that vary in length and origin [7, 8]. In addition, the RNAi pathways differ not only in the RNA precursor molecule, but also in genes, enzymes, and effector complexes involved throughout the process. However, some key steps are conserved. Briefly, RNA duplexes are processed into short RNA duplexes, which are then used to guide the recognition of their target, either to cleave a complementary mRNA, or to repress their target translation at a posttranscriptional silencing level, or to modify the chromatin structure at the transcriptional level [7, 8].

The RNA precursor molecules from the RNAi pathways, all of which are already identified in insects, are small RNAs, categorized into three classes [8, 10]: the first two classes are small interfering RNAs (siRNAs; 20–25 nucleotides) and microRNAs (miRNAs; 21–24 nucleotides) [7] (Figure 1). Both miRNAs and siRNAs share a common RNase-III processing enzyme, Dicer, and closely related effector complexes and both can regulate gene expression at the posttranscriptional level [8, 10, 11]. Conversely, the third class of small RNAs, the PIWI-interacting RNAs (piRNAs; 24–30 nucleotides), are generated independent of the Dicer activity [12]. piRNAs have been reported to play an essential role in germ-line development, stem cell renewal, transposon silencing, and epigenetic regulation [13-16]. These piRNAs originate from a diversity of sequences, including repetitive DNA and transposons, and they seem to act both at the posttranscriptional and chromatin levels [10]. The mechanism that generates and amplifies piRNAs is not well-understood, but involves slicer activities (Argonaute proteins associated with cleaving activity) [8, 10, 17]. Considered a specialized subclass of piRNAs, **r**epeat-**a**ssociated **si**RNAs (rasiRNAs; 25-29 nucleotides) were identified in the *Drosophila* genome [18], and suggested by Meister and Tuschl [7] to be involved in guiding chromatin modification in this insect species (Figure 1).

The most recognized RNAi pathways are the siRNA and miRNA; despite being triggered by different molecules, both precursors are long double-stranded RNAs (dsRNAs). Naturally in a cell, long dsRNAs can derive from RNA virus replication, from the transcription of convergent cellular genes or mobile genetic elements, or from self-annealing cellular transcripts [8]. In the siRNA pathway, these long dsRNA are processed by Dicer into siRNA duplexes. By contrast, in the miRNA pathway, miRNAs are generated from endogenous transcripts (primary miRNAs; pri-miRNAs) that form stem–loop structures [19, 20]. In the nucleus, these hairpin regions are recognized and cleaved into precursor mirRNAs (pre-miRNAs) by Drosha, another RNase-III-family enzyme, and the pre-miRNAs are transported to the cytoplasm through the nuclear export receptor Exportin-5 (Expo-5) [19, 20]. Subsequently, the pre-miRNA undergoes another endonucleolytic cleavage, now catalyzed by Dicer, generating an miRNA duplex [19, 20] (Figure 1).

The siRNA and miRNAs duplex containing ribonucleoprotein particles (RNPs) are subsequently rearranged into effector complexes. Although it is difficult to assign distinct functional labels, an siRNA-containing effector complex is referred to as an "RNA-induced silencing complex" (RISC), and an miRNA-containing effector complex is referred to as an miRNP [7]. In these complexes, the regulation is at a posttranscriptional level and every RISC or miRNP contains a member of the Argonaute (Ago) protein family [7]. For the regulation at the transcriptional level as guided by rasiRNAs, a specialized nuclear Argonaute-containing complex, known as the RNA-Induced Transcriptional Silencing complex (RITS) mediates gene silencing [10]. In general, one strand of the short-RNA duplex (the guide strand) is loaded onto an Argonaute protein at the core of the effector complexes. During loading, the nonguide strand is cleaved by an Argonaute protein and ejected. The Argonaute protein then uses the guide RNA to associate with target RNAs that contain a perfectly complementary sequence

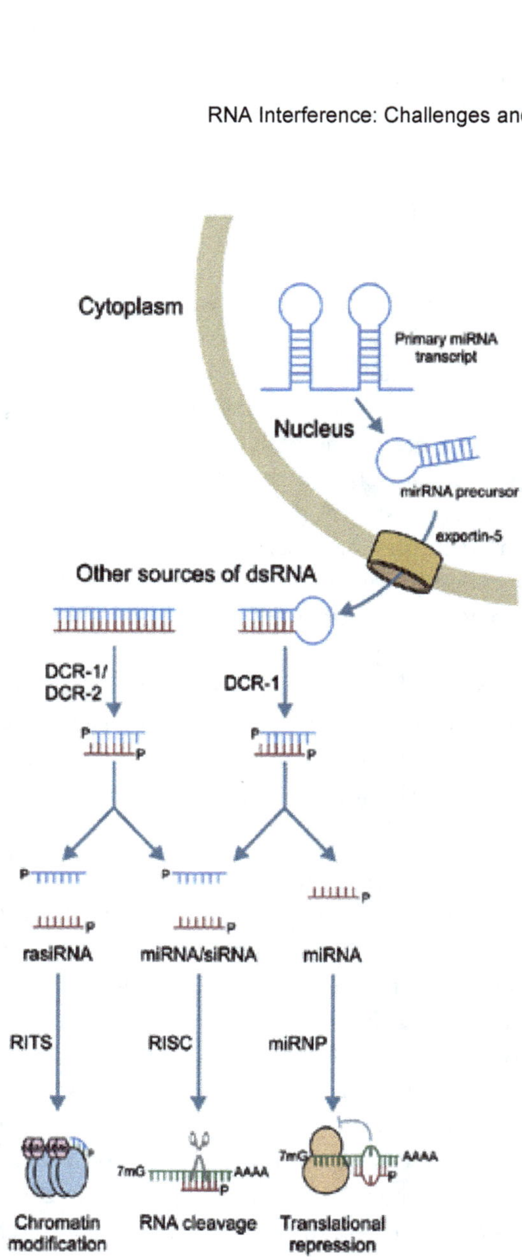

Figure 1. RNA-mediated gene silencing pathways. In the nucleus, primary miRNA transcripts (pri-miRNAs) are processed to mirRNA precursors (pre-miRNA) by the RNase-III-like enzyme Drosha. The pre-miRNA is exported through the export receptor Exportin-5 (Exp-5) to the cytoplasm, and then processed by Dicer to microRNA (miRNA). These miRNAs are unwound and assembled into miRNP (miRNA containing effector complex of RiboNucleo Protein particles) or RISC (RNA Induced Silencing Complex), triggering silencing responses by translational repression of target mRNAs or mRNA-target degradation, respectively. In the cytoplasm, long dsRNA are processed to siRNA (small interfering RNA) by the RNase-III-like enzyme Dicer. The short dsRNAs are unwound and assembled into RISC or RITS (RNA-Induced Transcriptional Silencing) complexes. The siRNA guides the RNA cleavage by the RISC complex, while rasiRNA (repeat-associated short interfering RNA) guides the condensation of heterochromatin by the RITS complex. 7mG: 7-methyl guanine; AAAA: poly-adenosine tail; Me: methyl group; P: 5′- phosphate. (Adapted from [7])

and then catalyzes the slicing of these targets, either to be cleaved by RISC, to be blocked for translation in miRNP or by inducing histone modifications in RITS [7] (Figure 1). The mechanism of miRNA-guided translational regulation is not as well-understood in the case of target-

RNA cleavage, and to make things more complicated, miRNAs can act as siRNAs, and siRNAs can act as miRNAs [7].

Dicer is one of the enzymes involved in RNAi mechanism that is encoded by a variable number of genes and presents distinct specificity among organisms [21]. For instance, mammals and *Caenorhabditis elegans,* the best characterized animal for RNAi, have each a single Dicer responsible for functions in both siRNA and miRNA pathways [12], while *Drosophila melanogaster* has two paralogues: Dicer-1 (Dcr-1) that preferentially processes miRNA precursors, and Dicer-2 (Dcr-2) required to process long dsRNA into siRNAs [22]. However, in *Tribolium castaneum*, a model organism among insects for systemic silencing by RNAi, Dcr-2 showed an important role at the RNAi pathway, whereas Dcr-1 is suggested to have an involvement in wing development, most likely through the miRNA pathway [23].

Another gene family involved in RNAi pathways is the Argonaute proteins (Ago). Ago is a central protein component of silencing complexes (RISC, RITS, miRNP) that acts in mediating target recognition and silencing [24]. Argonaute proteins contain two domains: a PAZ domain involved in dsRNA binding, and a PIWI-domain responsible for RNase activity [23]. In *Drosophila,* Ago-1 is involved in the miRNA pathway; Ago-2 in the siRNA pathway; while Piwi, Aubergine (Aub), and Ago-3 are associated in transcriptional silencing [13, 25-27]. In *Tribolium,* a single class of Argonaute was identified (Tc-Ago-1) in the miRNA pathway, while two classes of Ago-2 paralogues (Tc-Ago-2a and Tc-Ago-2b) were found in the siRNA pathway, probably deriving from gene duplication in the beetle lineage [23]. This duplicated Tc-Ago-2 might lead to higher amounts of Ago-2 protein, potentially with the enhancement of the RNAi response [23]. In the silkmoth *Bombyx mori,* a Lepidoptera species in which the RNAi response is considered much less robust [28, 29], *AGO* genes from all three main RNAi pathways were identified (*BmAGO-1* – miRNA; *BmAGO-2* – siRNA; *BmAGO-3* – piRNA), which were shown to be involved in the RNAi response in Bm5 cells [30]. Taken together, these findings, and other reviews [29], support the idea of a function overlap of the three main RNAi pathways in *B. mori* [29].

2.1. Systemic RNAi

Systemic RNAi is described as a silencing signal transmitted widely throughout a treated organism [5, 31]. The knowledge about the systemic RNAi mechanism in insects is important as it may affect the approaches adopted to develop "RNAi-mediated pest control" because the systemic mechanism is not conserved among those organisms. Systemic RNAi has two important steps to be considered: the uptake of dsRNA by the cells and the systemic spreading of the signals. Some of the main genes involved in systemic RNAi are presented below and discussed for the model organisms.

2.1.1. dsRNA uptake

In insects, two types of dsRNA uptake mechanisms have been identified [32]. The first one involves a multi-transmembrane domain protein, Systemic Interference Defective (Sid). In *C. elegans,* Sid-1 is essential and sufficient to mediate uptake and systemic spread of RNAi signal in both somatic and germ-line cells [33, 34]; conversely, in insects, Sid-1-like (Sil) proteins appear to be variable across orders [32]. For instance, Diptera do not present *SIL* genes, while *Tribolium* and *B. mori* presented three *SIL* homologues [23, 35]. However, these *Tribolium* genes share more identity with another *C. elegans* gene, *TAG-130*, not required for systemic RNAi in *C. elegans* compared to that with *SID-1* [23]. The second dsRNA uptake mechanism involves endocytosis, specific for dsRNAs acquired from the environment, known as environmental RNAi [5, 31]. First discovered in *Drosophila* S2 cells and later in *C. elegans*, this uptake of dsRNA by endocytosis appears to be evolutionary-conserved [36-38]. However, we should be cautious to conclude that all organisms have a dsRNA uptake mechanism based on endocytosis. For instance, Ulvila and colleagues [38] working with *Drosophila* S2 cells, which are hemocyte-like, described high rates of endocytosis as compared to the majority of other cell types in this species [39].

Other important proteins for systemic RNAi were identified in *C. elegans* but are specific only to germ-line cells, such as Rsd-2, Rsd-3, and Rsd-6 [40]. The Rsd-2 protein contains no particular known motifs but interacts with Rsd-6 that has a Tudor domain, suggesting that these two proteins act together [40]. The *RSD-3* gene encodes a protein that contains an epsin amino-terminal homology (ENTH) domain, found in proteins involved in vesicle trafficking, suggesting the involvement of endocytosis in systemic RNAi [40]. In *Tribolium*, a homologue for *RSD-3* (*Tc-RSD3*) has been found, but in *Drosophila*, which does not exhibit a systemic silencing response, a homologous Rsd-3 protein (Epsin-like) was identified [23]. So, the presence of Rsd-3 does not seems to determine whether or not systemic RNAi occurs in insects, and it is possible that the expression level and/or tissue specificity of this gene may affect the degree of RNAi efficiency and the dsRNA uptake from the environment [23].

2.1.2. RNAi systemic spreading: amplification and maintenance of dsRNA

Once the dsRNA overcomes all the uptake barriers, the silencing signal should be transported from treated cell to other cells, and spread to other tissues. Further, dsRNA should be constantly produced, e.g., either by the amplification of dsRNA by an RNA-dependent RNA polymerase (RdRP), and/or constantly acquired for the maintenance of the silencing responses.

In *C. elegans*, primary siRNAs processed by Dicer are used as a template for an RdRP activity to produce secondary dsRNAs [41]. The RdRP activity is key for the RNAi signal amplification. However, so far in insects, no RdRP-related protein has been found [21, 23], suggesting that strong RNAi response in insects does not rely on amplification of the trigger dsRNA, and it must be based on a different mechanism yet to be identified. Alternatively, constant supply of dsRNA may be provided by RNAi-plants to provide continuous effects.

The presence of the main genes involved in systemic RNAi and amplification in *Drosophila* and *Tribolium* fail to explain the respective absence and presence of systemic RNAi [23]. Nevertheless, the several differences in the number of these core component genes found between species suggests an interesting avenue for further investigation [23]. For instance, Ago protein that have already been shown to determine RNAi efficiency [42], was found to be duplicated in the *Tribolium* genome, while *Drosophila* carries only a copy of *AGO-2* gene, suggesting a relationship between number of *AGO* copies and RNAi response [23].

Another component that might affect RNAi efficiency in different insects are the proteins containing the dsRNA-binding motif (dsRBM), which help small molecules to properly load inside of the silencing complexes [23]. These proteins act together with Dicer, and seem to be responsible for determining Dicer specificity in *Drosophila* [23]. In the *T. castaneum* genome, two *R2D2-like* genes (a particular dsRBM) were found (*TcR2D2* and *TcC3PO*), which might help *Tribolium* to be hypersensitive to dsRNA molecule uptake by the cells [23]. However, in the *Anthonomus grandis* transcriptome, only an *R2D2* contig was identified [21]. The presence of an additional R2D2-like protein in *Tribolium* might also allow a longer-lasting RNAi effect, once dsRBM proteins are known to bind to dsRNAs, and might be involved in the maintenance of dsRNA in cells [23].

3. Factors affecting the silencing effect and RNAi efficiency as an insect control method

The RNAi approach to control insect pests had been considered for many years, but application of this technology was just realized after it was shown that ingestion of dsRNA would trigger RNAi. The concept of RNAi-plant mediated pest control was demonstrated in 2007 by the development of transgenic plants producing dsRNAs against specific insect genes, with the consequent effect on the target species [43, 44]. The main prerequisites to generate successful RNAi insect-resistant transgenic plants are: (i) identification of a specific gene with an essential function in the insect that can cause developmental deformities and/or larval lethality when knocked down or knocked out; and (ii) dsRNA delivery by oral ingestion that must be uptaken by the insect cells, and spread systemically.

The insect must uptake the dsRNA version of a target gene region by feeding. To silence the target gene, this specific dsRNA must be taken up from the gut lumen into the gut cells as what is considered as "environmental RNAi." If the target gene is expressed in a tissue distinct from the digestive system, the silencing signal should successfully spread via cells and tissues as a systemic RNAi. Both environmental and systemic RNAi are considered noncell-autonomous RNAi, which means that the interfering effect takes places in tissues/cells different from the location of application or production of the dsRNA. Conversely, in the cell-autonomous RNAi, the silencing process is limited to the cell in which the dsRNA is introduced [5]. However, the mechanism of ingested dsRNA uptake and systemic spreading of the silencing signal in the insect have yet to be fully characterized and understood.

Some factors can affect the efficiency of the dsRNA uptake and systemic silencing spread in different insects. Here, we highlight important points that must be considered in developing an RNAi approach against insect pests.

3.1. Target gene

The choice of the target gene should be carefully considered. Each gene requires particular effort to be silenced. Terenius and colleagues [28] reviewed more than 150 RNAi experimental results from RNAi of lepidopterans involving 130 genes, from which only 38% were silenced at a satisfactory level, while 48% failed to be silenced, and 14% were silenced at insufficient levels. Among the target genes, those involved in immunity were more effectively silenced, and, in contrast, genes expressed in epidermal tissues seem to be most difficult. Differences for RNAi sensitivity among genes in the same tissue was described in [28].

3.2. dsRNA design

The design of the dsRNA determines the one particular target gene to be silenced, but off-target effects can occur if siRNAs have some sequence similarity with unintended genes. Tobacco plants expressing *Helicoverpa armigera* ecdysone receptor (*EcR*) dsRNA improved resistance to another insect, *Spodoptera frugiperda*, due to the high identity shared between the nucleotide sequence of *HaEcR* and *SeEcR* genes [45]. Although this result implies that an RNAi-plant can control two or even more lepidopteran pests, this can also affect nontarget insects, becoming a biosafety issue.

3.3. dsRNA length

The length of the dsRNA fragments plays an essential role in the effectiveness of molecular uptake in insects, which is directly involved in the success of the target gene silencing. In most of the RNAi experiments, the insects are fed with long dsRNAs [5]. Some experiments showed that long dsRNAs are more efficiently uptaken than siRNAs [37, 46]. This may be due to the fact that a long dsRNA, with 100% match of the target mRNA, after processing into siRNA will provide a greater diversity of siRNAs available to cause specific suppression of target gene and increase the desired effect, and, additionally, reduce the likelihood of developing resistance [47]. In contrast, other studies reported suppression of genes in different insects via incorporation of siRNA in diet instead of dsRNA [48, 49].

3.4. dsRNA concentration

Optimal concentration of dsRNA delivered to the insect is required to induce sufficient gene target silencing. It is noteworthy to mention that exceeding the optimal dsRNA concentration may not result in more silencing [50, 51]. However, higher concentration of dsRNA decreased the duration of dsRNA exposure to reach 50% mortality of *Diabrotica virgifera virgifera* [46], suggesting an inverse relationship between dsRNA concentration and duration of exposure. In cricket (*Gryllus bimaculatus*), the highest concentrations of dsRNA yielded more efficient gene knockdown [52]. The amount of dsRNA sufficient to significantly reduce mRNA levels of *PER* and *CLK* genes were one and two μM, respectively. These concentrations reduced the expression level of the targets, but a higher concentration (20 μM) for the *CYC* gene was required, suggesting that the sensitivity to dsRNAs also depends specifically on the gene [52].

3.5. Controls

Empty vector, empty cassette, buffer only, irrelevant or nonspecific control (such as dsGFP – Green Fluorescent Protein gene region), or any other kind of negative control are essential to discriminate specific gene silencing from the simple induction of siRNA processing machinery by exposure to a dsRNA. Mainly, a negative control should demonstrate the specificity of the dsRNA designed for a target, not interfering in specific target expression, and even unspecific effects. Also, any control should have similar size and concentration of the used dsRNA [53].

3.6. Molecular silencing confirmation

An efficient molecular confirmation of the RNAi silencing should be conducted, which includes target RNA expression, and analyses of protein amount and/or enzyme activity. In RNA analysis, additional care should be taken for expression analysis. The method of choice for RNA expression analysis is the quantitative amplification of reversed transcripts or RT-qPCR, considered a very sensitive and accurate method. To provide precision in RT-qPCR, some essential care is required, such as the choice of appropriate stable reference genes and primer pair design with sufficient amplification efficiency. The reference genes should exhibit stable expression among experimental conditions, providing reliable estimate of gene expression results [54]. Additionally, primers should be designed flanking the region used to design the dsRNA to ensure that the initial cleavage of the mRNA could be detected, thus avoiding false-positives [55]. Conventional care of RT–qPCR reactions defined by the Minimum Information for Publication of Quantitative Real-Time PCR Experiments (MIQE) guidelines must be strictly followed [56].

3.7. Protein stability and phenotype analysis

Proteins can exhibit a long half-life and interfere with the phenotypic changes. However, phenotype changes are not totally related to small decrease of protein levels; haplo-sufficient genes produce proteins capable of performing the biological processes normally, even at half of the protein levels [53]. Phenotype changes could be more difficult to be observed in RNAi responses if the protein product of the target gene has a long half-life. For example, the reduction of *Da6* (nicotinic acetylcholine receptor subunit) expression in both *D. melanogaster* and *T. castaneum* exhibited weak phenotype responses [57], which may be explained based on the long stability of the nicotinic acetylcholine receptors (nAChRs) [58]. Nevertheless, for most of the genes, mRNA turnover and protein half-life are unknown and this lack of information presents one of the principal challenges for the RNAi experiments [39].

3.8. Insect issues, life stage, nucleases, and gut pH

Some insect characteristics should also be considered before starting an RNAi experiment including the developmental stage of insects. Although handling advanced developmental stages of insects is more efficient, silencing effects are more prominent in earlier stages. For instance, in second instar larvae of *Rhodnius prolixus*, the gene *nitropin 2* was knocked down for 42%, but no silencing was observed in the fourth instar individuals, even though both larval stages were treated with the same concentration of dsRNA [59]. In *Spodoptera frugiperda*, fifth instar larvae presented higher gene silencing as compared to adult moths [60].

Another consideration that can affect the RNAi silencing efficiency is the presence of insect nucleases and gut pH. For instance, feeding assays with *Lygus lineolaris* showed no mortality effects because the saliva of *L. lineolaris* contains dsRNA-degrading activity. Thus, dsRNA ingested did not result in siRNA fragments, rather were completely digested to monomers [61]. Also, dsRNA degradation is reduced during molting period and further reduced by starvation in some insects [62]. The stability of the dsRNA in the midgut could be affected not only by enzymatic but also by chemical hydrolysis [63]. In both cases, gut pH is an important factor; particularly, it is quite variable among insect orders, with variation even among gut regions [64]. For example, in general, lepidopterans exhibit a strong alkaline gut (up to pH 10.5 in some species), which provides a highly hostile environment for dsRNA [64]; therefore, this order is particularly recalcitrant to gene silencing by RNAi.

4. Overview on the use of RNAi to control insects by transgenic plants

Most of the current transgenic crops with specific control against insect pests are based on *Bacillus thuringiensis* (Bt) toxins, which act in gut epithelial cell membrane in susceptible insects. Bt toxins are highly specific against certain orders of insects, where the most successful use was achieved against Lepidoptera and Coleoptera. However, continuous exposure of those insects to Bt crops evolved field-resistance, affecting the efficiency in controlling those pests [4, 65]. Also, there are limitations of Bt transgenics to manage some other important agricultural pests, such as the sap-sucking insects (Hemiptera). This encouraged the development of new strategies to help in controlling agricultural pests.

In 2007, two studies demonstrated the concept of plants expressing dsRNAs derived from hairpin vectors that directed dsRNAs to target gene regions of economically important agricultural pests: the cotton bollworm (*Helicoverpa armigera;* Lepidoptera; [44]) and the Western corn rootworm (WCR; *Diabrotica virgifera virgifera;* Coleoptera; [43]). After the demonstration of plants resistant to insects, the application of RNAi by transgenic plants became a potential new approach to control important agricultural pests, which led to the flourishing of a new field of research. So far, searches on the publication database "Web of Science" from Thomson Reuters (August 2015), identified 543 published studies based on the combination of the topics "RNAi," "plant" and "insect," and only one quarter was published before 2008.

To implement RNAi in agricultural pest control, the target insect should uptake the dsRNA autonomously, e.g., from transgenic plants expressing dsRNA. This feeding should be continuous, since insects lack an amplification mechanism based on RdRP, such as *C. elegans*. Many of the main agricultural pest species have already been targeted by RNAi technology using various genes and delivery methods [66]. However, three orders have been the major focus of the development of transgenic plants expressing target gene regions for RNAi: Coleoptera, Hemiptera, and Lepidoptera. Here, we list some of the most recently published RNAi transgenic plants studies performed against those insect orders (Table 1).

Specie	Order	Crop	Target Gene	Remarks	Reference
Diabrotica v. virgifera	Coleoptera	*Zea mays*	*vATPase*	Mortality	[67]
Leptinotarsa decemlineata	Coleoptera	*Solanum tuberosum*	*β-actin, Shrub*	Mortality	[68]
Helicoverpa armigera *Spodoptera exigua*	Lepidoptera	*Nicotiana tabacum*	Nuclear receptor complex of 20-hydroxyecdysone (*HaEcR*)	Molting defect and larval lethality	[45]
Helicoverpa armigera	Lepidoptera	*Nicotiana tabacum*	Molt-regulating transcription factor gene (*HR3*)	Developmental deformities and larval lethality	[70]
Helicoverpa armigera	Lepidoptera	*Arabidopsis thaliana*	*HaAK*	Developmental Deformities and larval lethality	[71]
Myzus persicae	Hemiptera	*Arabidopsis thaliana and Nicotiana benthamiana*	*MpC001, Rack1*	Progeny reduced	[72]
Myzus persicae	Hemiptera	*Arabidopsis thaliana*	*serine protease*	Progeny reduced	[73]
Myzus persicae	Hemiptera	*Nicotiana tabacum*	*hunchback(hb)*	Inhibited reproduction	[74]
Bemisia tabaci	Hemiptera	*Nicotiana rustica*	*vATPase*	Mortality	[75]

Table 1. Overview of the recently published studies on the use of plant-RNAi against different insect pests

4.1. Coleoptera

The coleopterans are likely to be the first target to be controlled by the new generation of transgenics, the "RNAi-plants." *Diabrotica virgifera virgifera* (Western corn rootworm, WCR) is one of the most important agricultural pests, and this species, along with other coleopterans, requires little effort to have genes silenced by RNAi, independent of the delivery method and gene target. The significant breakthrough was demonstrated when WCR presented significant larval stunting and mortality, causing less injury to maize roots that express a hairpin version of *V-ATPase A* [43]. Since then, many studies have been conducted using various target genes, while not focusing only on pest control, but also to characterize the mechanism of action of the RNAi [46]. A recent study with WCR demonstrated that long dsRNAs of *Dv V-ATPase C* expressed in maize provides highly efficient root protection, but the siRNA population generated in the transgenic plant does not lead to lethal RNAi responses when consumed by the insect [67].

Studies have also been performed in other species, such as the important potato pest *Leptinotarsa decemlineata* (Colorado potato beetle, CPB). So far, this is the first study to compare efficacy at controlling pest insects by dsRNAs expressed either in the chloroplast or in the cytoplasm. Transgenic potato plants expressing hairpin versions of *β-actin* and *Shrub* genes (both insectidal dsRNAs) in the chloroplasts (transplastomic plants) conferred the most potent insecticidal activity (insects died after 5 days), while the conventional expression from nuclear transgenics did not affect the beetles [68].

An explanation for this result is that since choroplasts do not have cellular RNAi machinery [69], the dsRNAs produced inside these organelles are not cleaved by a plant Dicer and the beetles ingest almost entirely long dsRNA. In contrast, beetles fed on nuclear-transformed plants consumed mostly siRNAs; previous dsRNA-feeding studies already indicated that ingested long dsRNAs were much more effective than ingested siRNAs. It should be highlighted that all the other studies have been based on an efficient cytoplasm-derived dsRNA in various crops, indicating that possibly potato plants process long dsRNA more effective than the plants from those other studies (Table 1 [69]).

4.2. Lepidoptera

Plants producing *Bt* proteins were the first generation of transgenic plants to control insects, and most of the lepidopterans were successfully managed by Bt crops for years. However, the durability of Bt technology appears to be unsure. The number of pest species that evolved Bt resistance in the field, reducing transgenic efficacy, increased from one in 2005 to five in 2010 [4]. Among those five species, four are lepidopterans [4]. The lepidopterans could be the first and main targets for RNAi crops if they were not as recalcitrant to gene silencing, without any definite explanation for the limited and unstable RNAi responses [28, 29]. For instance, the concentration of dsRNA necessary to knock down a specific gene by feeding *Diatraea saccharalis* (Lepidoptera) neonate larvae is much higher than the one required for the same larval stage of *D. v. virgifera* (Coleoptera).

The first successful RNAi plant protected against a lepidopteran (*Helicoverpa armigera*) was demonstrated by silencing the *CYP6AE14* gene, necessary for detoxifying gossypol from cotton (*Gossypum hirsutum*) [44]. Studies have been conducted to explore alternative target genes to control and understand the RNAi mechanism in lepiopterans. Larval lethality and molting defects were detected in *H. armigera* fed with transgenic tobacco plants expressing dsRNA targeted to the nuclear ecdysone receptor complex (*HaEcR*), absolutely required for insect development [45]. The transgenic tobacco expressing dsRNA of *HaEcR* had an improved resistance to another lepidopteran pest, *Spodoptera exigua*. This cross-species effect might indicate a risk to affect nontarget insects, highlighting the importance of biosafety studies that should be carefully conducted [45].

The expression of dsRNA in both *Escherichia coli* and transgenic tobacco plants to silence a molt-regulating transcription factor gene (*HR3*) of *H. armigera* resulted in developmental deformity and larval lethality [70]. Transgenic *Arabidopsis thaliana* plants expressing dsRNA targeted to *arginine kinase* (*AK*) of *H. armigera* (*HaAK*) led to a 55% mortality rate in first instar larvae, while retarding growth in surviving larvae [71]. However, no lethal phenotypes were observed for the third instar larvae, although transcript levels of *HaAK* were distinctly suppressed [71].

4.3. Hemiptera

Hemipterans are characterized as piercing/sucking insects, representing major agricultural pests that inflict direct damages by sucking sap, or indirectly by acting as a vector of several viruses and bacterial infections. Since hemipterans feed through sucking the phloem, only systemic chemical insecticides are effective against these insects, resulting in high residual toxicity. The problem is further aggravated as no Bt toxin has been identified as exhibiting adequate insecticidal effects against hemipterans. Transgenic crops based on RNAi offer a large potential to control hemipteran, requiring expression of target gene dsRNAs on the phloem. One first report was published in 2011 about developing transgenic *Nicotiana benthamiana* and *A. thaliana* expressing dsRNA targeting genes expressed in *Myzus persicae* gut (*RACK1*) and salivary glands (*MpC002*) [72]. A reduction of the expression level of the target genes and a decrease in *M. persicae* fecundity were observed, but no lethal effects [72].

The same phenotype was observed when *M. persicae* fed on *A. thaliana* expressing dsRNA of a serine protease gene (*MySP*), with no lethal effects, but reduced fecundity [73]. Once again, reduced reproduction, but no lethal phenotype was observed when *M. persicae* was fed on tobacco plants expressing dsRNA targeting the *hunchback* gene [74]. A possible explanation for not achieving the expected phenotypes (mortality) after target gene depletion is that the dsRNA level produced by RNAi transgenic plants could not be sufficient for an efficient uptake of dsRNA or siRNA by sap-sucking insects [74]. However, more recently, mortality rates were observed in *Bemisia tabaci* fed in tobacco plants expressing dsRNA of *v-ATPaseA* [75]. This result provides a proof-of-concept that plants expressing dsRNA, at an efficient level and targeting crucial genes, could resist the attack of Hemipteran pests [75].

5. Conclusion and future perspectives

Since the concept of a transgenic plant expressing dsRNA targeted to a specific essential gene in the insect that affects its viability was first demonstrated in 2007, the technology has been extended to a large number of insect species from various orders. Elucidating the various mechanisms and components of the RNA interference pathway has progressed, but many aspects remain to be clarified. Many differences in components and mechanisms among insect orders and between insects and other organisms still need to be worked out. Some of these differences (e.g., genes involved, gene number, and level of expression) may explain variation in recalcitrance among insect species and need to be further investigated. Of particular interest are the mechanisms of dsRNA uptake, signal amplification, and systemic spread in the major pest species. Additional insect- or order-specific characteristics, such as gut pH, presence of dsRNA-degrading activity in digestive system, among others that could be associated with differences in recalcitrance to RNAi need to be dissected and clarified.

Due to the variety of RNAi response to RNAi in insects, no single protocol is suitable for all species. Issues related to the choice of effective target genes, including determining the size of optimal dsRNA length and ideal gene region. Assuming that the method of choice to deliver dsRNA is transgenic plants, a major question still to be addressed is the impact of plant dsRNA processing in the effective RNAi-induced silencing. There is still a need for investigation in this area. The choice of a suitable inducible promoter for expressing the dsRNA construct is another point barely explored.

Based on the recent publications reviewed in this chapter, the progress in developing "RNAi-plants" to control important insect pests widely demonstrated the potential of this technology to complement or replace Bt crops, providing resistance against a broad variety of insect pests. However, to be applied on a commercial level, several issues related to the RNAi mechanism and biosafety still need to be addressed. As a new technology, risk assessments and government regulations still have to be developed. However, RNAi transgenic crops are expected to have wider acceptance and reduced biosafety requirements for RNAi traits, in comparison to a protein incorporated into a plant, such as a Bt transgenic [39]. Thus, RNAi-mediated pest control will open a new paradigm in insect pest management.

Author details

Thais Barros Rodrigues* and Antonio Figueira

*Address all correspondence to: thaisbarros.bio@gmail.com

Centro de Energia Nuclear na Agricultura (CENA), Universidade de São Paulo, Piracicaba, SP, Brazil

References

[1] Bravo A, Soberon M. How to cope with insect resistance to Bt toxins? *Trends Biotechnol.* 2008;26:573-9. DOI: 10.1016/j.tibtech.2008.06.005

[2] Kos M, van Loon JJA, Dicke M, Vet LEM. Transgenic plants as vital components of integrated pest management. *Trends Biotechnol.* 2009;27:621-7. DOI: 10.1016/j.tibtech.2009.08.002

[3] Wu K-M, Lu Y-H, Feng H-Q, Jiang Y-Y, Zhao J-Z. Suppression of cotton bollworm in multiple crops in China in areas with Bt toxin-containing cotton. *Science.* 2008;321:1676-8. DOI: 10.1126/science.1160550

[4] Tabashnik BE, Brevault T, Carriere Y. Insect resistance to Bt crops: lessons from the first billion acres. *Natur Biotechnol.* 2013;31:510-21. DOI: 10.1038/nbt.2597

[5] Huvenne H, Smagghe G. Mechanisms of dsRNA uptake in insects and potential of RNAi for pest control: A review. *J Insect Physiol.* 2010;56:227-35. DOI: 10.1016/j.jinsphys.2009.10.004

[6] Whyard S, Singh AD, Wong S. Ingested double-stranded RNAs can act as species-specific insecticides. *Insect Biochem Mol Biol.* 2009;39:824-32. DOI: 10.1016/j.ibmb.2009.09.007

[7] Meister G, Tuschl T. Mechanisms of gene silencing by double-stranded RNA. *Nature.* 2004;431:343-9. DOI: 10.1038/nature02873

[8] Jinek M, Doudna JA. A three-dimensional view of the molecular machinery of RNA interference. *Nature.* 2009;457:405-12. DOI: 10.1038/nature07755

[9] Obbard DJ, Gordon KHJ, Buck AH, Jiggins FM. The evolution of RNAi as a defence against viruses and transposable elements. *Philo Trans Royal Soc B-Biologic Sci.* 2009;364:99-115. DOI: 10.1098/rstb.2008.0168

[10] Moazed D. Small RNAs in transcriptional gene silencing and genome defence. *Nature.* 2009;457:413-20. DOI: 10.1038/nature07756

[11] Choudhuri S. Small Noncoding RNAs: Biogenesis, Function, and Emerging Significance in Toxicology. *J Biochem Mol Toxicol.* 2010;24:195-216. DOI: 10.1002/jbt.20325

[12] Ghildiyal M, Zamore PD. Small silencing RNAs: an expanding universe. *Natur Rev Genet.* 2009;10:94-108. DOI: 10.1038/nrg2504

[13] O'Donnell KA, Boekel JD. Mighty piwis defend the germline against genome intruders. *Cell.* 2007;129:37-44. DOI: 10.1016/j.cell.2007.03.028

[14] Castaneda J, Genzor P, Bortvin A. piRNAs, transposon silencing, and germline genome integrity. *Mutat Res – Fund Mol Mech Mutagen.* 2011;714:95-104. DOI: 10.1016/j.mrfmmm.2011.05.002

[15] Shpiz S, Olovnikov I, Sergeeva A, Lavrov S, Abramov Y, Savitsky M, et al. Mechanism of the piRNA-mediated silencing of *Drosophila* telomeric retrotransposons. *Nucleic Acids Res.* 2011;39:8703-11. DOI: 10.1093/nar/gkr552

[16] Pillai RS, Chuma S. piRNAs and their involvement in male germline development in mice. *Dev Growth Different.* 2012;54:78-92. DOI: 10.1111/j.1440-169X.2011.01320.x

[17] Aravin AA, Hannon GJ, Brennecke J. The Piwi-piRNA pathway provides an adaptive defense in the transposon arms race. *Science.* 2007;318:761-4. DOI: 10.1126/science.1146484

[18] Saito K, Nishida KM, Mori T, Kawamura Y, Miyoshi K, Nagami T, et al. Specific association of Piwi with rasiRNAs derived from retrotransposon and heterochromatic regions in the *Drosophila* genome. *Genes Dev.* 2006;20:2214-22. DOI: 10.1101/gad.1454806

[19] Pasquinelli AE, Hunter S, Bracht J. MicroRNAs: a developing story. Current Opinion in Genetics & Development. 2005;15:200-5. DOI: 10.1016/j.gde.2005.01.002

[20] Hammond SM. Dicing and slicing – The core machinery of the RNA interference pathway. *Febs Lett*. 2005;579:5822-9. DOI: 10.1016/j.febslet.2005.08.079

[21] Firmino AAP, de Assis Fonseca FC, Pepino de Macedo LL, Coelho RR, Antonino de Souza JD, Jr., Togawa RC, et al. Transcriptome Analysis in Cotton Boll Weevil (*Anthonomus grandis*) and RNA Interference in Insect Pests. *Plos One*. 2013;8: e85079. DOI: 10.1371/journal.pone.0085079

[22] Lee YS, Nakahara K, Pham JW, Kim K, He ZY, Sontheimer EJ, et al. Distinct roles for *Drosophila* Dicer-1 and Dicer-2 in the siRNA/miRNA silencing pathways. *Cell*. 2004;117:69-81. DOI: 10.1016/s0092-8674(04)00261-2

[23] Tomoyasu Y, Miller SC, Tomita S, Schoppmeier M, Grossmann D, Bucher G. Exploring systemic RNA interference in insects: a genome-wide survey for RNAi genes in *Tribolium*. *Genome Biol*. 2008;9. DOI:10.1186/gb-2008-9-1-r10

[24] Peters L, Meister G. Argonaute proteins: Mediators of RNA silencing. *Mol Cell*. 2007;26:611-23. DOI: 10.1016/j.molcel.2007.05.001

[25] Pal-Bhadra M, Leibovitch BA, Gandhi SG, Rao M, Bhadra U, Birchler JA, et al. Heterochromatic silencing and HP1 localization in *Drosophila* are dependent on the RNAi machinery. *Science*. 2004;303:669-72. DOI: 10.1126/science.1092653

[26] Brennecke J, Aravin AA, Stark A, Dus M, Kellis M, Sachidanandam R, et al. Discrete small RNA-generating loci as master regulators of transposon activity in *Drosophila*. *Cell*. 2007;128:1089-103. DOI: 10.1016/j.cell.2007.01.043

[27] Lin H. piRNAs in the germ line. *Science*. 2007;316:397. DOI: 10.1126/science.1137543

[28] Terenius O, Papanicolaou A, Garbutt JS, Eleftherianos I, Huvenne H, Kanginakudru S, et al. RNA interference in Lepidoptera: An overview of successful and unsuccessful studies and implications for experimental design. *J Insect Physiol*. 2011;57:231-45. DOI: 10.1016/j.jinsphys.2010.11.006

[29] Kolliopoulou A, Swevers L. Recent progress in RNAi research in Lepidoptera: intracellular machinery, antiviral immune response and prospects for insect pest control. *Curr Opin Insect Sci*. 2014;6:28–34. DOI: http://dx.doi.org/10.1016/j.cois.2014.09.019

[30] Kolliopoulou A, Swevers L. Functional analysis of the RNAi response in ovary-derived silkmoth Bm5 cells. *Insect Biochem Mol Biol*. 2013;43:654-63. DOI: 10.1016/j.ibmb.2013.05.001

[31] Whangbo JS, Hunter CP. Environmental RNA interference. *Trends Genet*. 2008;24:297-305. DOI: 10.1016/j.tig.2008.03.007

[32] Gu L, Knipple DC. Recent advances in RNA interference research in insects: Implications for future insect pest management strategies. *Crop Protect.* 2013;45:36-40. DOI: 10.1016/j.cropro.2012.10.004

[33] Winston WM, Molodowitch C, Hunter CP. Systemic RNAi in *C. elegans* requires the putative transmembrane protein SID-1. *Science.* 2002;295:2456-9. DOI: 10.1126/science.1068836

[34] Feinberg EH, Hunter CP. Transport of dsRNA into cells by the transmembrane protein SID-1. *Science.* 2003;301:1545-7. DOI: 10.1126/science.1087117

[35] Kobayashi I, Tsukioka H, Komoto N, Uchino K, Sezutsu H, Tamura T, et al. SID-1 protein of *Caenorhabditis elegans* mediates uptake of dsRNA into *Bombyx* cells. *Insect Biochem Mol Biol.* 2012;42:148-54. DOI: 10.1016/j.ibmb.2011.11.007

[36] Jose AM, Hunter CP. Transport of sequence-specific RNA interference information between cells. *Annu Rev Genet.* 2007;41:305-30. DOI: 10.1146/annurev.genet.41.110306.130216

[37] Saleh M-C, van Rij RP, Hekele A, Gillis A, Foley E, O'Farrell PH, et al. The endocytic pathway mediates cell entry of dsRNA to induce RNAi silencing. *Natur Cell Biol.* 2006;8:793-U19. DOI: 10.1038/ncb1439

[38] Ulvila J, Parikka M, Kleino A, Sormunen R, Ezekowitz RA, Kocks C, et al. Double-stranded RNA is internalized by scavenger receptor-mediated endocytosis in *Drosophila* S2 cells. *J Biologic Chem.* 2006;281:14370-5. DOI: 10.1074/jbc.M513868200

[39] Scott JG, Michel K, Bartholomay LC, Siegfried BD, Hunter WB, Smagghe G, et al. Towards the elements of successful insect RNAi. *J Insect Physiol.* 2013;59:1212-21. DOI: 10.1016/j.jinsphys.2013.08.014

[40] Tijsterman M, May RC, Simmer F, Okihara KL, Plasterk RHA. Genes required for systemic RNA interference in *Caenorhabditis elegans. Curr Biol.* 2004;14:111-6. DOI: 10.1016/j.cub.2003.12.029

[41] Sijen T, Fleenor J, Simmer F, Thijssen KL, Parrish S, Timmons L, et al. On the role of RNA amplification in dsRNA-triggered gene silencing. *Cell.* 2001;107:465-76. DOI: 10.1016/s0092-8674(01)00576-1

[42] Yigit E, Batista PJ, Bei Y, Pang KM, Chen C-CG, Tolia NH, et al. Analysis of the *C. elegans* argonaute family reveals that distinct argonautes act sequentially during RNAi. *Cell.* 2006;127:747-57. DOI: 10.1016/j.cell.2006.09.033

[43] Baum JA, Bogaert T, Clinton W, Heck GR, Feldmann P, Ilagan O, et al. Control of coleopteran insect pests through RNA interference. *Natur Biotechnol.* 2007;25:1322-6. DOI: 10.1038/nbt1359

[44] Mao Y-B, Cai W-J, Wang J-W, Hong G-J, Tao X-Y, Wang L-J, et al. Silencing a cotton bollworm P450 monooxygenase gene by plant-mediated RNAi impairs larval tolerance of gossypol. *Natur Biotechnol.* 2007;25:1307-13. DOI: 10.1038/nbt1352

[45] Zhu J-Q, Liu S, Ma Y, Zhang J-Q, Qi H-S, Wei Z-J, et al. Improvement of pest resistance in transgenic tobacco plants expressing dsRNA of an insect-associated gene EcR. *Plos One.* 2012;7: e38572. DOI: 10.1371/journal.pone.0038572

[46] Bolognesi R, Ramaseshadri P, Anderson J, Bachman P, Clinton W, Flannagan R, et al. Characterizing the mechanism of action of double-stranded RNA activity against Western corn rootworm (*Diabrotica virgifera virgifer*a LeConte). *Plos One.* 2012;7: e47534. DOI: 10.1371/journal.pone.0047534

[47] Auer C, Frederick R. Crop improvement using small RNAs: applications and predictive ecological risk assessments. *Trends Biotechnol.* 2009;27:644-51. DOI: 10.1016/j.tibtech.2009.08.005

[48] Kumar M, Gupta GP, Rajam MV. Silencing of acetylcholinesterase gene of *Helicoverpa armigera* by siRNA affects larval growth and its life cycle. *J Insect Physiol.* 2009;55:273-8. DOI: 10.1016/j.jinsphys.2008.12.005

[49] Upadhyay SK, Chandrashekar K, Thakur N, Verma PC, Borgio JF, Singh PK, et al. RNA interference for the control of whiteflies (*Bemisia tabaci*) by oral route. *J Biosci.* 2011;36:153-61. DOI: 10.1007/s12038-011-9009-1

[50] Meyering-Vos M, Mueller A. RNA interference suggests sulfakinins as satiety effectors in the cricket *Gryllus bimaculatus*. *J Insect Physiol.* 2007;53:840-8. DOI: 10.1016/j.jinsphys.2007.04.003

[51] Shakesby AJ, Wallace IS, Isaacs HV, Pritchard J, Roberts DM, Douglas AE. A water-specific aquaporin involved in aphid osmoregulation. *Insect Biochem Mol Biol.* 2009;39:1-10. DOI: 10.1016/j.ibmb.2008.08.008

[52] Uryu O, Kamae Y, Tomioka K, Yoshii T. Long-term effect of systemic RNA interference on circadian clock genes in hemimetabolous insects. *J Insect Physiol.* 2013;59:494-9. DOI: 10.1016/j.jinsphys.2013.02.009

[53] Pereira TC. *Introdução à Técnica de Interferência por RNA – RNAi.* 1st ed. Ribeirão Preto: Sociedade Brasileira de Genética; 2013. 170p.

[54] Rodrigues TB, Khajuria C, Wang HC, Matz N, Cardoso DC, Valicente FH, et al. Validation of reference housekeeping genes for gene expression studies in Western corn rootworm (*Diabrotica virgifera virgifera*). *Plos One.* 2014;9: e0124187. DOI: doi:10.1371/journal.pone.0124187

[55] Holmes K, Williams CM, Chapman EA, Cross MJ. Detection of siRNA induced mRNA silencing by RT-qPCR: considerations for experimental design. *BMC Res Notes.* 2010;3. DOI: 1756-0500/3/53

[56] Bustin SA, Benes V, Garson JA, Hellemans J, Huggett J, Kubista M, et al. The MIQE guidelines: Minimum information for publication of quantitative real-time PCR experiments. *Clin Chem*. 2009;55:611-22. DOI: 10.1373/clinchem.2008.112797

[57] Rinkevich FD, Scott JG. Limitations of RNAi of a6 nicotinic acetylcholine receptor subunits for assessing the in vivo sensitivity to spinosad. *Insect Sci*. 2013;20:101-8. DOI: 10.1111/j.1744-7917.2012.01523.x

[58] Lomazzo E, Hussmann GP, Wolfe BB, Yasuda RP, Perry DC, Kellar KJ. Effects of chronic nicotine on heteromeric neuronal nicotinic receptors in rat primary cultured neurons. *J Neurochem*. 2011;119:153-64. DOI: 10.1111/j.1471-4159.2011.07408.x

[59] Araujo RN, Santos A, Pinto FS, Gontijo NF, Lehane MJ, Pereira MH. RNA interference of the salivary gland nitrophorin 2 in the triatomine bug *Rhodnius prolixus* (Hemiptera : Reduviidae) by dsRNA ingestion or injection. *Insect Biochem Mol Biol*. 2006;36:683-93. DOI: 10.1016/j.ibmb.2006.05.012

[60] Griebler M, Westerlund SA, Hoffmann KH, Meyering-Vos M. RNA interference with the allatoregulating neuropeptide genes from the fall armyworm *Spodoptera frugiperda* and its effects on the JH titer in the hemolymph. *J Insect Physiol*. 2008;54:997-1007. DOI: 10.1016/j.jinsphys.2008.04.019

[61] Allen ML, Walker WB. Saliva of Lygus lineolaris digests double stranded ribonucleic acids. *J Insect Physiol*. 2012;58:391-6. DOI: 10.1016/j.jinsphys.2011.12.014

[62] Rodriguez-Cabrera L, Trujillo-Bacallao D, Borras-Hidalgo O, Wright DJ, Ayra-Pardo C. RNAi-mediated knockdown of a *Spodoptera frugiperda* trypsin-like serine-protease gene reduces susceptibility to a *Bacillus thuringiensis* Cry1Ca1 protoxin. *Environ Microbiol*. 2010;12:2894-903. DOI: 10.1111/j.1462-2920.2010.02259.x

[63] Price DRG, Gatehouse JA. RNAi-mediated crop protection against insects. *Trends Biotechnol*. 2008;26:393-400. DOI: 10.1016/j.tibtech.2008.04.004

[64] Katoch R, Sethi A, Thakur N, Murdock LL. RNAi for insect control: Current perspective and future challenges. *Appl Biochem Biotechnol*. 2013;171:847-73. DOI: 10.1007/s12010-013-0399-4

[65] Gordon KHJ, Waterhouse PM. RNAi for insect-proof plants. *Natur Biotechnol*. 2007;25:1231-2. DOI: 10.1038/nbt1107-1231

[66] Zhang H, Li H-C, Miao X-X. Feasibility, limitation and possible solutions of RNAi-based technology for insect pest control. *Insect Sci*. 2013;20:15-30. DOI: 10.1111/j.1744-7917.2012.01513.x

[67] Li H, Khajuria C, Rangasamy M, Gandra P, Fitter M, Geng C, et al. Long dsRNA but not siRNA initiates RNAi in western corn rootworm larvae and adults. *J Appl Entomol*. 2015;139:432-45. DOI: 10.1111/jen.12224

[68] Zhang J, Khan SA, Hasse C, Ruf S, Heckel DG, Bock R. Full crop protection from an insect pest by expression of long double-stranded RNAs in plastids. *Science*. 2015;347:991-4. DOI: 10.1126/science.1261680

[69] Whyard S. Insecticidal RNA, the long and short of it. *Science*. 2015;347:950-1. DOI: 10.1126/science.aaa7722

[70] Xiong Y, Zeng H, Zhang Y, Xu D, Qiu D. Silencing the HaHR3 Gene by transgenic plant-mediated RNAi to disrupt *Helicoverpa armigera* development. *Int J Biologic Sci*. 2013;9:370-81. DOI: 10.7150/ijbs.5929

[71] Liu F, Wang X, Zhao Y, Li Y, Liu Y, Sun J. Silencing the HaAK gene by transgenic plant-mediated RNAi impairs larval growth of *Helicoverpa armigera*. *Int J Biologic Sci*. 2015;11:67-74. DOI: 10.7150/ijbs.10468

[72] Pitino M, Coleman AD, Maffei ME, Ridout CJ, Hogenhout SA. Silencing of aphid genes by dsRNA feeding from plants. *Plos One*. 2011;6:e25709. DOI: 10.1371/journal.pone.0025709

[73] Bhatia V, Bhattacharya R, Uniyal PL, Singh R, Niranjan RS. Host generated siRNAs attenuate expression of serine protease gene in *Myzus persicae*. *Plos One*. 2012;7: e46343. DOI: 10.1371/journal.pone.0046343

[74] Mao J, Zeng F. Plant-mediated RNAi of a gap gene-enhanced tobacco tolerance against the *Myzus persicae*. *Transg Res*. 2014;23:145-52. DOI: 10.1007/s11248-013-9739-y

[75] Thakur N, Upadhyay SK, Verma PC, Chandrashekar K, Tuli R, Singh PK. Enhanced whitefly resistance in transgenic tobacco plants expressing double stranded RNA of v-ATPase A gene. *Plos One*. 2014;9: e87235. DOI: 1756-0500/3/53

8

RNA Interference – Natural Gene-Based Technology for Highly Specific Pest Control (HiSPeC)

Eduardo C. de Andrade and Wayne B. Hunter

Abstract

RNAi technologies are more environmentally friendly, as the technology provides greater specificity in pest targeting, while reducing the potential negative effects on ecosystems and leaving beneficial insects and other organisms unharmed in crop ecosystems. Consequently, the increase in native fauna improves the efficacy of biological control agents against pests and pathogens. A growing understanding of the ubiquitous nature of RNAi, along with evidence for efficient, non-transgenic, topical applications has already begun to garner support among organic and industry producers. Designing solutions to agricultural problems based upon the same mechanisms used in nature provides newer, safer solutions to pests and pathogens for all agricultural industries.

Keywords: Future, Crops, Organic, Non-transgenic, RNAi

1. Introduction

A phenomenon initially reported in plants [1] called the attention of the scientific community, leading to the discovery of a sophisticated mechanism of gene regulation and protection against invasive nucleic acids [2–4]. Furthermore, the mechanism described in plants, referred to as post-transcriptional gene silencing (PTGS), or virus-induced gene silencing (VIGS), had been described in the 1990s [5] and was often referred to as pathogen-derived resistance [6].

RNAi is a natural process of gene regulation and antiviral defense system of eukaryotic cells. RNAi is a mechanism that functions as a "gene silencer" by targeting specific RNA sequences. RNAi results in degradation, and in some situations, translation inhibition, resulting in a reduction or complete elimination of the expression of a targeted RNA [7]. RNAi is also linked to suppressing gene expression at transcriptional level by directing epigenetic alterations on chromatin [8].

The basic RNAi process consists of the trigger molecule, a long endogenous or exogenous double-strand RNA (dsRNA) molecule that is expressed in, or introduced into, the cell, which is processed by Dicer, a ribonuclease III (RNase III) enzyme into small RNA duplexes of 21–23 nucleotides in length. These duplexes are separated with one strand (the guide strand), producing a protein complex known as the RNA-induced silencing complex (RISC). The RISC complex uses the specific sequence of the guide strand to determine potential target messenger RNAs (mRNA). Once bound to the mRNA, the guide strand directs a RISC-bound endonuclease [called "slicer", an Argonaute (AGO) protein] to cleave the mRNA which has homology to the guide strand [9]. Thus, the RISC complex can target the messenger RNA (mRNA), an invasive virus RNA, or a transposable element transcript (Please note that RNAi cannot eliminate transposons itself, but its transcripts.) [10]. These components appear to be cosmopolitan in their distribution across the RNAi spectrum of the eukaryotic phyla. This implies that a common ancestor had a functional RNAi pathway [11], estimated to have occurred over a billion years or more ago [12].

The generation of virus-resistant transgenic plants, by expressing fragments of viral genomes, was the first demonstration of the beneficial use of the RNAi [13,14]. However, with the demonstration that ingestion of dsRNAs can robustly silence genes in *Caenorhabditis elegans* [7], RNAi became not only an important tool in genetic studies to identify gene function but also opened a new field of application in plant protection against insects, arthropods, and pathogens.

In this chapter, we outlined some aspects on the development of RNAi-based strategies to control insects, presenting some considerations and research steps that are important to be addressed.

2. RNAi-based products for agricultural management of insect pest

Advances in genomics and initiatives to sequence genomes of agriculturally important organisms created big breakthroughs within the entomology fields of study, including taxonomy, insect physiology, toxicology, immunology, pest management, and microbe–host interactions. This new paradigm affected how research could be conducted, to make discoveries and increase the speed by which these could be accomplished. With these breakthroughs, entomologists, pathologists, and biologists are rapidly advancing toward better, safer, and more specific pest and pathogen management. Development of gene-based methods was dependent upon having the knowledge to understand how the cells in a living organism respond to the threats from viral pathogens, how they regulate their own gene expression, and how they maintain these natural complex systems throughout their lives.

The initial genomes which were sequenced and annotated to elucidate these very complicated interactions from: the nematode – *C. elegans*, the fruit fly – *Drosophila melanogaster*, the red flour beetle – *Tribolium castaneum*, the silkworm – *Bombyx mori*, the pea aphid – *Acyrthosiphon pisum*, the honey bee – *Apis mellifera*, to bumble bee – *Bombus terrestris* and including a few more examples from the world of agriculture [15]. Current genome initiatives, like the i5K

Arthropod initiative [15] and the Beijing Institute of Genomics, BGI, China, plan to sequence thousands of arthropod and plant genomes. The enormous amount of new information produced will also increase the understanding of the genetic basis of the mechanisms nature uses to solve problems at the cellular and organismal levels.

The number of arthropod species which have had successful RNAi reports continues to increase, and this trend will carry agriculture into the future, covering five Classes, in four Subphyla of the Arthropoda phylum, which includes eight insect orders and over 30 insect species [16–17].

3. Pitfalls and solutions – Relevant considerations for development of RNAi in insects

Though the use of RNAi strategies to control a desired insect pest seems to be very straightforward; however, some issues should be taken into considerations: (1) for oral treatments the dsRNA must survive ingestion, then be absorbed by the epithelial cells, and depending upon the target translocated through the hemolymph to reach other tissues. In insects, the dsRNA is mainly introduced through feeding, but dermal application has already been reported to possibly bypass gut issues [18–21]; (2) once inside the body, the dsRNA must enter into the cell to activate the RNAi mechanism. In insects, cell uptake of dsRNA varies widely between species, because there are different mechanisms of systemic absorption and translocation of dsRNAs within and between cells, respectively, leading to differences in response and influencing the efficiency in silencing the target gene [17,22]; (3) once the RNAi mechanisms are triggered in a group of cells, it has been demonstrated that a systemic spread of silencing may also occur, so that other tissues / cells are also affected, which may increase the RNA effect. Successful studies have shown that dsRNA can circulate in the hemolymph, and cause a suppression of genes in tissues distant from initial entry sites in the insect gut, affecting cuticle formation, the nervous system, or ovaries[23–26]. However, in insects results can be highly variable and research efforts continue to elucidate the effects of systemic signaling.

In theory, any cellular mRNA can be inactivated in a precise and controlled manner. With this in mind, the use of the RNAi mechanism to manage an insect pest relies on the capacity to design the dsRNA. The sequence of the dsRNA provides specificity and the researcher must determine the active concentration needed to obtain the desired RNAi outcome; thus, proper design and evaluation of the dsRNA becomes critical.

Identification of vitally important (i.e., with high mortality) target genes of a particular insect is a crucial step toward development of RNAi-based control strategy. Thanks to world science development and increasing efforts of the research community, the identification of an essential target can be achieved by an extended literature search and analyses of available DNA/RNA sequence databases [27]. Once identified, "candidate" target sequences are used to design potent "RNAi causing structures". Then, the dsRNAs must be experimentally validated for functionality, specificity, and stability, toward the specific RNAi target of interest. Furthermore, the development of an efficient delivery system for "RNAi causing structures" is another key step. There are several methods available that include, but are not limited to: microinjection [28], soaking (for mosquito larvae, and nematodes) [29,30], and feeding (chewing and piercing-sucking insects) [17,17,27,31,32].

One approach to identify potential target genes which will function under field conditions is to perform bioassays that closely mimic the conditions in the field, for example, using a bioassay that mimics the feeding of a hemipteran insect acquiring the dsRNA during the natural feeding process performed on the crop plant. One problem with delivering dsRNA through feeding is that, depending on the bioassay, it may be difficult to measure the dose of dsRNA ingested, from the dose absorbed by the gut cells and the target cells [33].

Oral delivery of dsRNA through feeding can be performed by using artificial diet, detached plant parts (leaves, buds, roots), or intact plants [17,24,34,35]. Delivering dsRNA through the diet provides an easy procedure to screen large numbers of dsRNAs in insect larvae and adults [23,24,34,37]. In addition, it allows addressing different issues, such as effective length of dsRNA, determine regions of the gene to be target which may provide better suppression, and to determine the effective lethal concentration (LC50) [23,38].

Although oral feeding provides a more natural screening system, it is important to take into consideration that for some insect species from across all taxonomic orders, they may not provide an effective RNAi response when conducting oral feeding bioassays regardless of the dosage of dsRNA, as the dsRNA may not enter, or be detected in the insect's body [22]. In contrast, in these same insects when dsRNA was injected directly into the insect's body, a potent RNAi response was observed [23,39,40]. Indeed, lack of positive results using feeding bioassays does not necessarily indicate that the insect is insensitive to RNAi, but in a majority of the situations, insects have nucleases in the saliva, in the midgut, or even in the hemolymph that degrades dsRNA before it can be absorbed by the cells [40–42].

Wynant et al. [40] discussed the interactions of enzymes and RNAi-causing dsRNAs in the alimentary tract and hemolymph of insects and other arthropods using oral delivery. The elucidation of the roles of microbes and host enzymes on RNAi efficacy across arthropod species continues to be a challenging field of research [43].

Where information about absorption of dsRNA or presence of nucleases is not available for a particular insect species, the use of reporter dsRNAs molecules are useful to clarify possible issues. It is essential that the dsRNAs sequence should not match with any insect's transcript sequence. The dsRNA "movement" can be monitored (detected), or quantified in the insect's body by RT-qPCR, showing that the insect has acquired the potent, fully functional, systemically spreading dsRNA during feeding (plant, diet, drop of water, etc.) (Figure 1).

When conducting a RT-PCR detection of reporter dsRNA after insect feeding, it is important to sample a tissue other than the gut such as the hemolymph, fat body, or ovary. Careful collection of tissues which are not in direct contact with the gut provides evidence that the dsRNA was truly absorbed by the cells, and you are not just detecting dsRNA just in the digestive tract.

With small insects, as the Asian Citrus Psyllid (ACP) *Diaphorina citri* (whitefly or aphids), collection of material can be difficult without bringing in gut tissues, so another option is to

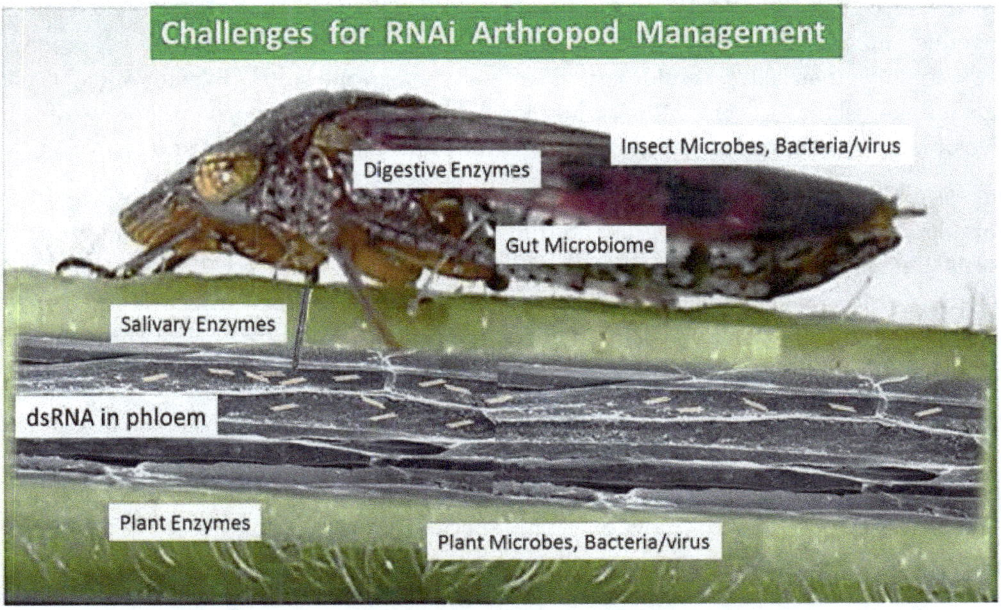

Figure 1. Topically applied RNA, provides long dsRNAs for insect ingestion. If absorbed into the plant, then long dsRNA persists in plant vascular tissues, xylem, and phloem, for several weeks due to lower metabolic activity, fewer enzymes, and microbes. Once the dsRNA enters a plant or insect cell, the RNAi mechanism is triggered, and the dsRNA processed [Image: Hunter, W.B., USDA-ARS, 2015].

let the insects feed on the source of the dsRNA (plant, diet, etc.) for a period of 24–48 h, then transfer them to an untreated food source. After feeding for 36 h, or more, the insect should excrete any food residue from the treated food source, which contains dsRNA. After this period, proceed with sample collection for dsRNA detection.

The reporter dsRNA is designed so that the sequence does not match with any known mRNA transcript in your insect. This is to avoid off target of other transcripts in the insect. Some commonly used dsRNAs which are used as negative controls in RNAi experiments are: green fluorescent protein (GFP), β-glucuronidase (GUS), and enhanced yellow fluorescent protein (EYFP) [44].

When designing RNAi experiments, important questions arise regarding the design of dsRNA, including: the length of the molecule and the region targeted within the mRNA. The minimal required length to achieve an RNAi effect will vary depending on insect species [45]. For example, in *Tribolium castaneum*, analysis showed that the dsRNA length had a strong influence on the efficacy of the RNAi response, with longer dsRNA proven to be more effective on curtailing gene expression [46]. In *T. castaneum* dsRNA, it was observed that length was crucial for cellular uptake; a minimum of 70 nucleotides were necessary to achieve the desired interference. However, other studies in the potato/tomato psyllid, *Bactericera cockerelli* [47], the pea aphid *Acyrthosiphon pisum* [48], and the lepidopteran *Manduca sexta* [49] have reported gene suppression using shorter dsRNAs, between 21 and 27 nucleotides in length. These molecules are called small interfering RNAs (siRNA). Overall, the majority of studies demonstrate success with dsRNA ranging from 140 to 520 nucleotides in length. Interestingly, Huvenne and Smagghe [31] reported success using a dsRNA 1,842 nucleotides in length. dsRNAs longer than 200 nucleotides provide the advantage of resulting in many siRNAs, post-cleavage against the targeted mRNA, thus maximizing the RNAi response and preventing the development of individuals with "resistance" due to the natural genetic variation.

There is no consensus on the mRNA region that the dsRNA should match to (e.g., 5′ or 3′). For example, in the pea aphid, *A. pisum,* no difference in mortality was observed in groups of insects that received dsRNA matching the 5′ or 3′ end of the *hunchback* (hb) gene [27]. In the mosquito, *Aedes aegypti* greater RNAi effects were achieved when insect larvae ingested dsRNA targeting the 3′ end versus 5′ end of an apoptosis gene, *AaeIAP1* [18]. These different results highlight the need to screen several dsRNA molecules across the entire mRNA [50].

In the context of field applications of RNAi for insect management, dsRNAs can be designed to be highly specific to both the target gene and the insect species. If desired, the RNAs can be designed to have a broader spectrum to affect several pest species. For example, RNAi strategies can be designed to remove one aphid species from a cropping system, or be designed to remove multiple aphid species from that same ecosystem [24,38].

4. Bioassays for dsRNA screening

For RNAi research attempting the development of a viable pest management product. It is of utmost importance to identify the best delivery mechanisms (i.e., topical sprays, baits, or transgenic plants) as early as possible; this will expedite the entire process and can cut years off of the development and commercialization timeline.

The example outlined below highlights RNAi bioassays directed toward two citrus insect pests, each one with different feeding behaviors: piercing-sucking plant-feeding (the Asian citrus psyllid *Diaphorina citri,* Hemiptera) and a chewing beetle pest (the weevil *Diaprepes abbreviatus,* Coleoptera). In both situations, the bioassays were designed to evaluate the efficacy of oral ingestion of dsRNAs under "natural feeding conditions" which mimic conditions the insects will encounter in the field.

4.1. Bioassays for piercing-sucking insects

The artificial feeding bioassay is being widely used for studies on insect nutrition, pathogen acquisition, toxicity, and RNAi (Figure 2A) [51–53].

It is notable that liquid feeding bioassays (dsRNAs mixed in a liquid diet or a sucrose solution) frequently result in high mortality levels in the controls, and increased degradation of dsRNA in the solution due to bacterial or fungal contaminations [42,57]. In addition, these bioassays require significantly high dsRNA concentrations to achieve insect mortality. Concentrations up to 1µg/µL [58–60] cannot be reproduced inside plant vascular tissues.

Hemipteran pests in citrus (psyllids, leafhoppers, aphids, whiteflies) have piercing-sucking mouthparts that are inserted into the plant vascular system to feed. The development of an

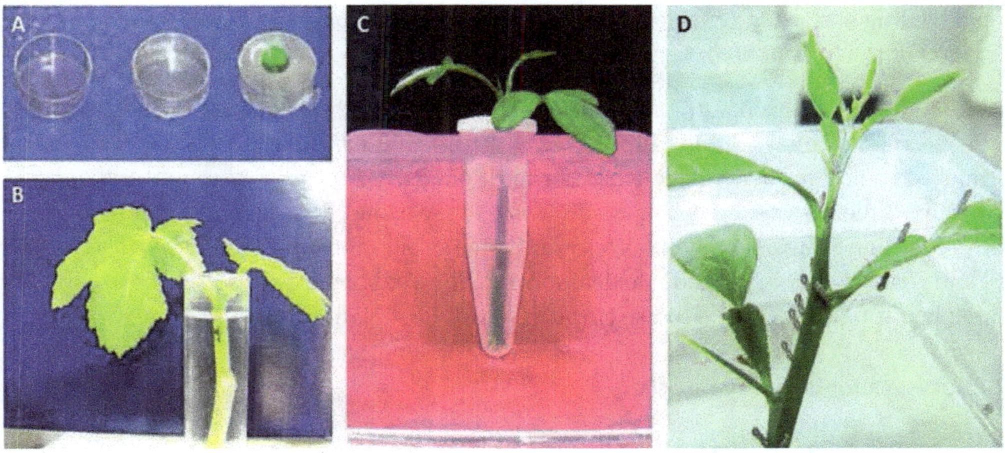

Figure 2. RNAi feeding assays used at the USDA lab, ARS, Ft. Pierce, FL (2007-2014), to successfully screen dsRNA constructs rapidly and under controlled conditions: (A) sucrose solutions within artificial membranes (5 ng dsRNA/μL) [54], (B) rooted okra plant cuttings, (C) citrus flush (5 ng to 100 ng dsRNA/ 0.25 g plant tissue). Plant cuttings absorb dsRNA directly providing systemic movement of dsRNA, (D) insects are given a feeding access period to ingest the dsRNA across 10 days to observe mortality (Hunter and Andrade, USDA-ARS 2015) [54–56].

RNAi control strategy against these insects relies on effective delivery of the dsRNA through the vascular tissues.

Demonstration of the first dsRNA delivery into full-sized citrus trees and grapevines, without a delivery vector, expression vector, or transformation event was performed in 2008 [56]. These results showed that two hemipteran insects, the xylem-feeding leafhopper (*H. vitripennis*), and the phloem-feeding Asian citrus psyllid (*D. citri*), tested positive for ingested dsRNA after feeding from host plants treated with dsRNA as either a foliar spray or root drench. These results along with other studies that demonstrated successful RNAi through oral ingestion in insects [24,34,36,61,62] support the potential for exogenously delivered RNAi control strategies.

Use of cut plant feeding bioassays for hemipteran pests enables the screening of a large number of dsRNAs molecules at a reduced cost of materials and time. The bioassay, can use leaf disks, whole leaf, new growth leaves and stem, or rooted cuttings, to absorb and deliver dsRNAs. In citrus, the "flush", which are new growth foliar shoots, are collected from potted citrus seedlings grown in a glasshouse (USDA-ARS, Fort Pierce, FL). The leaves and stem material are about 7–8 cm long. The plant material is washed in 0.2% bleach water, for 10 min. Then the base of each stem is cut at a 45 degree angle while submerged in filtered water. The material is then placed into a 1.5 mL tube containing 0.5 mL water (Figure 2B and C). The dsRNA solution, 300 μL, is added to the water, the tube top is wrapped with plastic or Parafilm™ and placed under artificial lighting to stimulate absorption of dsRNA solution. The next day the tube is filled with water using a 26 gauge syringe needle and syringed filtered (0.45 μ). The treated cuttings are then placed into a cage and adult insects provided feeding access for 10 days (Figure 2D). The plant material can remain viable for up to 40 days on average. While most bioassays may terminate after eight to 10 days of observations for mortality, having a longer feeding access time enables observations on insect oviposition, egg viability, or nymph development.

Each dsRNA molecules has an optimal concentration. So each dsRNA molecule is evaluated across a range of total concentrations (i.e., 5, 20, 50, 100 nanograms/ tissue). The bioassay permits screening for synergistic effects of multiple dsRNAs and to screen a single dsRNA against multiple insect species. For example, the assay using citrus flush permits screening of dsRNAs designed against psyllids for off target effects in the citrus aphid (*Toxoptera citricidus*) and glassy-winged sharpshooter leafhopper (*Homalodisca vitripennis* (Germar), two closely related hemipterans, which also use citrus trees as a host plant.

4.2. Bioassays for chewing insects

For insects which are foliage feeders, the delivery of dsRNA can be achieved as a foliar topical spray. In this scenario, the dsRNAs are evaluated similarly as topical insecticides. The dsRNA solution is sprayed on leaves, and then fed to the insects. An example of the effectiveness of this approach was reported by Bolognesi [45] working with the coleopteran *Diabrotica virgifera,* in which dsRNA administered through feeding, silenced genes in tissues far from the gut epithelium.

Similar results were obtained while developing an RNAi strategy against the Diaprepes root weevil (DRW), *Diaprepes abbreviatus* L., (Curculionidae: Coleoptera) (Andrade and Hunter). The adults feed and oviposition on mature citrus leaves. Topically applied dsRNA was sprayed on a bouquet of citrus leaves for delivery to DRW adults (Figure 3A). RNA's have been shown to move through the plant xylem and phloem [6].

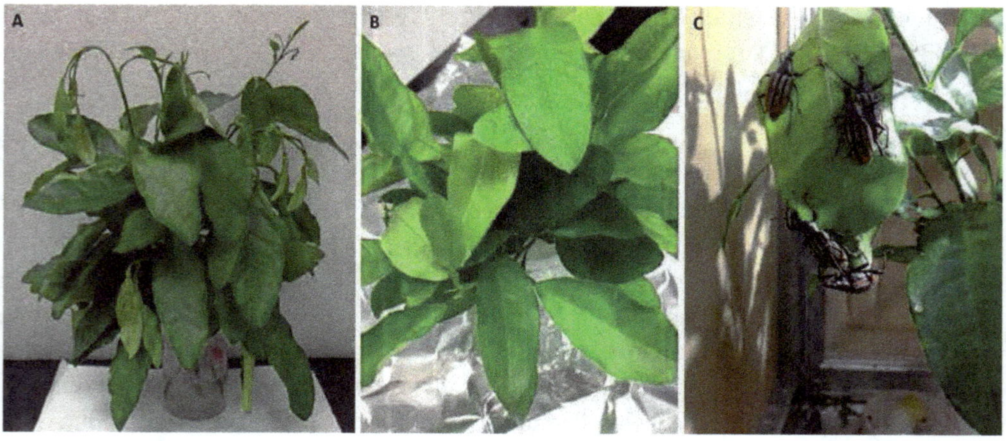

Figure 3. Citrus *"leaf bouquet"* feeding bioassay for *Diaprepes* root weevil. **(A)** Fresh stems with leaves are washed in 0.2% bleach water, rinsed with Nanopure™ filtered water, then the stems are freshly cut while submerged in water. The leaf bouquets are placed in water-filled containers and placed under artificial lighting for 24 h prior to use. **(B)** Topical foliar treatment: the dsRNA is mixed with water and applied using a low-volume aerosol sprayer. **(C)** After the leaves dry, the "bouquets" are caged with adult insects.

A test spray using only water established the volume needed to provide full coverage of leaf bouquets without excessive run off (Figure 3B). After the leaves have dried, they are caged with adult insects (Figure 3C). Freshly treated citrus leaf bouquets replaced previous bouquets every five to seven days for a 5-week period. The total amount of dsRNA to be sprayed over the leaf bouquet was determined by evaluating a range of concentrations in a pretest experiment for efficacy. The effects from RNAi in insects usually start to appear within 4 to 5 days post-ingestion, which suggests there may be a dose response [63]. Since foliage feeding insects tend to eat a lot of leaf material each day, a low-dose spray may be able to deliver a significant amount of dsRNA.

5. Final considerations on RNAi applied to agriculture

Efficient delivery and increased stability of dsRNA need to be developed if non-transgenic, topically delivered, RNAi strategies are to be established. Increased stability and superior delivery into some insects can be achieved using nanoparticle-mediated RNAi [63–65], traditional crop improvement strategies, in which plants express hairpin dsRNAs, will continue to be a mainstay of agricultural approaches [63,65,66].

Transgenic plants have successfully used RNAi strategies to produce crops with improved virus resistance, increased nutrition and fiber content [67]; biotechnology companies are trying to move towards a faster, more natural process of topically applied RNAi. dsRNA molecules are part of naturally occurring processes in all living organisms. They exist in our foods, and our bodies [66]. The short persistence time of dsRNA in the environment is demonstrated by the fact that analyses of soils and plant debris, treated with dsRNA have consistently shown rapid breakdown of dsRNAs within 2–3 days [68], also means less concerns about unintended contamination of water supplies, soils, or adverse air quality effects. Furthermore, since all living things have evolved to break down dsRNA and use the nucleic acids as cellular nutrients, this technology will be safer than conventional chemistries for those who apply RNAi products, or eat the produce [66–69].

RNAi technologies have greater specificity in pest targeting, which reduces negative impacts on crop ecosystems by leaving more insects and other organisms unharmed in the field. The increased fauna consequently improves the efficacy of pollination, and biological control agents that help suppress a broad range of pests. The increased understanding of the ubiquitous nature of RNAi, along with evidence of efficient topical application, has already begun to garner support for this technology among members of the organic grower's communities, which desperately need a truly natural, innovative breakthrough, to manage many of the pests and pathogens which plague the organic industries.

5.1. Cost-effective methods for the mass production and formulation of dsRNA

Cost-efficient methods for mass production of vast amounts of dsRNA are being developed, and include bacterial, plant, and synthetic production [65]. While small amounts of dsRNA can be easily produced in the laboratory for research purposes, commercially available kits are not a viable, cost-effective method for the production of large quantities of dsRNA [65]. The costs associated with the commercialization and implementation of RNAi products are decreasing rapidly. The costs of dsRNA production have dropped from $500,000 USD for 40 g in 2008 to less than $4,000 USD for 40 g today. *For example, see* [70]. As interests in commercialization of RNAi-based products increase, better production systems will be developed to meet the predicted demands of these growing markets [17,65,71]. One of the most cost-effective methods for production is in bacteria, since for most countries bacteria-produced dsRNA would provide an affordable production system which could advance RNAi as, "*The* novel biological insecticide of the future!" Most agricultural companies interested in the future of RNAi are working on developing their own technologies that will further reduce production costs predicted to be near $4 USD per one gram by the end of 2015. *For example, see* [72].

5.2. Other applications

Future applications of RNAi and other gene-based targeting biotechnologies will add value to existing beneficial insects (pollinators, predators, parasitoids). A real-world example is a study conducted over several years in which an RNAi product designed to reduce Israeli acute paralysis virus replication was fed to honey bees. The treated bees had significantly greater survival and produced significantly more honey [73]. RNAi strategies have also reduced honey bee parasites, like *Varroa* mites [74,75], and internal microsporidian parasites [76] without deleterious effects to the bees. The highly specific nature of RNAi approaches can be exploited to reduce pests with no harmful effects on non-target species. The use of RNAi in combination with beneficial pollinators and natural enemies has the potential to raise the level of all pest management efforts [17].

Biotechnology has demonstrated the safe production of plants which are more nutritious, less toxic, more resistant to drought, and more efficient for biofuel production [66, 67]. RNAi has already been successfully used to produce crops which are virus- and drought-resistant [66]. However, plants expressing dsRNAs while stable and safe take years to develop and millions of dollars to commercialize [65]. Development of topically applied RNAi, which is a non-transgenic approach improves crop traits and provides a major step forward for environmentally sound crop management [66, 67].

6. Conclusions

As more insects and mites develop chemical resistance to one or more insecticides, now estimated to be over 500 species with resistance to one or more products [77], it is imperative that new types of pest control are developed. The public would like the world to be filled with environmentally friendly technologies, safe for human and animal consumption, technologies which are safe for use around animals and beneficial insects, safe for each type of ecosystem, forest, field, crop, or backyard, a technology that will not endanger water or food quality, a more natural solution, with a natural approach toward problem-solving. So enters RNA interference!

RNA interference, or gene silencing, is a way to reduce specific mRNAs so that a particular protein is either not made or it is reduced. The RNAi mechanism is a natural one which occurs in the cells of humans, animals, insects, and plants, and appears to have evolved as a primary defense system against virus replication [78]. Andrew Fire and Craig Mello, won the Nobel Prize in 2006 [79] for explaining how the RNAi mechanism is triggered, when a cell encounters double-stranded RNA, and how this could be used to benefit humanity. Humanity's greatest discoveries have come from observing the natural world; while RNAi will not solve every problem, it certainly can help improve plant health, reduce insect pests and pathogens [17, 66, 67, 80]. Some of the benefits from developing RNAi as topically applied products are: 1) The rapid degradation of the molecules ensures low environmental risks. All cells have the capacity to degrade dsRNA, and the salvage pathways to recycle these bases and nucleosides to form new nucleotides. Thus, cells constantly breaking down DNA and RNA into recycled nucleotides [81]. 2) Topical RNAi applications do not insert genes, so do not produce proteins. RNAi reduces the expression of the targeted proteins, a modulation effect of the natural system. 3) RNAi can be designed and tested faster (in about 2–3 years) than producing transgenic crops, which can take 10 to 20 years and cost hundreds of millions of dollars [65]. 4) Finally, RNAi strategies as topical sprays would, for the first time, be able to remove one or two closely related insect species, while leaving all the other insects unharmed [38]. The ability to design RNAi as highly specific pest control will finally provide relief to biological control agents and beneficial insects [17, 44, 73], significantly improving integrated pest management programs.

The advantages and promises from RNAi technology sound amazing. However, serious efforts in outreach and education are needed to better inform the different stake holders including the general public, and agricultural industry, leaders as well as decision makers in the regulatory and political communities to help expedite the release and adoption of RNAi products and technology.

7. Disclaimer

Mention of trade names or commercial products herein is solely for the purpose of providing specific information and does not imply recommendation or endorsement, to the exclusion of other similar products or services by the U.S. Department of Agriculture. USDA is an equal opportunity provider and employer.

Acknowledgements

We thank Dr. Xiomara Sinisterra-Hunter, AgTec, LLC, Plant Biotechnology Consultant, Port St. Lucie, FL, for critical reviews of the manuscript, and Maria Gonzalez, Biological science technician, USDA, Fort Pierce, FL, for technical assistance.

Author details

Eduardo C. de Andrade[1] and Wayne B. Hunter[2]

*Address all correspondence to: eduardo.andrade@embrapa.br

1 Embrapa Cassava and Fruits, Rua Embrapa, s/n, Cruz das Almas,BA, Brasil

2 USDA, ARS, U.S. Horticultural Research Laboratory, Fort Pierce, FL, USA

References

[1] Napoli C, Lemieux C, Jorgensen, R. Introduction of a chimeric chalcone synthase gene into petunia results in reversible co-suppression of homologous genes in trans. Plant Cell 1990;2:279–89. DOI: http://dx.doi.org/10.1105/tpc.2.4.279.

[2] Voinnet O, Pinto YM, Baulcombe DC. Suppression of gene silencing: a general strategy used by diverse DNA and RNA viruses of plants. Proc Nat Acad Sci USA 1999;96:14147–52. DOI: 10.1073/pnas.96.24.14147.

[3] Voinnet O. Induction and suppression of RNA silencing: insights from viral infections. Nat Rev Genetics 2005;6:206–20. DOI: 10.1038/nrg1555.

[4] Sidahmed AM, Wilkie B. Endogenous antiviral mechanisms of RNA interference: a comparative biology perspective. Method Molecul Biol 2010;623:3–19. DOI: 10.1007/978-1-60761-588-0_1.

[5] Baulcombe DC. RNA as a target and an initiator of post-transcriptional gene silencing in trangenic plants. Plant Molecul Biol 1996;32:79–88. DOI 10.1007/BF00039378.

[6] Molnar A, Melnyk C, Baulcombe DC. Silencing signals in plants: a long journey for small RNAs. Genome Biol 2011;12:215. DOI 10.1186/gb-2010-11-12-219.

[7] Fire A, Xu S, Montgomery MK, Kostas SA, Driver SE, Mello CC. Potent and specific genetic interference by double-stranded RNA in *Caenorhabditis elegans*. Nature 1998;391:806–11. DOI: 10.1038/35888.

[8] Castel SE, Martienssen RA. RNA interference in the nucleus: roles for small RNAs in transcription, epigenetics and beyond. Nat Rev Genetics 2013;14:100–12. DOI: 10.1038/nrg3355.

[9] Tomari Y, Zamore PD. Perspective: machines for RNAi Genes Develop 2005;19:517–29. DOI: 10.1101/gad.1284105.

[10] Buchon N, Vaury C. RNAi: a defensive RNA-silencing against viruses and transposable elements. Heredity 2006;96:195–202. DOI:10.1038/sj.hdy.6800789.

[11] Cerutti H, Casas-Mollano, J.A. On the origin and functions of RNA-mediated silencing: from protists to man. Current Genetics 2006;50:81–99. DOI: 10.1007/s00294-006-0078-x.

[12] Roger AJ, Hug LA. The origin and diversification of eukaryotes: problems with molecular phylogenetics and molecular clock estimation. Philosoph Transac Royal Soc B 2006;361:1039–1054. DOI: 10.1098/rstb.2006.1845.

[13] Hamilton AJ, Baulcombe DC. A species of small antisense RNA in posttranscriptional gene silencing in plants. Science 1999;286:950–952. DOI: 10.1126/science.286.5441.950.

[14] Bonfim K, Faria JC, Nogueira EO, Mendes EA, Aragão FJL. RNAi-mediated resistance to bean golden mosaic virus in genetically engineered common bean (*Phaseolus vugaris*). Molecul Plant-Microbe Interact 2007;20:717–26. DOI: http://dx.doi.org/10.1094/MPMI-20-6-0717.

[15] i5K Consortium. The i5K initiative: advancing arthropod genomics for knowledge, human health, agriculture, and the environment. J Heredity 2013;104:595–600. DOI: 10.1093/jhered/est050.

[16] Zhang H, Li H, Miao X. Feasibility, limitation and possible solutions of RNAi-based technology for insect pest control. Insect Sci 2013:20:15–30. DOI 10.1111/j.1744-7917.2012.01513.x.

[17] Zotti M, Smagghe G. RNAi technology for insect management and protection of beneficial insects from diseases: lessons, challenges and risk assessments. Neotropic Entomol 2015;44. DOI 10.1007/s13744-015-0291-8.

[18] Pridgeon JW, Zhao L, Becnel JJ, Strickman DA, Clark GG, Linthicum KJ. Topically applied *AaeIAP1* double-stranded RNA kills female adults of *Aedes aegypti*. J Med Entomol 2008;45:414–20. DOI:http://dx.doi.org/10.1093/jmedent/45.3.414.

[19] Wang Y, Zhang H, Li H, Miao X. Second-generation sequencing supply an effective way to screen RNAi targets in large scale for potential application in pest insect control. PLoS One 2011;6:e18644. DOI: 10.1371/journal.pone.0018644.

[20] El-Shesheny I, Hajeri S, El-Hawary I, Gowda S, Killiny N. Silencing abnormal wing disc gene of the Asian citrus psyllid, *Diaphorina citri* disrupts adult wing development and increases nymph mortality. PLoS One 2013;8:e65392. DOI:10.1371/journal.pone.0065392.

[21] Killiny N, Hajeri S, Tiwari S, Gowda S, Stelinski LL. Double-stranded RNA uptake through topical application, mediates silencing of five *CYP4* genes and suppresses insecticide resistance in *Diaphorina citri*. PLoS One 2014;9:e110536. DOI:10.1371/journal.pone.0110536.

[22] Terenius O, Papanicolaou A, Garbutt JS, Eleftherianos I, Huvenne H, et al. RNA interference in Lepidoptera: an overview of successful and unsuccessful studies and

implications for experimental design. J Insect Physiol 2011;57:231–245. DOI: 10.1016/j.jinsphys.2010.11.006.

[23] Araujo RN, Santos A, Pinto FS, Gontijo NF, Lehane MJ, Pereira MH. RNA interference of the salivary gland nitrophorin 2 in the triatomine bug *Rhodnius prolixus* (Hemiptera: Reduviidae) by dsRNA ingestion or injection. Insect Biochem Molecul Biol 2006;36:683–93. ISSN 0965-1748; 0965-1748. DOI:10.1016/j.ibmb.2006.05.012

[24] Whyard S, Singh AD, Wong S. Ingested double-stranded RNAs can act as species-specific insecticides. Insect Biochem Molecul Biol 2009;39:824–32. DOI: 10.1016/j.ibmb.2009.09.007.

[25] Paim RM, Pereira MH, Di Ponzio R, Rodrigues JO, Guarneri AA, Gontijo NF, Araujo RN. Validation of reference genes for expression analysis in the salivary gland and the intestine of *Rhodnius prolixus* (Hemiptera, Reduviidae) under different experimental conditions by quantitative real-time PCR. BMC Res Notes 2012;5:128. DOI: 10.1186/1756-0500-5-128.

[26] Paim RM, Pereira MH, Araujo RN, Gontijo NF, Guarneri AA. The interaction between *Trypanosoma rangeli* and the nitrophorins in the salivary glands of the triatomine *Rhodnius prolixus* (Hemiptera; Reduviidae). Insect Biochem Molecul Biol 2013;43:229–36. DOI:10.1016/j.ibmb.2012.12.011.

[27] Mao J, Zeng F. Feeding-based RNA interference of a gap gene is lethal to the pea aphid, *Acyrthosiphon pisum*. PLoS One 2012;7:e48718. DOI:10.1371/journal.pone.0048718.

[28] Liu S, Ding Z, Zhang C, Yang B, Liu, Z. Gene knockdown by introthoracic injection of double-stranded RNA in the brown planthopper, *Nilaparvata lugens*. Insect Biochem Molecul Biol 2010;40:666–71. DOI: 10.1016/j.ibmb.2010.06.007.

[29] Singh AD, Wong S, Ryan CP, Whyard S. Oral delivery of double-stranded RNA in larvae of the yellow fever mosquito, *Aedes aegypti*: implications for pest mosquito control. J Insect Sci 2013;13:69. Available from: http://www.insectscience.org/13.69.

[30] Dutta TK, Banakar P, Rao U. The status of RNAi-based transgenic research in plant nematology. Front Microbiol 2015;5:1–7. DOI: 10.3389/fmicb.2014.00760.

[31] Huvenne H, Smagghe G. Mechanisms of dsRNA uptake in insects and potential of RNAi for pest control: a review. J Insect Physiol 2010;56:227–35. DOI:10.1016/j.jinsphys.2009.10.004.

[32] Pitino M, Coleman AD, Maffei ME, Ridout CJ, Hogenhout SA. Silencing of aphid genes by dsRNA feeding from plants. PLoS ONE 2011;6:e25709. DOI: 10.1371/journal.pone.0025709.

[33] Li H, Guan R, Guo H, Miao X. New insights into an RNAi approach for plant defence against piercing-sucking and stem-borer insect pests. Plant Cell Environ 2015:38:1–9. DOI: 10.1111/pce.12546.

[34] Baum JA, Roberts, J.K. Chapter Five- progress towards RNAi-mediated insect pest management. Adv Insect Physiol 2014;47:249–95. DOI: 10.1016/B978-0-12-800197-4.00005-1.

[35] Zhu F, Xu JJ, Palli R, Ferguson J, Palli S.R. Ingested RNA: interference for managing the populations of the Colorado potato beetle, *Leptinotarsa decemlineata*. Pest Manage Sci 2011;67:175–82. DOI: 10.1002/ps.2048.

[36] Turner CT, Davy MW, MacDiarmid RM, Plummer KM, Birch NP, Newcomb RD. RNA interference in the light brown apple moth, *Epiphyas postvittana* (Walker) induced by double-stranded RNA feeding. Insect Molecul Biol 2006;15:383–91. DOI: 10.1111/j.1365-2583.2006.00656.x

[37] Aronstein K, Oppert B, Lorenzen MD. RNAi in Agriculturally-Important Arthropods, RNA Processing, Prof. Paula Grabowski (Ed.), 2011, ISBN: 978-953-307-557-0, InTech, [Available from: http://www.intechopen.com/books/rna-processing/rnai-in-agriculturally-important-arthropods. Accessed 2015/08/25.

[38] Bachman PM, Bolognesi R, Moar WJ, Mueller GM, Paradise MS, et al. Characterization of the spectrum of insecticidal activity of a double-stranded RNA with targeted activity against western corn rootworm (*Diabrotica virgifera virgifera* LeConte). Transgenic Res 2013;22:1207–22. DOI: 10.1007/s11248-013-9716-5.

[39] Wynant N, Verlinden H, Breugelmans B, Simonet G, Vanden Broeck J. Tissue-dependence and sensitivity of the systemic RNA interference response in the desert locust, *Schistocerca gregaria*. Insect Biochem Molecul Biol 2012;42:911–7. DOI:10.1016/j.ibmb.2012.09.004.

[40] Wynant N, Santos D, Verdonck R, Spit J, Van Wielendaele P, Vanden Broeck, J. Identification, functional characterization and phylogenetic analysis of double stranded RNA degrading enzymes present in the gut of the desert locust, *Schistocerca gregaria*. Insect Biochem Molecul Biol 2014;46:1–8.DOI: http://dx.DOI.org/10.1016/j.ibmb.2013.12.008.

[41] Garbutt JS, Bellés X, Richards EH, Reynolds SE. Persistence of double-stranded RNA in insect hemolymph as a potential determiner of RNA interference success: evidence from *Manduca sexta* and *Blattella germanica*. J. Insect Physiology 2012. DOI: http://dx.doi.org/10.1016/j.jinsphys.2012.05.013.

[42] Christiaens O, Swevers L, Smagghe G. DsRNA degradation in the pea aphid (*Acyrthosiphon pisum*) associated with lack of response in RNAi feeding and injection assay. Peptides 2014;53:307–14. DOI: 10.1016/j.peptides.2013.12.014.

[43] Sharma P, Sharma S, Maurya RK, De TD, Thomas T, Lata S, Singh N, Pandey KC, Valecha N, Dixti R. Salivary glands harbor more diverse microbial communities than gut in *Anopheles culicificacies*. Parasites Vectors 2014;7:235. DOI: 10.1186/1756-3305-7-235.

[44] Scott JG, Michel K, Bartholomay LC, Siegfried BD, Hunter WB, Smagghe G, Zhu KY, Douglas AE. Towards the elements of successful insect RNAi. J Insect Physiol 2013;59:1212–21. http://dx.doi.org/10.1016/j.jinsphys.2013.08.014.

[45] Bolognesi R, Ramaseshadri P, Anderson J, Bachman P, Clinton W, Flannagan R, Ilagan O, Lawrence C, Levine S, Moar W, et al. Characterizing the mechanism of action of double-stranded RNA activity against western corn rootworm (*Diabrotica virgifera virgifera* LeConte). PLoS One 2012;7: e47534. DOI:10.1371/journal.pone.0047534.

[46] Miller SC, Miyata K, Brown SJ, Tomoyasu Y. Dissecting systemic RNA interference in the red flour beetle *Tribolium castaneum*: parameters affecting the efficiency of RNAi. PLoS One 2012;7:e47431. DOI:10.1371/journal.pone.0047431.

[47] Wuriyanghan H, Rosa C, Falk BW. Oral delivery of double-stranded RNAs and siRNAs induces RNAi effects in the potato/tomato psyllid, *Bactericerca cockerelli*. PLoS One 2011;6:e27736. DOI: 10.1371/journal.pone.0027736.

[48] Mutti NS, Park Y, Reese JC, Reeck GR. RNAi knockdown of a salivary transcript leading to lethality in the pea aphid, *Acyrthosiphon pisum*. J Insect Sci 2006;6:1–7. DOI: 10.1673/031.006.3801.

[49] Kumar P, Pandit SS, Baldwin I.T. Tobacco rattle virus vector: a rapid and transient means of silencing *Manduca sexta* genes by plant mediated RNA interference. PLoS One 2012;7:e31347. DOI:10.1371/journal.pone.0031347.

[50] Noh MY, Beeman RW, Arakane Y. RNAi-based functional genomics in *Tribolium castaneum* and possible applications for controlling insect pests. Entomol Res 2012;42:1–10. DOI: 10.1111/j.1748-5967.2011.00437.x.

[51] Hamilton MA. Further experiments on the artificial feeding of *Myzus persicae* (Sulz.) Annal Appl Biol 1935;32:243–58. DOI:10.1111/j.1744-7348.1935.tb07160.x.

[52] Li J, Wang W-P, Wang M-Q, Ma W-H, Hua H-X. Advances in the use of the RNA interference technique in Hemiptera. Insect Sci 2013;20:31–9. DOI 10.1111/j. 1744-7917.2012.01550.x.

[53] Christiaens O, Smagghe G. The challenge of RNAi-mediated control of hemipterans. Curr Opin Insect Sci 2014;6:15–21. DOI: http://dx.doi.org/10.1016/j.cois.2014.09.012.

[54] Hall DG, Shatters RG, Carpenter JE, Shapiro JP. Research toward an artificial diet for adult Asian Citrus Psyllid. Annal Entomol Soc Am 2010;03: 611–17. DOI:http://dx.doi.org/10.1603/AN10004.

[55] Hall DG, Richardson ML, Ammar E-D, Halbert SE. Asian citrus psyllid, *Diaphorina citri*, vector of citrus huanglongbing disease. Entomol Experiment Applic 2012;146:207–23. DOI: 10.1111/eea.12025.

[56] Hunter WB, Glick E, Paldi N, Bextine BR. Advances in RNA interference: dsRNA treatment in trees and grapevines for insect pest suppression. Southwest Entomol 2012;37:85–7. DOI: http://dx.doi.org/10.3958/059.037.0110.

[57] Upadhyay SK, Chandrashekar K, Thakur N, Verma PC, Borgio JF, Singh PK, Tuli R. RNA interference for the control of whiteflies (*Bemisia tabaci*) by oral route. J Biosci 2011;36:153–61. DOI:10.1007/s12038-011-9009-1.

[58] Borgio JF. RNAi mediated gene knockdown in sucking and chewing insect pests. J Biopesticides 2010;3:386–93. Available from: http://www.jbiopest.com/users/lw8/efiles/francis_borgio.pdf.

[59] Katoch R, Sethi A, Thakur N, Murdock LL. RNAi for insect control: current perspective and future challenges. Appl Biochem Biotechnol 2013;171:847–73. DOI:10.1007/s12010-013-0399-4.

[60] Tomizawa M, Noda H. High mortality caused by high dose of dsRNA in the green rice leafhopper *Nephotettix cincticeps* (Hemiptera: Cicadellidae). Appl Entomol Zoo 2013;48:553–59. DOI:10.1007/s13355-013-0211-5.

[61] Zhou X, Wheeler MM, Oi FM, Scharf ME. RNA interference in the termite *Reticulitermes flavipes* through ingestion of double-stranded RNA. Insect Biochem Molecul Biol 2008;38:805–15. DOI:10.1016/j.ibmb.2008.05.005.

[62] Zha W, Peng X, Chen R, Du B, Zhu L, He, G. Knockdown of midgut genes by dsRNA-transgenic plant-mediated RNA interference in the Hemipteran insect *Nilaparvata lugens*. PLoS One 2011;6(5):e20504. DOI:10.1371/journal.pone.0020504.

[63] Yu N, Christiaens O, Lui J, Niu J, Cappelle K, Caccia S, Huvenne H, Smagghe G. Delivery of dsRNA for RNAi in insects: an overview and future directions. Insect Sci 2013;20:4–40. Doi 10.1111/j.1744-7917.2012.01534.x.

[64] Zhang X, Zhang J, Zhu KY. Chitosan/double-stranded RNA nanoparticle-mediated RNA interference to silence chitin synthase genes through larval feeding in the African malaria mosquito (*Anopheles gambiae*). Insect Molecul Biol 2010;19:683–93. DOI: 10.1111/j.1365-2583.2010.01029.x

[65] Palli SR. RNA interference in Colorado potato beetle: steps toward development of dsRNA as a commercial insecticide. Curr Opin Insect Sci 2014;3. DOI: 10.1016/j.cois.2014.09.011.

[66] Petrick JS, Brower-Toland B, Jackson A, Kier LD. Safety assessment of food and feed from biotechnology-derived crops employing RNA-mediated gene regulation to achieve desired traits: a scientific review. Regul Toxicol Pharmacol 2013;66:167–76. DOI: http://dx.doi.org/10.1016/j.yrtph.2013.03.008.

[67] Koch A, Kogel K-H. New wind in the sails: improving the agronomic value of crop plants through RNAi-mediated gene silencing. Plant Biotechnol J 2014;12:821–31. DOI:10.1111/pbi.12226.

[68] Dubelman S, Fischer J, Zapata F, Huizinga K, Jiang CJ, et al. Environmental fate of double-stranded RNA in agricultural soils. PLoS ONE 2014;9. DOI:10.1371/journal.pone.0093155.

[69] Ivashuta SI, Petrick JS, Heisel SE, Zhang Y, Guo L, Reyholds TL, Rice JF, Allen E, Roberts JK. Endogenous small RNAs in grain: Semi-quantification and sequence homology to human and animal genes. Food Chem Toxicol 2009;47:353–60. DOI: 10.1016/j.fct.2008.11.025.

[70] AgroRNA, South Korea, [Internet]. Available from: http://www.agrorna.com/. Accessed: 2015/08/25.

[71] Nguyen TA, Fruehauf JH. *transkingdom* RNA interference (*tk*RNAi): a novel method to induce therapeutic gene silencing. T-Cell Protocols. Method Molecul Biol 2009;514:27–34. Available from: http://link.springer.com/protocol/10.1007%2F978-1-60327-527-9_3.

[72] APSE, LLC, [Internet]. Available from: http://www.apsellc.com/. Accessed: 2015/08/25.

[73] Hunter W, Ellis J, VanEngelsdorp D, Hayes J, Westervelt D, Glick E, Paldi N. Large-scale field application of RNAi technology reducing Israeli acute paralysis virus disease in honey bees (*Apis mellifera,* Hymenoptera: Apidae). PLoS Pathogens 2010;6:e1001160. DOI:10.1371/journal.ppat.1001160.

[74] Campbell EM, Budge GE, Bowman AS. Gene-knockdown in the honey bee mite *Varroa destructor* by a non-invasive approach: studies on a glutathione S-transferase. Parasites Vectors 2010;3:73. DOI:10.1186/1756-3305-3-73.

[75] Garbian Y, Maori E, Kalev H, Shafir S, Sela I. Bidirectional transfer of RNAi between honey bee and *Varroa destructor*: *Varroa* gene silencing reduces *Varroa* population. PLoS Pathogens 2012;8(12):e1003035. DOI: 10.1371/journal.ppat.1003035.

[76] Paldi N, Glick E, Oliva M, Zilberberg Y, Aubin L, Pettis JS, Chen YP, Evans JD. 2010. Effective gene silencing of a microsporidian parasite associated with honey bee (*Apis mellifera*) colony declines. Appl Environ Microbiol 2010;76:5960–4. DOI:10.1128/AEM.01067-10.

[77] Elzen GW, Hardee DD. United States Department of Agriculture–Agricultural Research Service, Research on managing insect resistance to insecticides. Pest Management Sci 2003;59:770–6.

[78] Blair CD, Olson KE. The role of RNA interference (RNAi) in Arbovirus-vector interactions. Viruses 2015;7:820–43. DOI: 10.3390/v7020820.

[79] The Nobel Prize in Physiology or Medicine 2006. Andrew Z. Fire and Craig C. Mello "For their discovery of RNA interference - gene silencing by double-stranded RNA". Available from: http://www.nobelprize.org/nobel_prizes/medicine/laureates/2006/. [Accessed: 2015-08-25].

[80] Whyard S. Insecticidal RNA, the long and short of it. Science 2015;347:950–91. DOI: 10.1126/science.aaa7722.

[81] Lane AN, Fan TW-M. Survey and summary. Regulation of mammalian nucleotide metabolism and biosynthesis. Nucleic Acids Res 2015;43:1–20. DOI: 10.1093/nar/gkv047.

9

In Search of New Methodologies for Efficient Insect Pest Control: The RNAi "Movement"

Anna Kourti, Luc Swevers and
Dimitrios Kontogiannatos

Abstract

The development of insecticide formulations with new mechanisms of action (modes of action, MOAs) is a huge priority for pesticide industry. This priority has become apparent during the last few years after (a) the observed increase in insect resistance for the most widely used active substances and (b) the harmful effects of the excessive use of pesticides on human health, environment, beneficial insects and fish. Silencing of genes by RNAi (RNA interference) technology provides an alternative, selective to species level, environmentally friendly strategy to combat insect pests. Double-stranded RNA molecules (double-stranded RNAs, dsRNAs) targeting important developmental genes are taken up by the digestive tract of the targeted insect speciesand induce RNAi, which results in inhibition of growth, development and reproduction of the targeted insect species. After the rapid development of RNAi technology in the past 10 years, biotech industry is seeking for new applications aimed at producing environmentally friendly genetic insecticides or genetically modified plants (GMPs) that induce environmental RNAi in the targeted insect species. These technologies are expected on the market at the end of this decade. In this chapter, we exploit established methods involving recent initiatives of RNAi technology with respect to the development of new bio-insecticidal formulations.

Keywords: modes of action, RNA interference, double-stranded RNAs, genetically modified plants, agricultural biotechnology

1. Introduction

Eukaryotic cells are equipped with a conserved mechanism by which exogenously added or endogenously expressed RNA duplexes (double-stranded RNA or dsRNA) are directly degradedin to their complementary endogenously encoded messenger RNA (mRNA), resulting in targeted gene silencing. This phenomenon is generally referred to as RNA interference (RNAi) [1, 2]. In plant and animal organisms, RNAi provides a line of defense against viruses and parasitic genetic elements (transposons) while a similar, but mechanistically separated, mechanism regulates tissue-specific gene expression at translational level [3]. Induction of RNAi begins when high-molecular-weight dsRNAs are selectively degraded by type III ribonucleases encoded by RNAse III-related genes known as Dicer or Dicer-like genes. The Dicer enzymes appear to specifically act on the dsRNAs leading to their degradation (digestion) by their 5'–3' ends resulting in the production of small 21–24 base (ds) ribonucleotides known as small interfering RNAs (siRNAs) [4]. The double-stranded siRNAs are incorporated into a multiprotein complex known as the RNA-induced-silencing complex (RISC) that is actually induced by the presence of the RNAs. In this complex, the "passenger" (sense) strand of siRNAs is degraded and the antisense or guide strand is directed to the mRNA target. The guide sequence enables Watson-Crick complementarity to the mRNA target which is enzymatically degraded by a family of proteins called "Argonauts" (Argonaute proteins), thereby preventing translation of the mRNA. Arguably, the mechanism of gene silencing is specialized and targeted at the nucleotide sequence level. The possibility of specific gene downregulation through RNAi has proven mainly in insects which lack methods for functional genomic analysis [5]. The extremely interesting observation that dsRNA molecules taken up through the digestive tract of the nematode *Caenorhabditis elegans* induce gene-specific downregulation [6, 7] created hopes that oral dsRNA uptake could regulate gene expression in other invertebrates as well, including insects. This technology could be used for the reasonable purpose of developing environmentally friendly pesticides to combat agricultural insect species.

The first-historical publications describing the use of RNAi technology in crop insect control were those of Baum et al. [8] and Mao et al. [9]. These researchers showed that genetically modified plants expressing dsRNAs of entomological origin could influence the development and growth of phytophagous insect species which were feeding on these plants. Corn plants expressing hairpin dsRNAs, which target the A subunit of the ATPase gene in *Diabrotica virgifera virgifera* (western corn rootworm, WCR), showed significant protection from the damage caused by this insect species [8]. Following previous discoveries, *Arabidopsis* plants expressing double-stranded RNA hairpins targeting the cytochrome P450 monooxygenase gene in the corn pest *Helicoverpa armigera* showed decreased resistance to the sesquiterpene gossypol [9]. The above developments in gene-targeting research gave birth to a new term known as environmental RNAi [10]. Environmental RNAi involves the phenomenon in which RNAi is induced after environmental exposure to insect dsRNAs by oral or topical administration. Successful environmental RNAi has been reported in a wide range of insect families belonging to the classes of Coleoptera, Diptera, Dictyoptera, Hemiptera, Hymenoptera, Isoptera, Lepidoptera, Neuroptera and Orthoptera [11]. The technology of environmental RNAi is the best candidate for replacing conventional insecticides and avoiding collateral damages to the ecosystem, beneficial insects and human health.

2. dsRNA delivery systems

2.1. dsRNA injection

The most widely used methodology for administrating dsRNA molecules in insect cells is by injecting volumes of *in vitro* synthesized dsRNAs into their hemocoel. This methodology was mostly used for functional analysis of genes in model and non-model insects from the early 2000s till date. DsRNAs could be *in vitro* synthesized using different approaches (there are many alternatives but we describe the one which was extensively used in our laboratory). In this approach, the gene of interest should be cloned in both sense and antisense directions in plasmids flanked with at least one T7 promoter. Then, the plasmids are linearized with restriction enzymes and transcribed in two different reactions (using T7 RNA polymerase) to synthesize sense and antisense ssRNAs. The complementary RNA molecules are then mixed and annealed. For the annealing step, the two transcripts should be mixed in precisely equimolar amounts (**Figure 1**). We have been using this methodology for synthesizing a wide range of targets for functional analysis of genes of the lepidopteron *Sesamia nonagrioides*. For the juvenile hormone esterase-related gene of *Sesamia*, we have targeted different parts of the full gene transcript by synthesizing *in vitro* three different dsRNAs, corresponding to a 472-bp part of its 5′-translated region, a 1276-bp part of its central translated, 3′-translated and part of its 3′ -untranslated region and a 1725-bp part encompassing both of the above regions, which spanned 94% of the total cDNA. All transcripts resulted in gene-specific knockdown of *SnJHER* but only the 1725 bp dsRNA was able to cause a significant phenotype [12]. In order to silence the 1276-bp part, we ligated a SnJHER 1276-bp fragment into the MCS of the RNAi L4440 vector (**Figure 2A**). The L4440/ SnJHER1276 plasmid was then linearized with either XhoI or NcoI (to create sense and antisense plasmids) and used as template for RNA synthesis. After DNase treatment (to destroy the DNA templates), sense and antisense ssRNAs were annealed to form dsRNA and analyzed in agarose gels before injection to insects (**Figure 2B**).

In other insect species, a wide range of successful experiments of intra-hemolymph RNAi have already been published and some of them will be described below:

- In adult fruit flies, RNAi could be induced by injecting dsRNAs into the abdomen of anesthetized individuals targeting genes which were expressed in their central nervous system (CNS) [13].
- In *Bombyx mori*, injection of double-stranded RNA corresponding to the silkworm white gene (Bmwh3) into preblastoderm eggs of wild-type silkworm induced phenotypes similar to those observed with mutants of the white egg 3 locus. The induced phenotypes were characterized by the presence of white eggs and translucent larval skin [14].
- Additionally, parental silencing of the hemolin gene from the Giant silkmoth, *Hyalophora cecropia*, demonstrated that hemolin is crucial for the normal development of embryos. When RNAi females were mated, no larvae emerged from their eggs and when dissected, the eggs revealed malformed embryos [15].

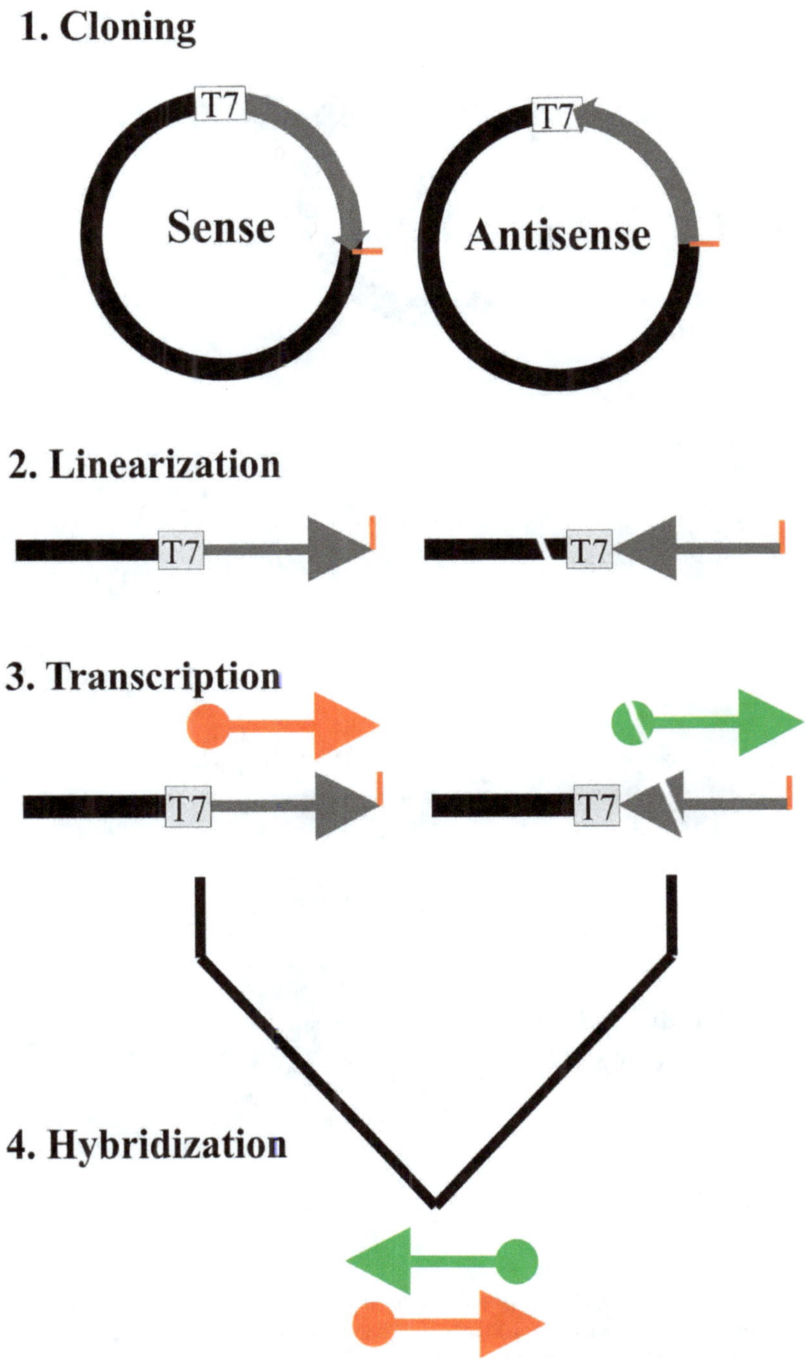

Figure 1. *In vitro* dsRNA synthesis strategy. Plasmid sequences are indicated in black while inserts for RNA productions downstream of the T7 promoter (cloned in two different orientations) are displayed in gray. Sense and antisense RNAs are indicated in red and green, respectively.

- In *Manducta sexta* injection of double-stranded integrin-beta1 RNA into larvae resulted in decreased integrin beta1 expression in plasmatocytes and significantly suppressed encapsulation [16].

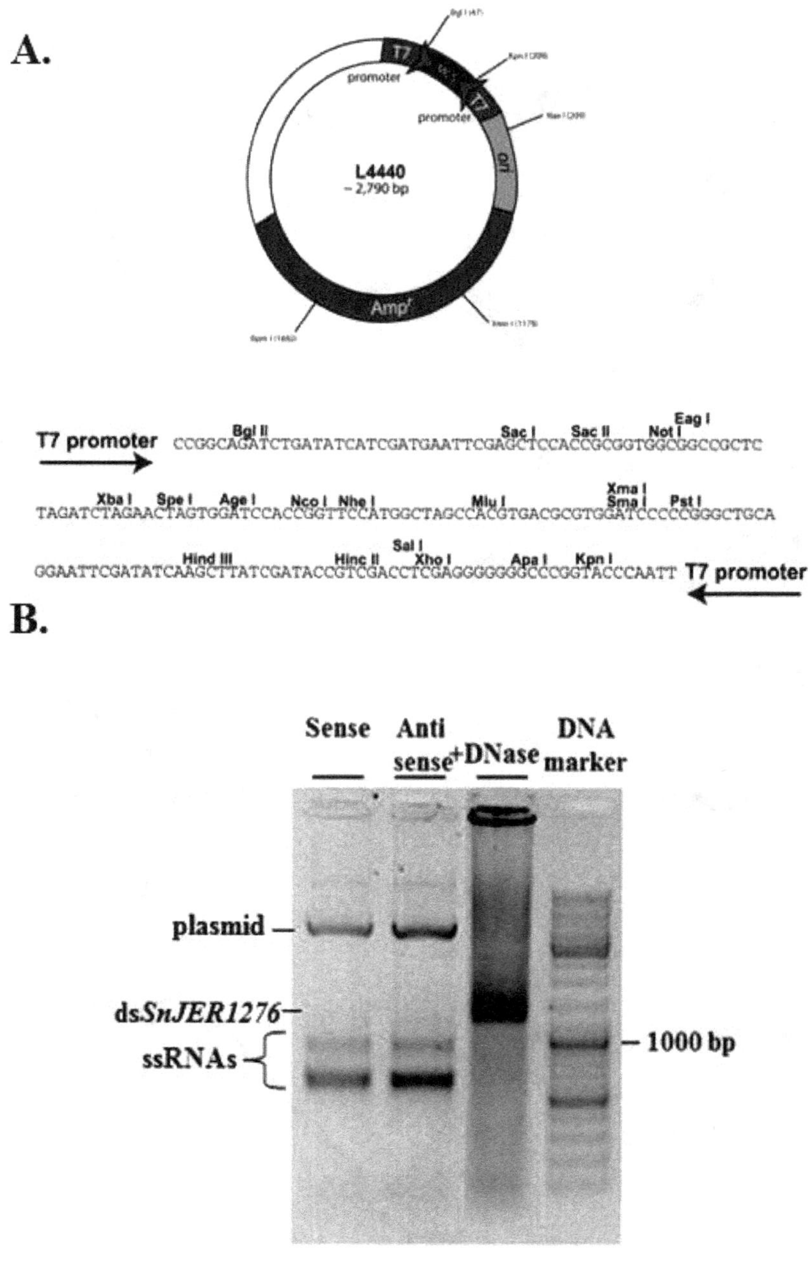

Figure 2. Production of dsRNA corresponding to the gene *SnJHER*. **A**. Schematic representation of L4440 plasmid and its polylinker for cloning gene fragments for dsRNA production (https://www.addgene.org/1654/). The polylinker is flanked on either side by a T7 RNA polymerase promoter for RNA synthesis. **B**. Synthesis of ds*SnJHER*1276. Sense and antisense ssRNAs running in 1% w/v agarose gel (first and second lanes counting from the left). The two ssRNAs were annealed and subjected to DNase treatment (third lane). DNA marker is being shown on the fourth lane.

- While in *Aedes aegypti* injection of double-stranded RNA corresponding to the broad gene (BR) isoform Z2 led to a significant decrease in the expression of the *Vitellogenin* (Vg) gene at 8 and 24 h post blood meal. Knockdown of Z1 or Z4 resulted in enhanced Vg expression beyond its normal expression time [17].

- Injection of both dsRNA/siRNA could induce the silence of chitin synthase gene A (CHSA), which is an important gene for the growth and development of cuticles and trachea in beet armyworm, *Spodoptera exigua*. The cuticle of CHSA-silenced insects was disordered and the epithelial walls of larval trachea did not expand. Moreover, injections significantly increased abnormalities relative to control larvae [18].
- In *Tribolium castaneum*, injection of dsRNA prepared using the common or isoform-specific regions of ecdysone receptor (EcR) and ultraspiracle (USP) genes as templates caused derailment of development [19].
- In *S. frugiperda*, silencing of the allatostatin AS-C-type (Spofr/Manse-AS) or the allatotropin AT 2 (Spofr-AT 2) genes after intra-hemolymph administration resulted in reduction of their transcript levels in brain and gut of last instar larvae and adults. This suppression led to an increased JH titer in larvae [20].
- In *Gryllus bimaculatus*, injection of the circadian clock gene period (*G. bimaculatus* period, Gb'per) dsRNA into the abdomen of third instar nymphs knocked down the mRNA levels to 25% of that in control animals. Most Gb'per dsRNA-injected nymphs lost their circadian locomotor activity rhythm, while those injected with DsRed2 dsRNA as a negative control clearly maintained the rhythm [21].
- The membrane-bound trehalase genes of *S. exigua SeTre-1 and SeTre-2* were analyzed by dsRNA injections. The RNA interference (RNAi) of either SeTre-1 or SeTre-2 was gene-specific and effective, with efficiency rates up to 83% at 72 h post injection. After RNAi of SeTre-1 and SeTre-2, significant higher mortality rates were observed during the larval-pupal and pupal-adult stages [13].
- In *D. virgifera virgifera* LeConte (Coleoptera: Chrysomelidae), injection of laccase 2 DvvLac2-specific double-stranded RNA resulted in the prevention of post-molt cuticular tanning, while injection of chitin synthase 2 DvvCHS2-specific dsRNA reduced chitin levels in midguts. Silencing of both DvvLac2 and DvvCHS2 was confirmed by real-time polymerase chain reaction (RT-PCR) and quantitative RT-PCR [22].
- DsRNA-based gene silencing resulted in a dramatic reduction in the levels of the corresponding mRNA in the *Locusta migratoria manilensis* (Meyen) nymphs injected with dsRNA of chitin synthase 1 LmCHS1, or either of its two variants, LmCHS1A and LmCHS1B. mortalities of 95, 88 and 51% were observed in the locusts injected with the LmCHS1, LmCHS1A and LmCHS1B dsRNA, respectively [23].
- In *Leptinotarsa decemlineata*, specific interference of Ldace1, an ortholog of *Anopheles gambiae Agace1* by means of dsRNA injection, resulted in a reduction of AChE activity to an approximate 50% compared to control, while interference of Ldace2 reduced AChE activity to an approximate 85%. Interference of Ldace1 in CPB adults caused a significant increase in mortality (43%) as early as 3 days post injection (p.i.). Interference of Ldace2 also caused a significant increase in mortality (29%) compared to control, although at seven days p.i. [24].
- In *G. bimaculatus* and the firebrat *Thermobia domestica*, a dose-dependent effect of dsRNA was observed to achieve knockdown of clock genes. However, this effect was affected by the particular gene that was silenced and the insect species (*Gryllus* versus *Thermobia*) [25].

- Injection of CHS dsRNA interfered with egg development in the ovary and the eggs that were laid were dark of color and not viable. Fluorescence microscopy demonstrated reduced deposition of chitin in previtellogenic and vitellogenic oocytes in the ovaries [26].
- In a later work, HSP70/HSC70 knockdown of *Rhodnius prolixus* insects showed lower resistance to prolonged starvation in comparison to appropriate controls, dying between 32 and 40 days after dsRNA injection. After blood feeding, the physiological effects of HSP70/HSC70 knockdown were more prominent and the insects died even earlier, within 14–20 days after feeding (21–27 days after dsRNA injection). These bugs showed impaired blood processing and digestion; reduced energetic metabolism and the midgut immune responses were compromised [27].

2.2. Oral delivery of dsRNAs

Oral delivery of dsRNAs aims to silence the selected gene after gut-mediated uptake and transport to the insect cells. If oral delivery is efficient, then much higher possibilities exist to formulate a dsRNA-based insecticide. For orally delivering dsRNAs, dsRNAs should be *in vitro* synthesized as described previously. Then, the dsRNAs are incorporated to the artificial diets of the insects or even sprayed in the plants which are used to be fed on. Important examples (highlights) from the literature are given below:

- Walshe et al. [28] first demonstrated specific gene knockdown by feeding in dipteran species. This was a first example of RNAi in a blood-sucking insect by including dsRNA in its blood meal. Delivery of dsRNA through the blood meal of *Glossina morsitans* was as effective as dsRNA injection with respect to the silencing of the midgut-expressed gene TsetseEP. By contrast, the gene 2A192 that is expressed in the fat body was only knocked down after dsRNA injection. Feeding of dsRNA reduced significantly the mortality rates of the flies compared with the injection treatment.
- Bautista et al. [29] silenced a P450 CYP6BG1 gene by dsRNA droplet feeding in *Plutella xylostella* in order to show its involvement in permethrin resistance. Quantitative real-time PCR showed efficient reduction of expression of CYP6BG1 transcripts in midgut and carcass after oral delivery, which was reflected in reduced total P450 activities of microsomal preparations and which resulted in significant reduction in resistance to the insecticide permethrin. The experiments indicate the participation of overexpressed CYP6BG1 in the resistance mechanism against permethrin [29].
- RNAi has been used successfully to silence endogenous honey bee genes by feeding [30]. This was the first successful large-scale real-world use of RNAi for insect-disease control. RNAi was shown to prevent bees from succumbing to infection from Israeli Acute Paralysis Virus, IAPV, under laboratory conditions. In this study, IAPV-specific homologous dsRNAs were used in the field, under natural beekeeping conditions in order to prevent mortality and improve the overall health of bees infected with IAPV [30].
- In the whitefly, *Bemisia tabaci* (Gennadius) (Homoptera: Aleyrodidae), Lü and Wan [31] explored the role of heat-shock protein (Hsp) genes in both male and female sexes by dsRNA feeding.

- Chen et al. [32] examined the effects of using a feeding-based RNAi technique to target the gene trehalose phosphate synthase (TPS) in the brown planthopper, *Nilaparvata lugens*. DsRNA feeding resulted in rapid and significant reduction in expression levels of TPS mRNA and enzymatic activity. Developmental abnormalities were observed in dsRNA-fed *N. lugens* larvae which resulted in lethal effects.
- Hunt et al. [33] developed an RNAi-mediated bioassay to explore proposed connections between expression of hexameric storage proteins and worker versus gyne (potential future foundress) castes in naturally founded colonies of the wasp genus *Polistes* (*P. metricus*). They targeted the hexamerin 2 gene in fifth (last) instar larvae by feeding with double-stranded hexamerin 2 RNA directly to larvae in naturally founded colonies in the field. Their results pave the way for functional genomic research that can contribute significantly to learning the interactions between environment and development and its significance for paper wasp evolution and behavioral ecology [33].
- Luan et al. [34] developed a new and high throughput methodology to silence whitefly genes using a leaf-mediated dsRNA-feeding method. A leaf-mediated dsRNA-feeding method was developed to test silencing of whitefly genes in high-throughput format. While silencing of ecdysone biosynthetic and regulatory genes had little effect on survival and fecundity of adult whiteflies, reduced survival and delayed development were observed during the treatment of the nymphal stages.
- Moreover, Mao and Zeng [35] performed RNAi at the second instar stage to knock down *hunchback* (*hb*) expression in the pea aphid, *Acyrthosiphon pisum*. Continuous feeding of *Aphb* dsRNA mixed in their artificial diet led to reduction of *Aphb* transcripts and rise of insect lethality. Their results indicated that the gene *hunchback* was an efficient RNAi target for managing populations of aphids.
- Li et al. [36] introduced dsRNAs of P450 CYP6CM1 genes corresponding to the B and Q biotypes into the insect body of *B. tabaci* adults through membrane feeding. RNAi of the P450 CYP6CM1 gene reduced gene expression, increased mortality and inhibited the ability to detoxify a pesticide or a plant secondary metabolite in both biotypes of *B. tabaci*, with better efficacy in B biotype than in Q biotype.
- Finally, Abd El Halim et al. [37] evaluated oral delivery of dsRNAs targeting sodium ion channel paralytic A *(TcNav)* gene in *T. castaneum* as a viable means of controlling this insect pest. Oral delivery of dsRNA caused dose-dependent mortalities between 19 and 51.34% accompanied by a significant knockdown in gene expression following 3 days of continuous feeding. The majority of larvae injected with, or fed, dsRNA died during the final larval stage prior to pupation. This work provided evidence of a viable RNAi-based strategy for insect control.

2.3. Bacterial-mediated RNAi

Bacterial dsRNA administration is based on the observations of Timmons and Fire [6] which showed that ingestion of bacterially expressed dsRNAs could produce specific and potent genetic interference in *C. elegans*. This approach uses an RNase III-deficient *Escherichia coli* strain known as HT115 (DE3) [F-, mcrA, mcrB, IN(rrnD-rrnE)1, rnc14::Tn10(DE3 lysogen: lavUV5 promoter -T7 polymerase]. In this methodology, the gene of interest is being cloned between two T7 promoters on a special RNAi plasmid known as L4440 (T7p, T7p, lacZN, OriF1) (**Figure 2A**). The plasmid is being transformed in HT115 cells and dsRNA production is achieved after induction with IPTG. The induced cells are then introduced in the worm's growth media and RNAi is achieved after a short period of incubation.

Similarly in insects the IPTG-induced bacteria are incorporated in their artificial diets or they are even sprayed in plant organs that insects are feeding on and RNAi is induced after a period of continuous feeding (**Figure 3**).

The successful application of bacterial-mediated RNAi has been reported in several cases:

- Tian et al. [38] showed that the growth and development of *S. exigua* larvae fed with HT115 cells expressing dsRNAs of the chitin synthase gene A (SeCHSA) was disturbed, resulting in lethality. The survival rates of fifth instar larvae, prepupal and pupal stages were significantly lower than those of controls.
- Similarly, Li et al. [39] used genetically engineered HT115 *E. coli* cells. Engineered bacteria were generated that produce specific dsRNAs targeting several essential genes in *Bactrocera dorsalis*, such as the ribosomal protein Rpl 19, the type V ATPase D subunit, the fatty acid elongase Noa and the small GTPase Rab11. Quantitative real-time PCR indicated

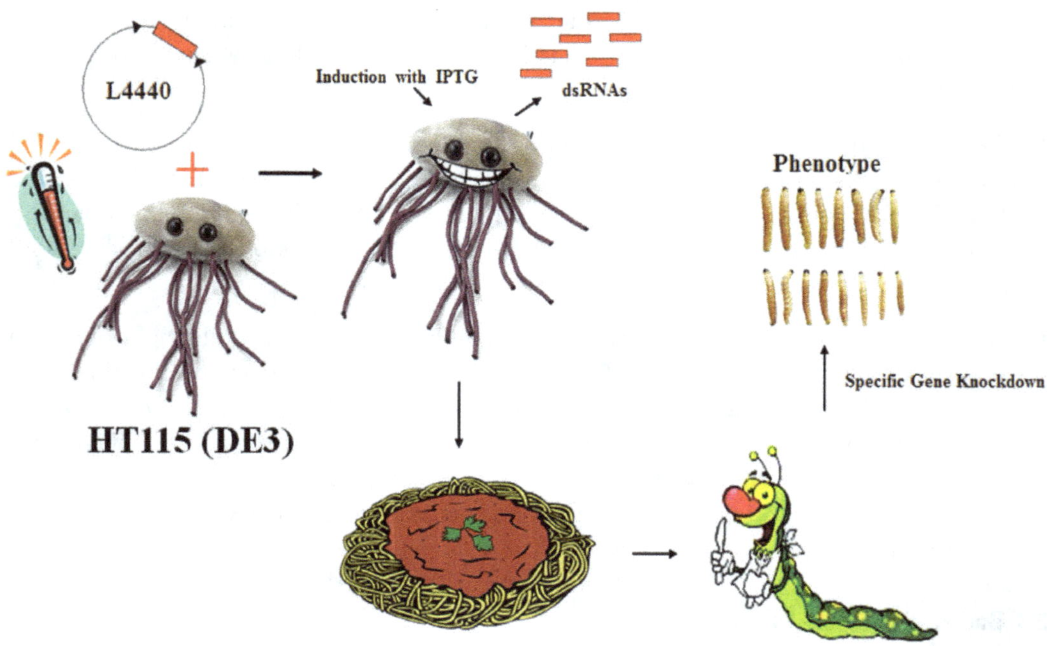

Figure 3. Strategy behind bacterial-mediated RNAi. The gene of interest is being cloned in the RNAi L4440 plasmid and transformed to competent HT115 cells. The transformed cells are then induced with IPTG and incorporated in insect's diet in order to induce RNAi.

that feeding of both engineered bacteria and isolated dsRNAs proved effective at silencing the four targeted genes when compared with nonspecific (EGFP) dsRNA.

- In the Colorado potato beetle, *L. decemlineata* (Say) (CPB), Zhu et al. [40] successfully triggered silencing of five target genes by dsRNA feeding resulting in significant mortality and reduced body weight gain in the treated beetles. These results suggested that the efficient induction of RNAi using bacteria to deliver dsRNA is a possible method for the management of CPB.
- Moreover, Zhang et al. [41] demonstrated the efficacy of RNAi in the cotton bollworm, *H. armigera,* using bacterial-mediated dsRNA expression of CYP6B6 gene. Gene and protein expression levels of CYP6B6 were reduced in *H. armigera* larvae fed with HT115 bacteria expressing CYP6B6 dsRNAs.
- Taracena et al. [42] silenced *R. prolixus* heme-binding protein (RHBP) and catalase (CAT) genes after feeding nymphs and adult triatomine insects with dsRNA expressing HT115 bacteria. The RNA interference effect was systemic and temporal. RHBP expression in the fat body was reduced by 99% three days after feeding and CAT expression was reduced by 99 and 96% in the ovary and the posterior midgut, respectively, 5 days after ingestion.

Essential for successful RNAi-feeding experiments is correct dsRNA induction before the oral administration step. A general protocol for bacterial-mediated dsRNA expression is given as follows. In this experiment, we cloned the 1276 bp part of *S. nonagrioides* juvenile hormone esterase-related gene in the L4440 plasmid and then we used it to transform HT115 (DE3)-competent cells. We used empty L4440-transformed HT115 cells as control. Single colonies of HT115/L4440-SnJHER1276 and HT115/L4440 cells were cultured in LB at 37°C with shaking at 220 rpm overnight. The cultures were diluted 50-fold in 100 ml LB supplemented with 100 μg/ml ampicillin plus 15 μg/ml tetracycline (Sigma) and cultured at 37°C to OD600 = 0.5. After induction of T7 RNA polymerase expression with 400 μM IPTG for 4 h with continuous shaking at 37°C, the bacteria were centrifuged (5000 g, 10 min) and the pellet was re-suspended with 0.5 ml of water. Total RNAs were extracted from bacterial cells using Trizol (Sigma). To remove excess ssRNA, RNA samples were treated with 1 μg of RNase-A (Sigma) in the presence of 0.3 M NaCl, which protects against digestion of dsRNA. The reaction occurred for 10 minutes at 37°C. The length and the quality of the produced dsRNAs were confirmed by electrophoresis on 1% agarose gel (**Figure 4**). As shown in **Figure 4** in the no RNase-A lane, no band was observed for the control L4440-transformed bacteria while a band running to ~1200 bp was observed in the L4440-SnJHER1276-transformed bacteria. After adding 1 μg of RNase-A, all RNAs were degraded leaving unaffected the DNA band. In the third lane after co-incubating dsRNAs with 1 μg of RNase-A in salinity of 0.3 M NaCl, only ssRNAs are degraded while dsRNAs remain unaffected. It was reported that RNase-A in high salinity buffers selectively digests ssRNAs leaving undigested the dsRNAs [43]. An alternative of the previous experiment was published in our laboratory by Kontogiannatos et al. [12]. In this experiment, we used a JHER hairpin expressed in pGEM T-easy plasmid which was used to transform HT115 cells and induce dsRNA expression.

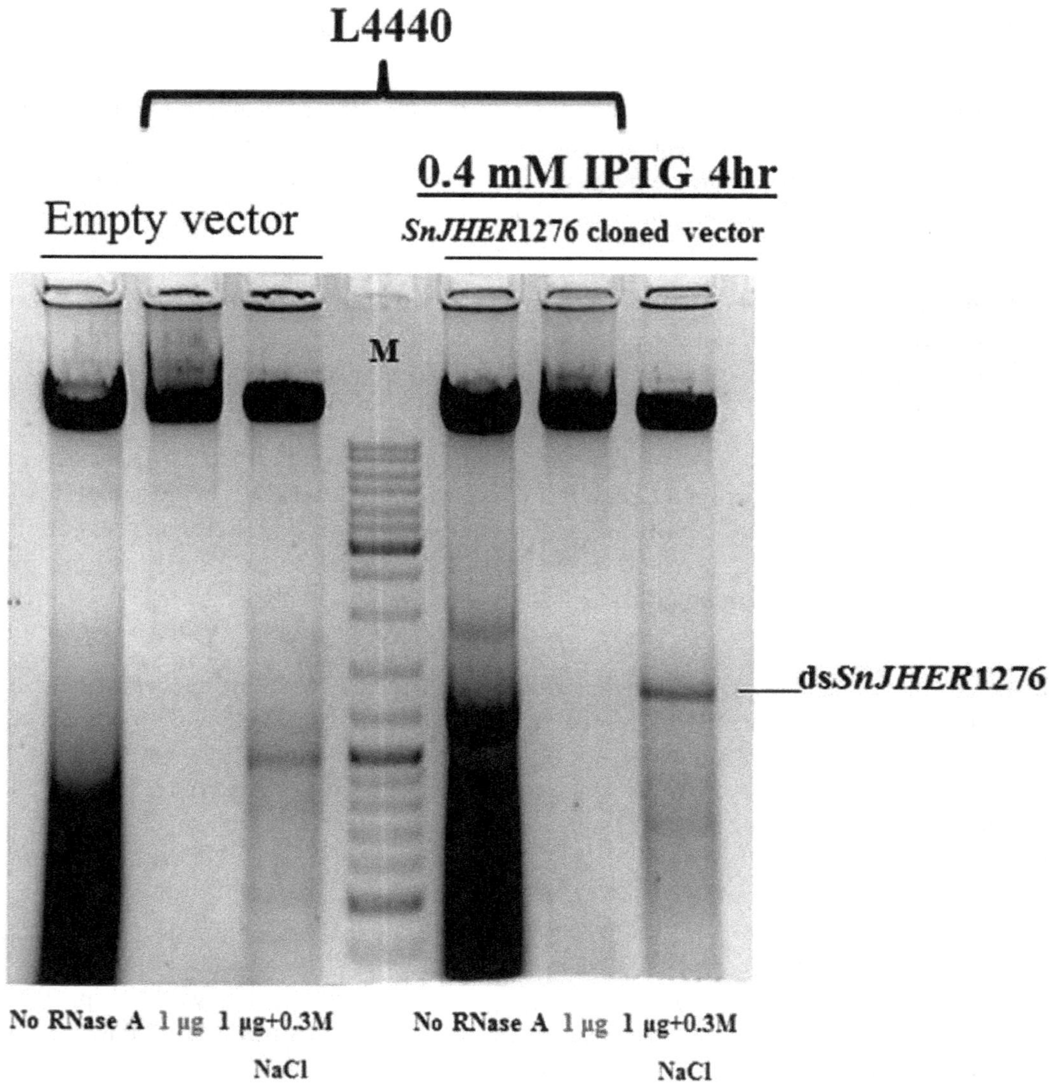

Figure 4. Bacterial-mediated production of SnJHER1276 in HT115 cells. Total RNA isolated from L4440 or L4440-SnJHER1276-transformed HT115 cells was analyzed in 1% w/v agarose gel. RNA extracts were treated with RNase A or RNase A+0.3 M NaCl. M: Molecular marker. Production of ds*SHER*1276 is indicated.

There is an alternative procedure for bacterial-mediated RNAi in which dsRNAs are first isolated from bacteria before injection into insects. In the following experiment, we silenced *S. nonagrioides ultraspiracle* gene after injecting bacterially expressed dsRNAs into its hemolymph. For doing that, we cloned a 689-bp fragment of *SnUSP* partial cDNA sequence (GenBank: JN704569) to the L4440 plasmid which was then used to transform competent HT115 cells. The protocol described previously was used to induce dsRNA expression. HT115 ds*SnUSP* expressing bacterial cells were Trizol treated and total RNAs were extracted and analyzed in 1% w/v agarose gels. In this case, we did not perform RNase-protection assay since dsRNAs were clearly visualized (**Figure 5B**). Note that in **Figures 4** and **5B**, a 1000-bp band exists in the empty L4440-transformed bacteria which disappear when the gene of interest is cloned. Total RNA extracts were purified and injected in fifth instar larvae at day 3 (L5d3) and specific phenotypes were observed (**Figure 5C**). A proportion of ds*SnUSP689*-injected animals died presenting a large range of developmental abnormalities. Gene-specific downregulation was observed after RT-PCR analysis (data not shown).

2.4. Plant-mediated RNAi

The observation that genetically modified plants expressing dsRNAs targeting specific insect genes could induce RNAi in the insect pests was first reported in independent publications of Baum et al. [8] and Mao et al. [9]. Baum et al. showed that corn plants expressing hairpin dsRNAs that target the A subunit of ATPase gene in the western corn rootworm were sig-

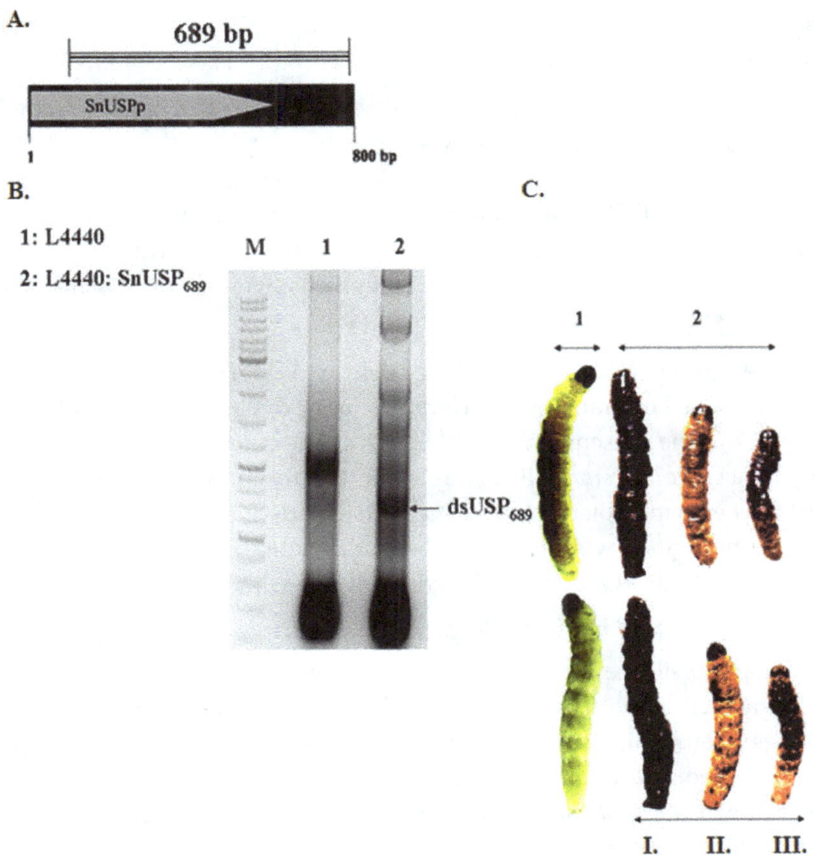

Figure 5. Phenotypes observed after knockdown of *SnUSP* by dsRNA produced in bacteria. **A.** Schematic representation of the partial cDNA sequence of *Sesamia nonagrioides ultraspiracle* gene (GenBank: JN704569). The bar above the sequence indicates the 689 bp fragment used for RNAi experiments. **B.** Confirmation of dsUSP689 synthesis in HT115 IPTG-induced bacteria. Total RNAs isolated from IPTG-induced HT115/L4440 (1) and HT115/L4440:SnUSP689 (2) bacteria were analyzed in 1% w/v agarose gels. C. Lethal phenotypes of L5d3-injected *S. nonagrioides* larvae injected with total RNAs isolated from the HT115/L4440:SnUSP689 (2) bacteria. Control HT115/L4440-injected animals are also indicated (1).

nificantly protected by the damage caused by this pest [8]. Furthermore, *Arabidopsis* plants expressing dsRNA hairpins targeting the cytochrome P450 monooxygenase gene in the corn pest *H. armigera* led to decreased resistance to the sesquiterpene gossypol to the feeding insects [9]. Following these publications of proof-of-principle, several other reports have documented the successful application of plant-mediated RNAi:

- In *H. armigera*, a molt-regulating transcription factor gene was selected to be used in plant-mediated RNAi experiments. Four different fragments covering the coding sequence of *HaHR3* were initially tested by bacterial-mediated RNAi. The most effective fragment (in terms of RNAi efficiency) was used for *Nicotiana tabacum* agrobacterium-mediated transformation. When *H. armigera* larvae were fed the *E. coli* or transgenic plants, the HaHR3 mRNA and protein levels dramatically decreased, resulting in developmental deformities and larval lethality [44].
- Similarly, dsRNAs of the gap gene hunchback (hb) of *Myzus persicae* were overexpressed in transgenic tobacco. Continuous feeding of neonate aphids on transgenic diet reduced *Mphb* mRNA level in the fed aphids and inhibited insect reproduction [35].
- In the brown planthopper *N. lugens*, a common 360-bp fragment between ecdysone receptor (EcR) NlEcR-A and NlEcR-B genes was used to construct a transgenic RNAi rice line. After newly hatched nymphs of *N. lugens* fed on the transgenic rice lines, effective RNAi was observed. The NlEcR expression levels were decreased in all lines compared with the controls. In all lines, survival rates of nymphal stages were nearly 90%, but the average number of offspring per pair in the treated groups was significantly less than that observed in the control, with a decrease of 44.18–66.27% [45].
- Efficient RNAi after plant-mediated dsRNA delivery was reported in the *Triticum-Sitobion* system. *S. avenae* fed on transgenic *T. aestivum* lines expressing dsRNAs of its carboxylesterase (CbE E4) gene presented reduced CbE E4 gene expression. The number of aphids grown on transgenic *T. aestivum* lines was lower than the number raised on non-transgenic plants. CbE E4 enzyme isolated from *S. avenae* fed on dsCbE plants hydrolyzed only up to 20–30% Phoxim solution within 40 min whereas a solution of the enzyme from CbE E4 fed on control plants hydrolyzed 60% of Phoxim solution within 40 min [46].
- Efficient plant-mediated RNAi was also reported in *H. armigera* [47]. Researchers used this technology to silence the *arginine kinase* (*AK*) gene of *H. armigera* (*HaAK*), encoding a phosphotransferase that plays a critical role in cellular energy metabolism in invertebrate species. Transgenic *Arabidopsis* plants producing *HaAK* dsRNAs were generated by *Agrobacterium*-mediated transformation. The feeding bioassays clearly showed that resistance of transgenic *Arabidopsis* plants to *H. armigera* was improved and levels of *HaAK* transcripts were drastically suppressed.
- Parental RNAi after plant-mediated dsRNA delivery was observed in *M. persicae*. DsRNA producing *A. thaliana* lines were constructed to target genes with different functions in the aphid. RNAi-mediated knockdown in aphids was achieved independently of gene identity and function and could reduce original expression levels by 70% between 4 and 8 days after feeding on dsRNA-producing transgenic *A. thaliana*. Target genes were also

downregulated in nymphs born from mothers exposed to dsRNA-producing transgenic plants and the RNAi effect lasted twice as long (12–14 days) in these nymphs [48].

2.5. Virus-mediated RNAi

The use of viruses is a less common methodology to transfer dsRNAs into the insect tissues. Virus-mediated-RNAi involves the expression of a dsRNA transgene into a virus which is then used to infect the insect cell or a tissue in order to express dsRNAs intracellularly. This methodology has not been used extensively because of the general viral interference with normal cell physiology; for instance, baculoviruses cause high lethality and potential phenotypes could not be distinguished between dsRNA-producing and control viruses. In addition, viruses can produce inhibitors of RNAi, thereby lowering silencing efficiency [49].

In order to successfully distinguish effects of virus-mediated RNAi, wild-type viruses should be somehow inactivated or at least should not cause highly toxic effects in the insect host. The first report of successful viral dsRNA delivery was made by Hajos et al. [50]. In this paper, the researchers used a recombinant baculovirus, *Autographa californica* multicapsid nucleopolyhedrovirus (AcMNPV), to express *Heliothis virescens* juvenile hormone esterase (JHE) gene in antisense orientation, driven by the viral p10 promoter. Infection with this recombinant virus greatly reduced the hemolymph JHE levels and resulted in aberrant morphogenesis of final-instar *H. virescens* larvae. This was the first time that baculovirus-mediated gene silencing could be accomplished and utilized to dissect insect development and to design a new class of baculovirus-based insecticides.

One of the most interesting virus-mediated RNAi reports is by Uhlirova et al. [51]. In this paper, researchers used a recombinant Sindbis virus as a tool to silence the gene encoding for the transcription factor Broad-Complex (BR-C) in *B. mori*. Sindbis virus with a BR-C antisense expression cassette reduced BR-C mRNA expression levels in infected tissues via an RNAi mechanism. BR-C silencing resulted in developmental arrest at the larval-pupal transition or in defective differentiation of adult compound eyes, legs and wings. Also the programmed cell death of the larval silk glands was prevented after RNAi of BR-C. *B. mori* nucleopolyhedrovirus (BmNPV)-mediated RNAi was demonstrated by our laboratory in a work by Kontogiannatos et al. [12]. Even if BmNPV's spectrum is extremely narrow, infection of the non-target species *S. nonagrioides* is feasible. In order to assess which kind of baculovirus is suitable for infection of *S. nonagrioides* larvae, we performed bioassays with genetically modified AcMNPV and BmNPV viruses expressing a GFP cassette under the control of *B. mori* actin promoter. Infected insects with 10^7 pfu/ml of the AcMNPV-BmA::GFP virus had significant higher mortality rates in almost 90% of the total injected animals. These animals presented all typical symptoms of polyhedrosis. In addition, the survived animals presented several developmental abnormalities, failing to complete normally their developmental cycle. In contrast to AcMNPV, infected insects with 10^7 pfu/ml of the BmNPV-BmA::GFP virus were able to proceed through their developmental stages and none of them presented signs of polyhedrosis. Both viruses were located mostly in the fat body tissues, in hemolymph (**Figure 6**), in epidermal cells and in tracheoles of the infected animals [12].

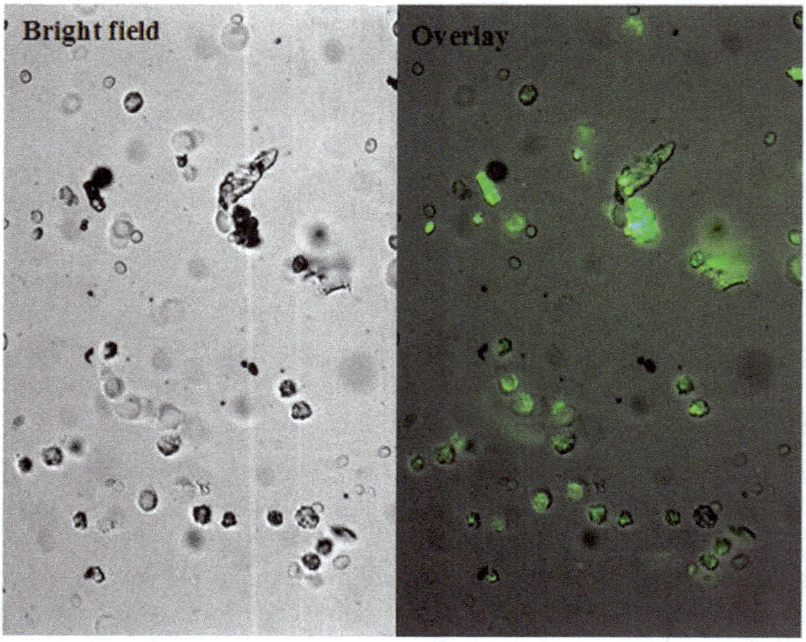

Figure 6. Hemolymph cells (20× magnification) of *S. nonagrioides* fifth instar larvae infected with the BmNPV-BmA::GFP virus, 7 days PI. Left. Bright field imaging of hemolymph cells infected with BmNPV-BmA::GFP. Right. Overlay of bright and fluorescence field images of infected *S. nonagrioides'* hemolymph cells.

The previous experiments showed that BmNPV should be the appropriate vector to transfer dsRNAs in *S. nonagrioides* cells. But this methodology should not be used for functional analysis of genes implicated in larval-pupal transformation since we observed that when insects were infected with either the AcMNPV-BmA::GFP or the BmNPV-BmA::GFP virus in the prepupal stage, larval-pupal transition was blocked while singular adults emerging from surviving pupae were also abnormal. Taking the above observations into consideration, it was nevertheless clear that the infection of *S. nonagrioides* larvae with a BmNPV-BmA::GFP-JHER472 hairpin-expressing virus resulted in specific gene downregulation with similar phenotypes than those after intra-hemolymph dsRNA administration [12].

Therefore, this methodology should be improved in order to create genetically modified baculoviruses that will cause even less physiological impact to the infected cells and to allow more clearly the distinction between infection-related effects and those caused by RNAi.

3. Two bottlenecks for efficient RNAi in insects: dsRNA stability and dsRNA uptake

Recently, several studies were published that focused directly on the causes for the variability of RNAi efficiency among different insect groups [52–54]. Beetles (Coleoptera) and cockroaches (Blattaria) are very sensitive to RNAi that is administered by injection or feeding;

locusts (Orthoptera) are sensitive to RNAi by injection but are refractory to RNAi by feeding, while caterpillars (Lepidoptera) are refractory to RNAi by both injection and feeding. A series of experiments with insects as well as derived cell lines investigated differences in cellular uptake of dsRNA as well as degradation of dsRNA among the different groups. One important finding was that dsRNA degradation correlated negatively with RNAi efficiency, that is, insects with low efficiency in RNAi (e.g. lepidopterans) degrade dsRNA faster in hemolymph and midgut than insects with high efficiency in RNAi (e.g. coleopterans) [52, 54]. The second important finding relates to the cellular uptake of dsRNA: while both lepidopteran and coleopteran cells can take up efficiently labeled dsRNA from the extracellular medium by endocytosis, this results in the production of siRNAs and silencing of target genes only in the coleopteran cells [52, 53]. The use of pH-sensitive dyes coupled to dsRNA molecules suggests that in lepidopteran cells endocytosis of dsRNA is followed by fusion of endosomes with lysosomes and subsequent degradation while in coleopteran cells presumably endosomal escape can occur and subsequent interaction of dsRNA with the RNAi machinery [53]. In lepidopteran cells, the core RNAi machinery works very efficiently [55] and the obstacle seems to be mainly the efficient arrival of the dsRNA trigger at the intracellular RNAi machinery.

These investigations indicate that the use of "naked" dsRNA to trigger RNAi by feeding will only work efficiently in beetles and cockroaches and that for other insects special delivery systems need to be developed. In the first instance, those delivery systems need to protect the dsRNA trigger from degradation in the midgut, an effort which is especially difficult to achieve for lepidopterans in which the alkaline gut content is prone to destabilize dsRNA even in the absence of nucleases [56]. Second, methods need to be developed for more efficient "functional" uptake of dsRNA in locusts and caterpillars in the sense that the internalized dsRNA is not degraded but efficiently presented to the RNAi machinery. Besides naked dsRNA, other delivery methods using bacteria, algae, plants, symbionts and viruses have been tested with variable efficiency [e.g. 36, 55, 57–59] but mechanistic details of how dsRNA escapes from the different vehicles to enter the cellular cytoplasm are lacking and should become an active area of research in the future.

Also synthetic nanoparticles are being tested for delivery of dsRNA in insects [23, 60]. Of note, chitosan dsRNA/siRNA nanoparticles have been reported to efficiently trigger RNAi in mosquito larvae [61, 62] and detailed protocols were published to achieve efficient gene silencing by this method [62]. In relevance to the discussion above, nanoparticles can be engineered to stimulate endosomal escape [63] and cell-penetrating peptides can be harnessed to deliver nucleic acid cargo directly to the cytoplasm [64, 65]. Moreover, fusions with viral capsid proteins have been used to deliver protein toxins to the hemocoel of insect pests [66]. Thus, research into the mode by which insect viruses can penetrate the midgut epithelium can lead to new biotechnological applications for efficient delivery of dsRNA/siRNA cargo to specific insect pests [67].

4. Commercialization of RNAi for crop protection

Because of the increasing burden of chemical pesticides (residual toxicity in the environment, pesticide resistance), interest for developing biological pesticides has expanded significantly during recent years. Biological pesticides are pesticides derived from natural materials such as animals, plants, bacteria and certain minerals [68, 69]. Biological pesticides include microbial pesticides (e.g. parasitoid wasps, predatory bugs), microbial pesticides (e.g. *Bacillus thuringiensis* (Bt) spores), semiochemicals (e.g. pheromones as attractants), natural products (e.g. fermentation products from bacteria such as *Streptomyces* and *Saccharopolyspora*) and plant-incorporated protectants (e.g. transgenic plants that produce Bt toxins). Advantages of biological pesticides are their reduced toxicity and reduced risk of persistence in the environment, increased specificity toward targeted pests and decreased risk for development of resistance. Biological pesticides often also represent a new mode of action and can thus be employed in combination with conventional pesticides to reduce their dose and environmental impact. The field of biological pesticides is now considered as a big opportunity for expansion since farming is becoming more and more environmentally responsible in the world. In the European Union, for instance, new guidelines are being developed for the promotion of the use of safer pesticides and biological pesticides are considered a major part for this solution [70].

RNAi technology is one of the most recent trends in the field of crop protection and conceptually approaches the "ideal" of the perfect pesticide: it targets only the intended pest and is predicted to have minimal impact on non-target organisms (pollinators, parasitoids, predators and vertebrates). Furthermore, it is biodegradable and therefore with minimal risk for human health and the environment. Because dsRNA is either produced enzymatically in vitro or in genetically transformed bacteria, it can be considered as a "natural product" (biological pesticide). However, RNAi technology, as with most biological pesticides, may be less effective than conventional chemical pesticides (slower killing may necessitate multiple applications) and associated with higher cost of production. Because of the "biological" nature, shelf life may be lower. Because of the novelty of the technology, delays can occur during registration for commercialization.

A major issue with RNAi technology so far concerns its efficiency. The success of RNAi to control pests seems to be mainly determined by the efficiency of delivery of dsRNA, the trigger of RNAi. Major obstacles in the success of RNAi are the uptake of dsRNA/siRNA by the cells and its stability (resistance to degradation) in the gut and the tissues [71–73]. Because of these issues, RNAi as an economically viable approach to control insect pests so far is limited to two coleopteran species, the western corn rootworm (*D. virgifera*) and the Colorado potato beetle (*L. decemlineata*), that are extremely sensitive to environmental RNAi [8, 74]. For other species, most notably non-coleopterans, it is perceived that the development of specialized "formulations" is necessary to deliver dsRNA with sufficient efficiency to cause an impact on larval growth and crop damage [75]. Specialized formulations could be tailored to the ecological and physiological characteristics of the targeted pests to stimulate oral uptake (e.g. food attractants), stability in the gut (e.g. chitosan nanoparticles) and interaction with gut epithelium (e.g. specific interaction with membrane proteins).

For the control of the two coleopteran pests mentioned above, two different strategies are used. A spray of dsRNA can be used to control infestation of potato plants by *Leptinotarsa*; this approach requires techniques for the (cheap) production of large amounts of dsRNA [74, 76]. For the control of *Diabrotica,* on the other hand, transgenic corn can be used that produces RNA hairpins targeting the genes of the pest [8]. Both approaches seem to be close for commercialization. While RNAi technology could be used as a method to directly affect insect growth and mortality, its use as a "synergist" to enhance the effects of other pesticides also can have important applications. For instance, RNAi is proposed as a "pyramided" insect protection trait in genetically modified crops [49]. In "pyramided" protection traits, different insecticidal compounds are employed that act with an independent mode of action in insect pests. RNAi technology and Bt toxins provide such an example because their mode of action is entirely different and also the dynamics of their toxicity is complementary: while Bt toxins act fast but are less persistent, dsRNA achieves its strongest effects after extended periods. Because of the decreased risk of development of pesticide resistance, the combination of two independent protection traits in a crop can be considered as an alternative to the high-dose approach of a single protection trait and will reduce the refugee requirements for genetically modified crops.

RNAi technology can also be used to increase the efficiency of conventional pesticides [77]. RNAi can be used to decrease the expression of both the targets (for instance, acetylcholinesterase in case of organophosphates and carbamates) and the detoxifying enzymes (for instance, cytochrome P450 enzymes, carboxylesterases and glutathione-S-transferases) of chemical insecticides to increase their effectivity. In combination with RNAi, chemical pesticides might be employed effectively at lower doses, thereby increasing the safety of their applications. Thus, the employment of RNAi technology in pesticide formulations is an important area for further applied research with potential for commercialization.

5. Conclusion

RNAi has been successfully applied in entomological research to analyze gene function in homeostasis, development, immunity and reproduction of insects. Furthermore, the potential of RNAi to control agricultural insect pests and vectors of human disease was revealed. In this review, an overview was presented of the success of the main methods of RNAi delivery (injection and feeding) and the use of different delivery vehicles was discussed (naked dsRNA versus bacterial-, plant- and virus-mediated RNAi) together with highlights of our own experiences with the lepidopteran pest *S. nonagrioides*. Our experiences and a survey of the literature indicate the usefulness to try different approaches for the delivery of dsRNA to achieve successful gene silencing. Regarding injections of dsRNA, we observed much more efficient gene silencing and phenotypic effects in the prepupal stage than in the larval stage and this effect was dependent on the length of the injected dsRNA fragment [12]. Thus, the success of the method of dsRNA injection may be dependent on the size of the dsRNA and the developmental stage of the insect. For feeding of bacteria expressing dsRNA, silencing of targeted genes was observed but phenotypic effects were limited, indicating insufficient delivery of the dsRNA trigger in our experimental system. Finally, in our work [12], we have pioneered the method of virus-mediated RNAi. Baculoviruses that express an RNA hairpin directed against the *JHER* gene could induce specific developmental phenotypes during metamorphosis in *Sesamia*. This approach, however, needed large groups of animals for evaluation since common effects on metamorphosis were observed after infection with baculoviruses that express specific (targeting *JHER*) and non-specific (targeting *luciferase*) hairpins. Engineered baculoviruses that are deficient in genes targeting the insect hormonal system (e.g. ecdysteroid glucosyltransferase) could be tested in future experiments to allow easier evaluation of phenotypes.

While clear successes in RNAi-mediated gene silencing were achieved and commercial application is expected for pest control in a few instances before the end of the decade, it is equally clear that much needs to be learned about the RNAi process in insects. Further research should focus on the deeper understanding of the process of RNAi in insects, especially with respect to the uptake of dsRNA from the environment. Recent research indeed indicates that efficient delivery of dsRNA is essential for robust RNAi-mediated-silencing effects. Improvements in RNAi should focus on increased stability of dsRNA in the environment, gut content and insect tissues and the development of efficient vehicles for effective release of dsRNA in the cytoplasm (as opposed to endocytotic vesicles) of the targeted cells. Only detailed understanding of the process of RNAi in insects, taking into account their different physiology and ecology, will allow us to develop the tools for robust triggering of gene silencing and to realize its full potential for insect pest control.

Author details

Anna Kourti[1]*, Luc Swevers[2] and Dimitrios Kontogiannatos[1]

*Address all correspondence to: akourti@aua.gr

1 Department of Biotechnology, School of Food, Biotechnology and Development, Agricultural University of Athens, Athens, Greece

2 Insect Molecular Genetics and Biotechnology Group, Institute of Biosciences & Applications, National Centre for Scientific Research "Demokritos", Athens, Greece

References

[1] Fire A, Xu S, Montgomery MK, Kostas SA, Driver SE, Mello CC. Potent and specific genetic interference by double-stranded RNA in *Caenorhabditis elegans*. Nature 1998; 391:806–11.

[2] Hannon GJ. RNA interference. Nature 2002; 418:244–51.

[3] Bartel, DP. MicroRNAs: target recognition and regulatory functions. Cell 2009; 136 (2):215–33.

[4] Elbashir SM, Lendeckel W, Tuschl T. RNA interference is mediated by 21- and 22 nucleotide RNAs. Genes Dev. 2001; 15 (2):188–200.

[5] Belles, X. Beyond Drosophila, RNAi in vivo and functional genomics in insects. Annu. Rev. Entomol. 2010; 55:111–28.

[6] Timmons L, Fire A. Specific interference by ingested dsRNA. Nature 1998; 395:854.

[7] Timmons L, Court DL, Fire A. Ingestion of bacterially expressed dsRNAs can produce specific and potent genetic interference in *Caenorhabditis elegans*. Gene 2001; 263:103–12.

[8] Baum JA, Bogaert T, Clinton W, Heck GR, Feldmann P, Ilagan O, Johnson S, Plaetinck G, Munyikwa T, Pleau M, Vaughn, T, Roberts J. Control of coleopteran insect pests through RNA interference. Nat. Biotechnol. 2007; 25:1322–6.

[9] Mao YB, Cai WJ, Wang JW, Hong GJ, Tao XY, Wang LJ, Huang YP, Chen XY. Silencing a cotton bollworm P450 monooxygenase gene by plant-mediated RNAi impairs larval tolerance of gossypol. Nat Biotechnol. 2007; 25(11):1307–13.

[10] Kupferschmidt K. A lethal dose of RNA. Science 2013; 341:732–3.

[11] Baum JA, Roberts JK. Progress towards RNAi-mediated insect pest management. Adv. Insect Physiol. 2014; 47:249–95.

[12] Kontogiannatos D, Swevers L, Maenaka K, Park EY, Iatrou K, Kourti A. Functional characterization of a juvenile hormone esterase related gene in the moth *Sesamia nonagrioides* through RNA interference. PLoS One. 2013; 8(9):e73834. doi: 10.1371/journal.pone.0073834

[13] Dzitoyeva S, Dimitrijevic N, Manev H. Intra-abdominal injection of double-stranded RNA into anesthetized adult Drosophila triggers RNA interference in the central nervous system. Mol. Psychiatry. 2001; 6(6):665–70.

[14] Quan GX, Kanda T, Tamura T. Induction of the white egg 3 mutant phenotype by injection of the double-stranded RNA of the silkworm white gene. Insect Mol. Biol. 2002;11(3):217–22.

[15] Bettencourt R, Terenius O, Faye I. Hemolin gene silencing by ds-RNA injected into *Cecropia* pupae is lethal to next generation embryos. Insect Mol. Biol. 2002;11(3):267–71.

[16] Levin DM, Breuer LN, Zhuang S anderson SA, Nardi JB, Kanost MR. A hemocyte-specific integrin required for hemocytic encapsulation in the tobacco hornworm, *Manduca sexta*. Insect Biochem Mol Biol. 2005; 35(5):369–80.

[17] Zhu J, Chen L, Raikhel AS. Distinct roles of broad isoforms in regulation of the 20-hydroxyecdysone effector gene, Vitellogenin, in the mosquito *Aedes aegypti*. Mol. Cell Endocrinol. 2007; 267(1–2):97–105.

[18] Chen X, Tian H, Zou L, Tang B, Hu J, Zhang W. Disruption of *Spodoptera exigua* larval development by silencing chitin synthase gene A with RNA interference. Bull Entomol Res. 2008; 98(6):613–9. doi: 10.1017/S0007485308005932

[19] Tan A, Palli SR. Ecdysone [corrected] receptor isoforms play distinct roles in controlling molting and metamorphosis in the red flour beetle, *Tribolium castaneum*. Mol Cell Endocrinol. 2008; 291(1–2):42–9. doi: 10.1016/j.mce.2008.05.006

[20] Griebler M, Westerlund SA, Hoffmann KH, Meyering-Vos M. RNA interference with the allatoregulating neuropeptide genes from the fall armyworm *Spodoptera frugiperda* and

its effects on the JH titer in the hemolymph. J Insect Physiol. 2008; 54(6):997–1007. doi: 10.1016/j.jinsphys.2008.04.019

[21] Moriyama Y, Sakamoto T, Matsumoto A, Noji S, Tomioka K. Functional analysis of the circadian clock gene period by RNA interference in nymphal crickets *Gryllus bimaculatus*. J Insect Physiol. 2009; 55(2):183–7. doi: 10.1016/j.jinsphys.2008.11.005

[22] Alves AP, Lorenzen MD, Beeman RW, Foster JE, Siegfried BD. RNA interference as a method for target-site screening in the Western corn rootworm, *Diabrotica virgifera virgifera*. J Insect Sci. 2010; 10:162. doi: 10.1673/031.010.14122

[23] Zhang J, Liu X, Zhang J, Li D, Sun Y, Guo Y, Ma E, Zhu KY. Silencing of two alternative splicing-derived mRNA variants of chitin synthase 1 gene by RNAi is lethal to the oriental migratory locust, *Locusta migratoria manilensis* (Meyen). Insect Biochem Mol Biol. 2010; 40(11):824–33. doi: 10.1016/j.ibmb.2010.08.001

[24] Revuelta L, Ortego F, Díaz-Ruíz JR, Castañera P, Tenllado F, Hernández-Crespo P. Contribution of Ldace1 gene to acetylcholinesterase activity in Colorado potato beetle. Insect Biochem Mol Biol. 2011; 41(10):795–803. doi: 10.1016/j.ibmb.2011.06.001

[25] Uryu O, Kamae Y, Tomioka K, Yoshii T. Long-term effect of systemic RNA interference on circadian clock genes in hemimetabolous insects. J Insect Physiol. 2013; 59(4):494–9. doi: 10.1016/j.jinsphys.2013.02.009

[26] Mansur JF, Alvarenga ES, Figueira-Mansur J, Franco TA, Ramos IB, Masuda H, Melo AC, Moreira MF. Effects of chitin synthase double-stranded RNA on molting and oogenesis in the Chagas disease vector *Rhodnius prolixus*. Insect Biochem Mol Biol. 2014;51:110–21. doi: 10.1016/j.ibmb.2013.12.006

[27] Paim RM, Araujo RN, Leis M, Sant'anna MR, Gontijo NF, Lazzari CR, Pereira MH. Functional evaluation of Heat Shock Proteins 70 (HSP70/HSC70) on *Rhodnius prolixus* (Hemiptera, Reduviidae) physiological responses associated with feeding and starvation. Insect Biochem Mol Biol. 2016; 77:10–20.

[28] Walshe DP, Lehane SM, Lehane MJ, Haines LR. Prolonged gene knockdown in the tsetse fly *Glossina* by feeding double stranded RNA. Insect Mol Biol. 2009; 18(1):11–9.

[29] Bautista MA, Miyata T, Miura K, Tanaka T. RNA interference-mediated knockdown of a cytochrome P450, CYP6BG1, from the diamondback moth, *Plutella xylostella*, reduces larval resistance to permethrin. Insect Biochem Mol Biol. 2009; 39(1):38–46.

[30] Hunter W, Ellis J, Vanengelsdorp D, Hayes J, Westervelt D, Glick E, Williams M, Sela I, Maori E, Pettis J, Cox-Foster D, Paldi N. Large-scale field application of RNAi technology reducing Israeli acute paralysis virus disease in honey bees (*Apis mellifera*, Hymenoptera: Apidae). PLoS Pathog. 2010; 26(12):e1001160. doi: 10.1371/journal.ppat.1001160.

[31] Lü ZC, Wan FH. Using double-stranded RNA to explore the role of heat shock protein genes in heat tolerance in *Bemisia tabaci* (Gennadius). J Exp Biol. 2011; 214(Pt 5):764–9.

[32] Chen J, Tang B, Chen H, Yao Q, Huang X, Chen J, Zhang D, Zhang W. Different functions of the insect soluble and membrane-bound trehalase genes in chitin bio-

synthesis revealed by RNA interference. PLoS One. 2010; 5(4):e10133. doi: 10.1371/journal.pone.0010133

[33] Hunt JH, Mutti NS, Havukainen H, Henshaw MT, Amdam GV. Development of an RNA interference tool, characterization of its target and an ecological test of caste differentiation in the eusocial wasp polistes. PLoS One. 2011; 6(11):e26641. doi: 10.1371/journal.pone.0026641

[34] Luan JB, Ghanim M, Liu SS, Czosnek H. Silencing the ecdysone synthesis and signaling pathway genes disrupts nymphal development in the whitefly. Insect Biochem Mol Biol. 2013; 43(8):740–6.

[35] Mao J, Zeng F. Plant-mediated RNAi of a gap gene-enhanced tobacco tolerance against the *Myzus persicae*. Transgenic Res. 2014; 23(1):145–52.

[36] Li X, Zhang M, Zhang H. RNA interference of four genes in adult *Bactrocera dorsalis* by feeding their dsRNAs. PLoS One. 2011; 18:6(3):e17788.

[37] Abd El Halim HM, Alshukri BM, Ahmad MS, Nakasu EY, Awwad MH, Salama EM, Gatehouse AM, Edwards MG. RNAi-mediated knockdown of the voltage gated sodium ion channel TcNav causes mortality in *Tribolium castaneum*. Sci Rep. 2016; 14: 29301.

[38] Tian H, Peng H, Yao,Q, Chen H, Xie Q, Tang B and Zhang W. Developmental control of a lepidopteran pest *Spodoptera exigua* by ingestion of bacteria expressing dsRNA of a non-midgut gene. PLoS One 2009; 4:e6225. http://dx.doi.org/10.1371/journal.pone.0006225

[39] Li J, Li X, Bai R, Shi Y, Tang Q, An S, Song Q, Yan F. RNA interference of the P450 CYP6CM1 gene has different efficacy in B and Q biotypes of *Bemisia tabaci*. Pest Manag Sci. 2015; 71(8):1175–81.

[40] Zhu F, Xu J, Palli R, Ferguson J, Palli SR. Ingested RNA interference for managing the populations of the Colorado potato beetle, *Leptinotarsa decemlineata*. Pest Manag Sci. 2011; 67(2):175–82.

[41] Zhang X, Liu X, Ma J, Zhao J. Silencing of cytochrome P450 CYP6B6 gene of cotton bollworm (*Helicoverpa armigera*) by RNAi. Bull Entomol Res. 2013; 103(5):584–91.

[42] Oliveira PL, Almendares O, Umaña C, Lowenberger C, Dotson EM, Paiva-Silva GO, Pennington PM. Genetically modifying the insect gut microbiota to control Chagas disease vectors through systemic RNAi. PLoS Negl Trop Dis. 2015; 12:9(2):e0003358.

[43] Molnár A, Csorba T, Lakatos L, Várallyay E, Lacomme C, et al. Plant virus-derived small interfering RNAs originate predominantly from highly structured single-stranded viral RNAs. J Virol 2005; 79:7812–8.

[44] Xiong Y, Zeng H, Zhang Y, Xu D, Qiu D. Silencing the HaHR3 gene by transgenic plant-mediated RNAi to disrupt *Helicoverpa armigera* development. Int J Biol Sci. 2013; 9(4):370–81.

[45] Yu R, Xu X, Liang Y1, Tian H, Pan Z, Jin S, Wang N, Zhang W. The insect ecdysone receptor is a good potential target for RNAi-based pest control. Int J Biol Sci. 2014; 10(10):1171–80.

[46] Xu L, Duan X, Lv Y, Zhang X, Nie Z, Xie C, Ni Z, Liang R. Silencing of an aphid carboxylesterase gene by use of plant-mediated RNAi impairs *Sitobion avenae* tolerance of Phoxim insecticides. Transgenic Res. 2014; 23(2):389–96.

[47] Liu F, Wang XD, Zhao YY, Li YJ, Liu YC, Sun J. Silencing the *HaAK* gene by transgenic plant-mediated RNAi impairs larval growth of *Helicoverpa armigera*. Int J Biol Sci. 2015; 11(1):67–74.

[48] Coleman AD, Wouters RH, Mugford ST, Hogenhout SA. Persistence and transgenerational effect of plant-mediated RNAi in aphids. J Exp Bot. 2015; 66(2):541–8.

[49] Swevers L, Smagghe G. Use of RNAi for control of insect crop pests. In: Arthropod-Plant Interactions, Novel Insights and Approaches for IPM, Progress in Biological Control, Volume 14. G. Smagghe & I. Diaz (Eds.), 2012; Springer-Verlag, Dordrecht, pp 177–197.

[50] Hajós JP, Vermunt AM, Zuidema D, Kulcsár P, Varjas L, de Kort CA, Závodszky P, Vlak JM. Dissecting insect development: baculovirus-mediated gene silencing in insects. Insect Mol Biol. 1999;8(4):539–44.

[51] Uhlirova M, Foy BD, Beaty BJ, Olson KE, Riddiford LM, et al. (2003) Use of Sindbis virus-mediated RNA interference to demonstrate a conserved role of Broad-Complex in insect metamorphosis. Proc Natl Acad Sci USA 100: 15607–15612.

[52] Ivashuta S, Zhang Y, Wiggins BE, Ramaseshadri P, Segers GC, Johnson S, Meyer SE, Kerstetter RA, McNulty BC, Bolognesi R, Heck GR. Environmental RNAi in herbivorous insects. *RNA (New York, N.Y.)*.2015; 21: 840–50. PMID 25802407 DOI: 10.1261/rna.048116.114

[53] Shukla JN, Kalsi M, Sethi A, Narva KE, Fishilevich E, Singh S, Mogilicherla K, Palli SR. Reduced stability and intracellular transport of dsRNA contribute to poor RNAi response in lepidopteran insects. RNA Biol. 2016; 13(7):656–69. doi: 10.1080/15476286.2016.1191728

[54] Wang K, Peng Y, Pu J, Fu W, Wang J and Han Z. Variation in RNAi efficacy among insect species is attributable to dsRNA degradation in vivo. Insect Biochem Mol Biol. 2016; 77:1–9.

[55] Kolliopoulou A, Swevers L. Functional analysis of the RNAi response in ovary-derived silkmoth Bm5 cells. Insect Biochem Mol Biol. 2013; 43:654–63. DOI: 10.1016/j.ibmb.2013.05.001

[56] Liu, J, Swevers L, Iatrou K, Huvenne H, Smagghe G. *Bombyx mori* DNA/RNA non-specific nuclease isoforms: expression in insect culture cells, subcellular localization and functional assays. J Insect Physiol. 2012; 58(8):1166–76. doi: 10.1016/j.jinsphys.2012.05.016

[57] Hajeri S, Killiny N, El-Mohtar C, Dawson WO, Gowda S. *Citrus tristeza* virus-based RNAi in citrus plants induces gene silencing in *Diaphorina citri*, a phloem-sap sucking

insect vector of citrus greening disease (Huanglongbing). J Biotechnol. 2014 20;176:42–9. doi: 10.1016/j.jbiotec.2014.02.01C

[58] Jin S, Singh ND, Li L, Zhang X, Daniell H. Engineered chloroplast dsRNA silences cytochrome p450 monooxygenase, V-ATPase and chitin synthase genes in the insect gut and disrupts *Helicoverpa armigera* larval development and pupation. Plant Biotechnol J. 2015; 13(3):435–46. doi: 10.1111/pbi.12355

[59] Whitten MMA, Facey PD, Del Sol R, Fernández-Martínez LT, Evans MC, Mitchell JJ, Bodger OG and Dyson PJ. Symbiont-mediated RNA interference in insects. Proc R Soc B 2016; 283:20160042.

[60] Taning CNT, Christiaens O, Berkvens N, Casteels H, Maes M, Smagghe G. Oral RNAi to control *Drosophila suzukii*: laboratory testing against larval and adult stages. J Pest Sci. (2016); 89: 803. doi:10.1007/s10340-016-0736-9

[61] Singh AD, Wong S, Ryan CP, Whyard S. Oral delivery of double-stranded RNA in larvae of the yellow fever mosquito, *Aedes aegypti:* implications for pest mosquito control. J Insect Sci. 2013; 13:69. doi: 10.1673/031.013.6901

[62] Zhan Q, Hua G, Adang MJ. Chitosan/DsiRNA nanoparticle targeting identifies AgCad1 cadherin in Anopheles gambiae larvae as an in vivo receptor of Cry11Ba toxin of *Bacillus thuringiensis* subsp. jegathesan. Insect Biochem Mol Biol. 2015; 60:33–8.

[63] Eguchi A, Meade BR, Chang YC, Fredrickson CT, Willert K, Puri N, Dowdy SF. Efficient siRNA delivery into primary cells by a peptide transduction domain–dsRNA binding domain fusion protein. Nature Biotechnol. 2009; 27:567–71.

[64] Endoh T, Ohtsuki T. Cellular siRNA delivery using cell-penetrating peptides modified for endosomal escape. Adv Drug Deliv Rev. 2009; 61:704–709.

[65] Huang YW, Lee HJ, Tolliver LM, Aronstam RS. Delivery of nucleic acids and nanomaterials by cell-penetrating peptides: opportunities and challenges. Biomed Res Central. 2014; Article ID 834079

[66] Bonning BC, Pal N, Liu S, Wang Z, Sivakumar S, Dixon PM, King GF, Miller WA. Toxin delivery by the coat protein of an aphid-vectored plant virus provides plant resistance to aphids. Nat Biotechnol. 2014; 32:102–5.

[67] Bonning BC, Chougule NP. Delivery of intrahemocoelic peptides for insect pest management. Trends Biotechnol. 2014; 32: 91–8.

[68] Thacker JRM. An Introduction to Arthropod Pest Control. Cambridge University Press, 2002; Cambridge, UK.

[69] Glare T, Caradus J, Gelernter W, Jackson T, Keyhani N, Köhl J, Marrone P, Morin L, Stewart A. Have biopesticides come of age? Trends Biotechnol. 2012; 30(5):250–8. doi: 10.1016/j.tibtech.2012.01.003.

[70] Villaverde JJ, Sevilla-Morán B, Sandín-España P, López-Goti C, Alonso-Prados JL Biopesticides in the framework of the European Pesticide Regulation (EC) No. 1107/2009. Pest Manag Sci 2014; 70:2–5.

[71] Scott JG, Michel K, Bartholomay LC, Siegfried BD, Hunter WB, Smagghe G, Zhu KY. Towards the elements of successful insect RNAi. J Insect Physiol. 2013; 59(12):1212–21. doi: 10.1016/j.jinsphys.2013.08.014

[72] Swevers L, Ioannidis K, Kolovou M, Zografidis A, Labropoulou V, Santos D, Wynant N, Broeck JV, Wang L, Cappelle K, Smagghe G. Persistent RNA virus infection of lepidopteran cell lines: interactions with the RNAi machinery. Insect Physiol. 2016; 93–94:81–93. doi: 10.1016/j.jinsphys.2016.09.001

[73] Christiaens O, Swevers L, Smagghe G. (2014). DsRNA degradation in the pea aphid (*Acyrthosiphon pisum*) associated with lack of response in RNAi feeding and injection assay. Peptides U. 2014; 307–314.

[74] Palli SR. RNA interference in Colorado potato beetle: steps toward development of dsRNA as a commercial insecticide. Curr Opin Insect Sci. 2014; 6:1–8.

[75] Das A, Dickinson DJ, Wood C, Goldstein B. Slep KC. Crescerin uses a TOG domain array to regulate microtubules in the primary cilium. Mol Biol Cell. 2015; doi:10.1091/mbc.E15-08-0603 DOI:10.1091/mbc.E15-08-0603#_blank

[76] San MK, Scott JG. The next generation of insecticides: dsRNA is stable as a foliar-applied insecticide. Pest Manag Sci. 2015; 72:801–9.

[77] Kim YH, Issa MS, Cooper A, Zhu KY. RNA interference: Applications and advances in insect toxicology and insect pest management. Pesticide Biochem Physiol. 2015; 120:109–17.

10

RNA Interference – A Powerful Functional Analysis Tool for Studying Tick Biology and its Control

Remil Linggatong Galay, Rika Umemiya-Shirafuji, Masami Mochizuki, Kozo Fujisaki and Tetsuya Tanaka

Abstract

Ticks (Acari: Ixodida) are blood-sucking arthropods globally recognized as vectors of numerous diseases. They are primarily responsible for the transmission of various pathogens, including viruses, rickettsiae, and blood parasites of animals. Ticks are second to mosquitoes in terms of disease transmission to humans. The continuous emergence of tick-borne diseases and acaricide resistance of ticks necessitates the development of new and more effective control agents and strategies; therefore, understanding of different aspects of tick biology and their interaction with pathogens is very crucial in developing effective control strategies. RNA interference (RNAi) has been widely used in the area of tick research as a versatile reverse genetic tool to elucidate the functions of various tick proteins. During the past decade, numerous studies on ticks utilized RNAi to evaluate potentially key tick proteins involved in blood feeding, reproduction, evasion of host immune response, interaction with pathogens, and pathogen transmission that may be targeted for tick and pathogen control. This chapter reviewed the application of RNAi in tick research over the past decade, focusing on the impact of this technique in the advancement of knowledge on tick and pathogen biology.

Keywords: Acari, ticks, Ixodidae, RNA interference, tick-borne diseases

1. Introduction

Ticks belong to the class of Arachnida together with spiders, scorpions, and mites. To date, there are about 900 species of ticks, majority of which are hard ticks belonging to the Ixodidae family, as well as about 200 species are soft ticks belonging to the Argasidae family, and a single species belonging to the Nuttalliellidae family [1]. Most of the ticks of medical and veterinary importance are hard ticks. Through their blood-feeding behavior, ticks can directly affect their host by causing anemia, irritation, and allergic reactions particularly in heavy infestation. The saliva of some tick species may also contain neurotoxic substances that may cause the condition termed "tick paralysis" [2]. Additionally, the transmission of pathogens including viruses, bacteria, and parasitic protozoa also occurs during blood feeding [1]. Ticks are considered second to mosquitoes in terms of their impact on public health, but they are the most important vectors of different pathogens in both domestic and wild animals [3]. Tick infestation and tick-borne diseases (TBDs) continue to have great economic impact on livestock production, particularly on cattle and small ruminants, in several continents [2]. The annual loss in cattle production worldwide due to ticks and TBDs has been estimated to be worth billions of USD [4].

The complete dependence of ticks to host blood for the completion of their life cycle and generation of offspring is the reason for their notoriety as vectors of several diseases. Depending on the species, a tick may utilize one to three hosts during their life cycle. Most of the pathogens they transmit can be carried on throughout their life cycle through transstadial (from one stage to the next) transmission and to the next generation through transovarial (from adults to eggs) transmission [5]. A single tick may carry multiple pathogens [6], thereby having the potential of infecting a host with a cocktail of pathogens. Most tick-borne infections are zoonotic in nature, and more of these are being recognized in recent years [1, 7]. Among the TBDs that are well-known in the veterinary and medical field are anaplasmosis, borreliosis, rickettsiosis, ehrlichiosis, babesiosis, theileriosis, and tick-borne encephalitis.

The significant impact of ticks and TBDs underscores the importance of tick control. For several decades, the application of chemical acaricides has been the primary tick control method, and acaricides were used extensively in livestock production. However, the continuous emergence of resistant tick strains makes most chemical acaricides ineffective [8]. Moreover, the increasing concerns for animal product and environmental contamination set limitations for this control method. To search for new and more effective means of controlling ticks and TBDs, researchers have actively expanded the understanding on tick biology.

RNA interference (RNAi) is a reverse genetic approach for manipulation of genes that commonly utilizes double-stranded RNA (dsRNA) to induce post-transcriptional gene-specific silencing [9]. RNAi has been extensively employed in many studies on tick biology and pathogen interaction since the first report of RNAi application in the hard tick *Amblyomma americanum* [10]. In fact, it is evident that a number of laboratories in different countries working on tick research are routinely performing RNAi, as shown by an increasing number of recent publications utilizing this technique. Typically, functional studies using RNAi involve gene knockdown with subsequent infestation and evaluation of phenotypes, such as blood feeding and reproduction success (Figure 1). Indeed, RNAi has been particularly useful in searching for tick proteins that can be targeted for control of tick development and TBDs [11].

This chapter aims to show the extent of RNAi application in tick research, emphasizing the progress of advanced knowledge on tick biology and tick-pathogen interaction. We first discussed so far known RNAi mechanisms and the current RNAi inducing methods in ticks; then, briefly described the studies on tick physiology, immunity, and pathogen interaction that employed RNAi, highlighting the prospects of applications of RNAi in tick research.

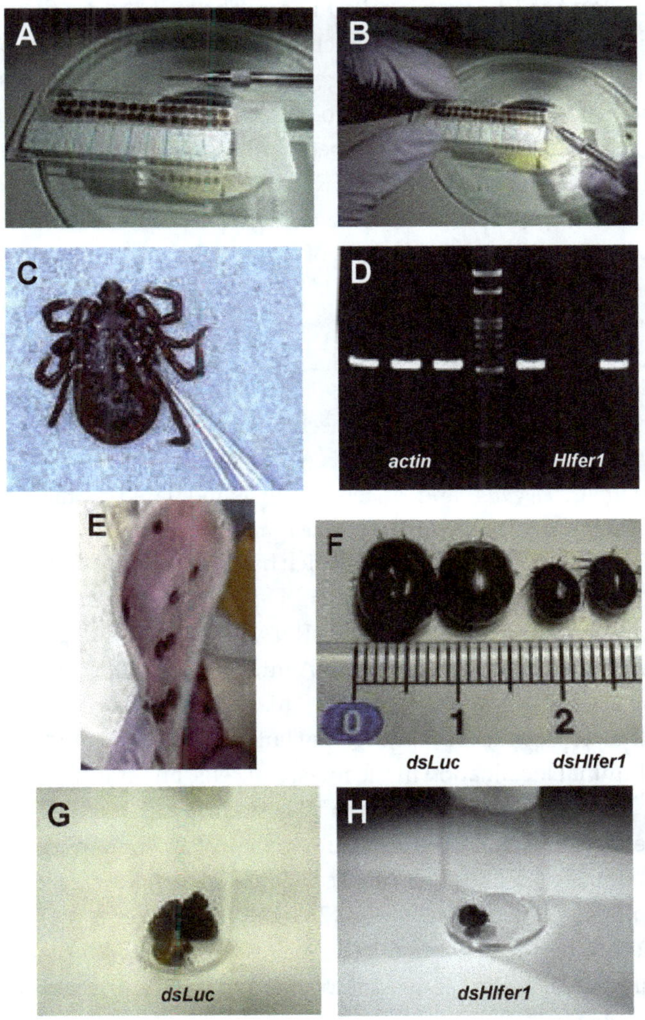

Figure 1. A typical RNAi experiment in the hard tick *Haemaphysalis longicornis*. The double-stranded RNA (dsRNA) is introduced to adult ticks by microinjection. Unfed adult ticks, placed on a double adhesive tape attached on a glass slide (A), are injected with dsRNA using a pointed microcapillary glass attached to a microinjector (B) through the membrane of the fourth coxa under a stereomicroscope (C). Successful silencing, as shown by the absence of a band for the target gene, such as *Hlfer1*, is confirmed around 4 d post-injection through RT-PCR after adjusting the cDNA level using an internal control, such as actin (D). Ticks were infested on a host and allowed to feed to repletion (E) and after dropping, parameters such as engorged body weight (F), survival, egg laying (G, H), and hatch were compared.

2. RNAi pathway in ticks

The mechanism of RNAi has been well studied in the nematode *Caenorhabditis elegans* and the fruit fly *Drosophila melanogaster* [9, 12]. RNAi begins with the uptake of dsRNA by the cell, followed by its cleavage to produce small interfering RNAs (siRNAs). Cleavage of dsRNA is accomplished by an RNAse III enzyme called Dicer. The siRNAs are then incorporated into RNA-induced silencing complex (RISC), which then drives the degradation or translational inhibition of the target mRNA that results to gene silencing. This silencing signal may spread among the cells and different tissues, leading to systemic gene silencing in the whole organism [13]. The mechanism of RNAi in ticks has not been fully elucidated, but the study of Kurscheid et al. [14] revealed that several components of RNAi machinery in other invertebrates are also present in the ticks, and they proposed a putative tick RNAi pathway. Here, we briefly describe the available knowledge on key components of RNAi machinery in ticks, in comparison of other invertebrates.

2.1. dsRNA uptake

There are two recognized dsRNA uptake mechanisms in invertebrates: a transmembrane channel-mediated uptake through systemic RNA interference defective (SID) transmembrane proteins described in *C. elegans*, and an endocytosis-mediated uptake described in most arthropods [15, 16]. Several SIDs identified in *C. elegans* have been shown to be involved in the spread of RNAi [17]. SID-1, SID-3, and SID-5, which have wide tissue distribution, are involved in the systemic spread of RNAi [18–20], whereas SID-2, localized mainly in the gut, is involved primarily in the intestinal uptake of ingested dsRNA [21]. The multi-domain SID-1 along the plasma membrane facilitates the traffic of dsRNA into and out of the cells. Homologs of SID-1 are present in some arthropods and vertebrates [18]. Both SID-3, a conserved tyrosine kinase, and SID-5 have intracytoplasmic localization, the latter being associated with late endosomes [19, 20]. SID-2 has luminal localization in the intestinal cells, and it was also found in the lower levels of excretory duct cells [21]. In addition to SIDs, endocytosis has also been also implicated as a dsRNA uptake mechanism in *C. elegans* through a protein containing an epsin N-terminal homology (ENTH) domain [22]. In *D. melanogaster*, dsRNA uptake in cells is facilitated mainly by scavenger receptor-mediated endocytosis [23]. Two scavenger receptors, Eater and Sr-CI, have been identified to be responsible for the majority of dsRNA uptake. These scavenger receptors are mainly expressed in the plasmatocytes and have a primary role in the phagocytosis of bacterial pathogens [24, 25].

SID homologues have not been identified in ticks. However, a homologue of ENTH, Epn-I, has been identified in the hard ticks *Rhiphicephalus* (*Boophilus*) *microplus* and *Ixodes scapularis* [14]. A class B scavenger receptor identified in *Haemaphysalis longicornis* (HlSRB) has been demonstrated to mediate systemic RNAi in this tick [26, 27]. Combined injection of dsRNA against *HlSRB* and other target genes, *Vitellogenin*-1 (*HlVg-1*) and *Vitellogenin Receptor* (*HlVgR*) effectively silenced these genes. However, silencing *HlSRB* prior to injection of dsRNA against *HlVg-1* and *HlVgR* inhibited the silencing of the latter two genes, suggesting that the uptake of the injected dsRNA is dependent on HlSRB in ticks. Similar to *D. melanogaster* scavenger receptors, HlSRB is also involved in the phagocytosis of bacteria [28], but it is expressed not only in the hemocytes but also in the other organs such as midguts, salivary glands, and ovary [26]. The presence of ENTH homologue and scavenger receptor indicates that the uptake of dsRNA in ticks is through endocytosis. Additionally, the presence of scavenger receptor in different tick tissues strongly implies its involvement in systemic RNAi, particularly after dsRNA injection. Introduction of dsRNA into the hemocoel of ticks directly exposes the different tick organs to dsRNA, and the scavenger receptor in these organs most likely mediates the entry of dsRNA into the cells.

2.2. dsRNA processing and RISC assembly

The recommended length of dsRNA to effectively induce silencing of the target gene in non-mammalian systems is more than 200 bp [15]. A study in *R. (B.) microplus* showed, however, that short dsRNAs between 100 and 200 bp were also effective in inducing silencing of *Ubiquitin-63E* homologue, with minimal off-target effects, but short hairpin dsRNAs were not able to induce silencing effects [29]. After cellular uptake, dsRNAs are cleaved into 21–25 nt siRNAs by an RNAse III enzyme called Dicer. In contrast to *C. elegans* and mammals that have only one Dicer, *D. melanogaster* and mosquitoes have two Dicers [15]. Dicer-2 is the one involved in the generation of siRNA, whereas Dicer-1 acts on stem loop RNA precursors to generate micro RNA (miRNA). Both, however, are required for siRNA-induced gene silencing due to their distinct roles in siRISC assembly [30]. Only a single putative Dicer has been identified so far in the hard tick *I. scapularis*, which is more similar to mammalian Dicer-1 [14].

The RNAi inhibition of a target mRNA is accomplished by RISC formed by siRNAs and Argonaute (AGO) proteins. AGO proteins are highly conserved between species, encoded by multiple genes in most organisms. All AGO proteins are characterized by two domains: the PAZ domain and the PIWI domain [31]. Upon ATP activation, AGO mediates RISC recognition of mRNA target that are homologous to siRNAs, subsequently leading to the cleavage of the mRNA target [9]. In most insects, including *D. melanogaster* and mosquitoes, five AGO genes have been identified [15, 31]. In ticks, a homologue of AGO-1 has been identified in *I. scapularis* and *R. (B.) microplus*, and a homologue of AGO-2 has been identified in *I. scapularis* [14]. However, the functions of these tick AGOs remains to be confirmed.

2.3. Amplification of RNAi signal

The ability to spread throughout the whole organism, inducing total systemic silencing of the target gene in spite of introducing only a relatively small amount of dsRNA, is an important aspect of RNAi observed in plants and invertebrates. This systemic RNAi-induced gene silencing in both plants and *C. elegans* involves RNA-directed RNA polymerase (RdRP) that amplifies the RNAi signal [9]. RdRP function in RNAi has not been found in arthropods, but a putative homologue of RdRP EGO-1 protein of *C. elegans* has been identified in the hard tick *I. scapularis*, and a partial sequence was also identified from *R. (B.) microplus* [14].

3. Methods of introducing dsRNA in ticks

3.1. Injection

Direct injection is the most widely used technique for introducing dsRNA for in vivo gene silencing, not only in ticks but also in insects [11, 32]. Through this method, dsRNA is usually introduced directly into the hemocoel of ticks allowing the dsRNA to circulate within the hemolymph. In most reports, a high concentration of at least 1 μg dsRNA per tick has been shown to be effective in inducing gene silencing [33], but in some reports, lower concentration has been found to be similarly effective [34–36]. Injection has been accomplished using a 33–36-gauge needle attached to a Hamilton syringe particularly in large tick species, such as *Amblyomma americanum*[37], *Dermacentor variabilis*, and *D. marginatus* [38], while microinjection using a microcapillary drawn to a fine point needle and inserted to a micromanipulator has been commonly employed in smaller tick species, including *Ixodes* [39], and *Haemaphysalis* [26] ticks. Different injection sites include the lower right quadrant of the ventral surface of the exoskeleton [40], the groove between the basis capituli and the scutum [37], the ventral torso of the idiosoma, away from the anal opening [39], and the coxal membrane in the fourth coxae [26, 41]. In some reports, dsRNA was injected through the spiracle [29, 42, 43] and anal pore; the latter inducing midgut-specific silencing of the target gene [44]. Injection of dsRNA has been commonly performed in unfed adult ticks, subsequently allowed to recover for at least 24 h before infestation or use in succeeding experiments. Exceptionally, dsRNA has been also injected in engorged *R.* (*B.*) *microplus* [42, 45-47], *A. americanum, I. scapularis,* and *D. variabilis* adults [43], which produced significant effects on the eggs and larvae, and microinjection has also been accomplished in *I. scapularis* [48-52] and engorged *O. moubata* nymphs [53].

3.2. Soaking

Soaking in dsRNA has been previously employed to study RNAi in the cell lines of *D. melanogaster* [23, 54]. In tick research, this method has been applied to induce in vitro RNAi not only in cell cultures [55-57], but also in some organs including whole salivary glands [36, 58-60] and midguts [61]. Soaking live *Varroa destructor* [62] and *Dermanyssus gallinae* [63] mites, as well as *Aedes aegypti* larvae [64] in a solution of dsRNA has been already demonstrated in producing effective silencing of the target genes in these organisms. However, soaking whole ticks in a solution of dsRNA has not been commonly performed. Soaking *Haemaphysalis longicornis* nymphs in a solution of dsRNA for 24 h resulted to significant transcript reduction of the target gene, although the effect on the phenotype was not observed in all the nymphs [65]. In our laboratory, we have attempted to soak *H. longicornis* larvae, nymphs, and adults in a dsRNA solution overnight, which resulted to a significant decrease in the mRNA level of a targeted gene (Galay et al., unpublished results). Soaking offers a simpler and less invasive method of introducing dsRNA without injuring the ticks and is applicable to immature tick stages. Furthermore, it does not require injection equipment; therefore, it is less laborious.

3.3. Electroporation

Electroporation is a technique that employs electric impulses to promote DNA uptake of cells and has been primarily used with in vitro cell transfection [66]. In tick research, this technique has been first applied to facilitate the introduction of dsRNA in *I. scapularis* eggs and nymphs [67]. After electroporation, fluorescein-labeled dsRNA was visualized all over the nymph's body and eggs, indicating the successful entry of dsRNA. In a more recent report, the wax coating of the eggs was first removed using heptane and hypochlorite prior to electroporation

[68]. Using heptane alone did not significantly decrease the hatching rate. Thus, heptane may be more helpful in evaluating the effect of a particular dsRNA to egg hatching. This technique also offers a less invasive method of dsRNA introduction that can be applied to immature tick stages and eggs.

3.4. Feeding

Feeding dsRNA in insects has been achieved in different species using diets mixed with dsRNA, liposome-embedded or lipophilic siRNAs, and bacteria and transgenic plants that can synthesize dsRNA [32, 69]. Although in vitro feeding assays have been shown to be useful in studying different tick molecules and tick-pathogen interaction [70], its application in RNAi study in ticks has been limited. A study on the Lyme disease vector *I. scapularis* employed capillary feeding of dsRNA to nymphs to suppress anticomplement gene *isac* [71]. In another study, adult *R. (B.) microplus* ticks were capillary fed with *ubiquitin* dsRNA mixed in whole blood or *Bm86* dsRNA mixed in bovine serum [72]. In both cases, ticks were pre-fed in an animal host before capillary feeding was performed. While this method may be advantageous over injection due to very minimal injury, drawbacks may arise from the uncertainty whether an individual tick will ingest the amount of dsRNA that will effectively induce silencing, and the possibility of variation in the amount of dsRNA ingested by the ticks within a treatment group. Furthermore, capillary feeding is difficult to perform and may not be applicable in ticks with short hypostome.

4. RNAi and study of tick physiology

4.1. Genes related to salivary functions

The saliva is an important arsenal of ticks containing hundreds of pharmacologically potent substances that facilitate attachment to their hosts and blood-sucking [73]. Different salivary proteins have redundant functions in counteracting the hemostatic [74], inflammatory, and immune mechanisms [75] of the host. Aside from its function in tick feeding, the salivary glands are also involved in osmoregulation and transmission of pathogens [76].

Many studies on characterization of salivary proteins in the recent years employed RNAi (Table 1). In fact, the first report on the application of RNAi in tick research described a tick inhibitor of inflammatory mediator, a salivary histamine-binding protein, wherein researchers induced in vitro RNAi by soaking salivary glands in dsRNA [10, 58]. Soluble N-ethylmaleimide-sensitive factor attachment receptors (SNARE) complex proteins, which mediate exocytosis in secretory pathways of the salivary glands, have been characterized in *Amblyomma* ticks. These include N-ethylmaleimide-sensitive fusion (NSF) protein, Synaptosomal Associated Protein of 25 kDa (SNAP-25) [77], Ykt6 [65], and vesicle transport through interaction with t-SNAREs (Vti) [78]. Silencing various genes such as Salp14, Salp9pac [39], Neuronal isoform munc18-1 (nSec1) [59], and synaptobrevin [36] affected the secretion of anticoagulant or the anticoagulant activity of salivary gland extracts, indicating that these genes are important in tick anti-hemostatic mechanism.

Longistatin [79] and acidic chitinases [80] have been found to be important in the formation of blood pool and tick cement cone, respectively. The attachment site of *longistatin*-silenced *H. longicornis* ticks did not show pathological changes, such as hemorrhagic lesions corresponding to the blood pool, while the attachment site of ticks simultaneously silenced acidic chitinases exhibited blood leakage and these ticks can be easily removed. Various protease inhibitors that have roles in anti-hemostatic, anti-inflammatory, and immunomodulatory mechanism have been also characterized using RNAi, including a cystatin, sialostatine L [81], a Kunitz type protease inhibitor, rhipilin [82], and serine protease inhibitors (serpin) [83, 84].

Other salivary proteins with immunomodulatory function, such as the anti-complement protein, isac [71], and two proteins that can inhibit neutrophil function, ISL 929 and 1373 [85], have also been knockdowned in *I. scapularis*. Silencing of *isac* in nymphs, induced by capillary feeding of dsRNA, not only reduced blood feeding, but also decreased the load of the spirochete *Borrelia burgdorferi* in the tick. Meanwhile, the saliva of ticks devoid of ISL 929 and 1373 had reduced ability in inhibiting host integrin. An osmoregulatory protein aquaporin, characterized in *I. ricinus* through RNAi, showed that suppression of this protein impaired the concentration of blood meal due to failure in removing water [86].

4.2. Genes related to digestion and midgut function

The midgut of ticks houses various kinds of enzymes that act on a large amount of ingested host blood, which contains great quantities of hemoglobin [151]. Functional studies on these enzymes and other midgut proteins using RNAi have expanded the understanding of tick digestive physiology (Table 1). Silencing hemoglobinolytic enzymes, such as leucine aminopeptidase [91, 92], longipain [95], and cathepsin L [96, 97] had negative impact on tick feeding. Moreover, the longipain of *H. longicornis* was found to have a protective role in *Babesia* infection through its babesiacidal activity [95]. Other proteins important in tick digestion that have been characterized using RNAi are thrombin inhibitors that prevent blood coagulation and serine proteinase, which induce erythrocyte degradation. Silencing of thrombin inhibitor hemalin from *H. longicornis* [93] and boophilin from *R. (B.) microplus* [47] prolonged the blood feeding period and decreased the oviposition of these ticks, respectively. Silencing serine protease reduced the weight of ticks after blood feeding due to impaired erythrocyte degradation [94].

4.3. Genes related to reproductive function

Ticks are known for their high fecundity, laying hundreds of eggs per batch in the case of soft ticks and up to thousands in the case of hard ticks. A series of physiological events takes place in female ticks during and after blood feeding that initiate ovarian maturation and subsequent oviposition. Vitellogenesis, the synthesis and oocyte deposition of the yolk protein precursor (vitellogenin), is a key process for ovarian development and oocyte maturation induced by blood meal in ticks [152]. Three genes encoding vitellogenin have been identified and characterized in *H. longicornis* [102].

Target gene	Tick species	RNAi Effect	Refs
Salivary proteins			
Histamine-binding protein (HBP)	*Amblyomma americanum*	Altered feeding pattern and longer feeding period; decreased histamine-binding activity in the salivary glands	[10, 58]
Salp14/ Salp9pac	*Ixodes scapularis*	Impaired feeding, decreased post-blood meal weight, decreased anticoagulant activity of salivary gland extract	[39]
Neuronal isoform munc18-1 (nSec1)	*A. americanum*	Decreased post-blood meal weight and prolonged feeding time, decreased anticoagulant secretion of salivary gland	[59]
Synaptobrevin	*A. americanum*	Inhibited secretion of anticoagulant stimulated by PGE	[36]
Cystatin	*A. americanum*	Decreased post-blood meal weight, mortality during feeding, low feeding success rate	[61]
Anticomplement protein (Isac)	*I. scapularis*	Decreased post-blood meal weight, decreased *Borrelia burgdorferi* infection	[71]
Sialostatin L (cystatin)	*I. scapularis*	Failure to feed on the host, decreased post-blood meal weight and failed oviposition	[77]
Aquaporin	*I. ricinus*	Decreased post-blood meal weight, decreased volume of ingested blood	[78]
HlYkt6 (SNARE)	*Haemaphysalis longicornis*	Decreased post-blood meal weight, high mortality, supressed salivary secretion and anticoagulant activity	[65]
ISL 929 and 1373	*I. scapularis*	Supressed PMN inhibitory activity of saliva from knockdowned ticks	[79]
Rhipilin (Kunitz type protease inhibitor)	*Rhipicephalus haemaphysaloides*	Prolonged attachment time, decreased post-blood meal weight	[80]
Longistatin	*H. longicornis*	Mortality after attachment, failure to engorge, poor blood pool formation	[81]
Serine protease inhibitor (serpin)	*A. americanum*	No effect on tick attachment, feeding and oviposition	[82]
	R. haemaphysaloides	Decreased attachment rate and engorgement weight	[83]
Reprolysin	*Rhipicephalus (Boophilus) microplus*	Decreased egg weight and egg conversion ratio	[84]
N-ethylmaleimide sensitive fusion protein (NSF)	*A. maculatum*	Inhibition of engorgement, failure of oviposition	[85]

Target gene	Tick species	RNAi Effect	Refs
Synaptosomal Associated Protein of 25 kDa (SNAP-25)	*A. maculatum*	Decreased post-blood meal weight, decreased egg weight, failure in hatching	[85]
Vti (SNARE)	*A. americanum, A. maculatum*	Decreased post-blood meal weight and survival, failed oviposition	[86]
Glutaminyl cyclase (QC)	*A. maculatum, I. scapularis*	Decreased post-blood meal weight, egg weight and hatch	[87]
AV422	*A. americanum*	Decreased post-blood meal weight	[88]
Acidic chitinase (Ach)	*A. americanum*	Leakage of blood from the mouthparts in late feeding phase, loose attachment in the host's skin	[89]
Digestive activity			
Longepsin	*H. longicornis*	No effects reported	[90]
Leucine aminopeptidase	*H. longicornis*	Extended pre-oviposition period, decreased egg weight and egg conversion ratio, morphological abnormalities in the oocytes	[91, 92]
Hemalin (thrombin inhibitor)	*H. longicornis*	Longer blood feeding period, failure to engorge, decreased inhibitory activity of fibrinogen clot formation in the midgut	[93]
Boophilin (thrombin inhibitor)	*R. (B.) microplus*	Decreased oviposition	[47]
Serine proteinase	*H. longicornis*	Suppressed erythrocyte degradation; decreased post-blood meal weight	[94]
Longipain	*H. longicornis*	Impaired blood feeding, decreased post-blood meal weight, increased *B. gibsoni* infection level and transovarial transmission	[95]
Cathepsin L	*I. ricinus*	Decreased weight gain	[96]
	H. longicornis	Decreased post-blood meal weight	[97]
Astacin	*R. (B.) microplus*	Decreased egg weight and egg conversion ratio	[84]
Tick reproduction			
Follistatin-related protein (FRP)	*H. longicornis*	Decreased egg conversion ratio	[98]
Vitellogenin receptor (VgR)	*Dermacentor variabilis*	Failure of Vg uptake by oocytes; failed oviposition	[34]
	H. longicornis	Suppressed oocyte maturation and failed oviposition, failure of *B. gibsoni* transovarial transmission	[99]

Target gene	Tick species	RNAi Effect	Refs
	A. hebraeum	Suppressed oocyte maturation, long pre-oviposition period,	[100]
Voraxin	*A. americanum*	Failure to engorge and lay eggs in females fed with males injected with a combination of subolesin and voraxin dsRNA	[101]
Vitellogenin (Vg)	*H. longicornis*	Decreased post-blood meal weight, abnormal oocytes, decreased egg conversion ratio	[102]
GATA factor	*H. longicornis*	Disrupted egg development	[103]
S6 kinase	*H. longicornis*	Disrupted egg development	[103]
Target of rapamycin (TOR)	*H. longicornis*	Decreased post-blood meal weight, mortality after engorgement, Failure of oocytes to mature and failure to lay eggs	[104]
Structural and metabolic function			
Glutamine:fructose-6-phosphate aminotransferase (HlGFAT)	*H. longicornis*	Decreased post-blood meal weight and survival	[105]
β-Actin	*I. scapularis*	Decreased post-blood meal weight and oviposition	[106]
Na^+K^+ATPase	*I. scapularis*	Decreased post-blood meal weight and oviposition	[106]
Valosin-containing protein (HlVCP)	*H. longicornis*	Decreased post-blood meal weight	[107]
Cyclophilins (Immunophilin)	*H. longicornis*	Lower post-blood meal weight, low survival after blood feeding and failure to lay eggs after silencing cyclophilin A	[108]
Ribosomal protein P0	*H. longicornis*	Decreased post-blood meal weight, low engorgement rate, and high mortality	[109]
Protein disulphide isomerases (PDI)	*H. longicornis*	Mortality after engorgement, leakage of blood from the midgut, little egg output	[110]
Organic anion transporter polypeptide (OATP)	*A. americanum*	Decreased post-blood meal weight, oviposition and egg conversion ratio	[37]
Ferritins (FER)	*I. ricinus*	Decreased post-blood meal weight, oviposition and hatch	[111]
	H. longicornis	Decreased post-blood meal weight, survival, oviposition and hatch	[112, 113]
Iron regulatory protein (IRP1)	*I. ricinus*	Decreased post-blood meal weight and hatching of eggs	[111]

Target gene	Tick species	RNAi Effect	Refs
Elongation factor 1-α	*R. annulatus, R. (B.) microplus*	High post-blood meal mortality, decreased post-blood meal weight and failure of oviposition	[45]
Lysine-ketoglutarate reductase/saccharopine dehydrogenase (LKR/SDH)	*H. longicornis*	Longer blood feeding period, decreased post-blood meal weight, longer pre-oviposition period, decreased oviposition and hatch after SDH silencing; higher volume of hemolymph after LKR silencing	[114]
Ubiquitin	*R. (B.) microplus*	Shorter post-blood meal survival, decreased or absence of egg output, impaired embryogenesis	[14, 29, 45, 72];
	R. annulatus	High mortality	[45]
Glycogen synthase kinase-3 (GSK-3)	*R. (B.) microplus*	Decreased oviposition and hatching	[115]
CD147 receptor	*A. americanum*	Inhibited feeding, low post-blood meal weight tender cuticle	[116]
Insulin-like growth factor binding protein-related proteins	*A. americanum*	Decreased post-blood meal weight	[117]
Putative 5.8S, ITS2 and 28S rRNA	*A. americanum*	High mortality and very low post-blood meal weight	[118]
Putative 2B7 60S ribosomal protein L13e	*A. americanum*	High mortality and very low post-blood meal weight	[118]
Putative interphase cytoplasm foci protein 45	*A. americanum*	High mortality and very low post-blood meal weight	[118]
Putative threonyl-tRNA synthetase	*A. americanum*	High mortality and very low post-blood meal weight	[118]
Putative 60S ribosomal protein L13a	*A. americanum*	100% mortality	[118]
Putative mitochondrial 12S rRNA	*A. americanum*	High mortality and very low post-blood meal weight	[118]
Chymotrypsin inhibitor (HlChI)	*H. longicornis*	Mortality after attachment, retarded blood feeding and longer feeding period, decreased post-blood meal weight, decreased egg weight and egg conversion ratio	[119]
Scavenger receptor	*H. longicornis*	Decreased post-blood meal weight, mortality after engorgement, decreased oviposition and hatch; inhibited bacterial phagocytosis of granulocytes	[26, 28]

Target gene	Tick species	RNAi Effect	Refs
4E-BP (eIF4E-binding protein)	*H. longicornis*	Decreased lipid accumulation in the midgut and fat bodies after long starvation period	[120]
Protein kinase B (AKT)	*H. longicornis*	Inhibition of engorgement and growth of organs during blood feeding; decreased expression of *longepsin*, *HlMIF* and *HlVg*s	[121]
	R. (B.) microplus	Decreased cell glycogen content and viability, and altered cell membrane permeability	[57]
Spook (Spo)	*Ornithodoros moubata*	Arrested development and molting	[53]
Shade (Shd)	*O. moubata*	Abnormal ecdysis and delayed molting	[53]
Cystatin (RHCyst)	*R. haemaphysaloides*	Decreased attachment and hatching rate	[122]
Tropomyosin	*H. longicornis*	Longer feeding time, decreased engorgement rate and post-blood meal weight, high mortality after blood feeding, failed oviposition	[123]
Protective antigens			
Subolesin (4D8)	*I. scapularis*	Decreased post-blood meal weight, oviposition and survival; failure of embryogenesis; silencing in eggs and larvae when dsRNA injected to engorged females	[43, 124]
	A. americanum	Decreased post-blood meal weight, oviposition and survival	[43, 101, 124]
	D. marginatus	Decreased post-blood meal weight, oviposition and survival	[124]
	D. variabilis	Decreased post-blood meal weight, oviposition and survival; decreased fertility; silencing in eggs and larvae when dsRNA injected to engorged females	[43, 124]
	R. sanguineus	Decreased post-blood meal weight, oviposition and survival; more dramatic effect when simultaneously silenced with Rs86	[124, 125]
	R. (B.) microplus	High mortality, decreased post-blood meal weight, oviposition and hatch in dsRNA-injected adults and progeny of dsRNA-injected adults	[42, 45, 46]
	R. annulatus,	Decreased post-blood meal weight	[45, 126]
	O. erraticus	Decreased egg output	[127]
	O. moubata	Decreased egg output	[127]

Target gene	Tick species	RNAi Effect	Refs
Midgut protein Rs86	*R. sanguineus*	Decreased post-blood meal weight and oviposition	[125]
Midgut protein Hl86	*H. longicornis*	Decreased post-blood meal weight	[128]
Midgut protein Bm86	*R. (B.) microplus*	Decreased number of engorging ticks, lower post-blood meal body weight and survival after feeding in *B. bovis*-infected host, decreased egg weight	[129]
Midgut protein Ree86	*R. evertsi evertsi*	No significant effect	[130]
Midgut protein ReeATAQ	*R. evertsi evertsi*	No significant effect	[130]
Longicin	*H. longicornis*	Decreased post-blood meal weight, increased *B. gibsoni* infection in the midgut and ovary, and transmission in the eggs	[131]
α2-macroglobulin proteins	*I. ricinus*	Decreased phagocytic action of hemocytes	[132, 133]
Macrophage migration inhibitory factor	*A. americanum*	No effect on phenotypes	[134]
Janus kinase (JAK)–signaling transducer activator of transcription (STAT) pathway	*I. scapularis*	Increased *A. phagocytophilum* infection level	[135]
Dual oxidase (Duox)	*I. scapularis*	Decreased level of *B. burgdorferi*	[136]
Peroxidase ISCW017368	*I. scapularis*	Decreased level of *B. burgdorferi*	[136]
Glutathione S-transferase	*R. (B.) microplus*	Decreased tick attachment and post-blood meal weight	[45]
	R.sanguineus	Increased susceptibility to permethrin	[137]
Selenoprotein W	*R. (B.) microplus*	Decreased tick attachment and post-blood meal weight	[45]
Selenoprotein K	*A. maculatum*	Decreased oviposition	[138]
Selenoprotein M	*A. maculatum*	Decreased oviposition	[138, 139]
Thioredoxin reductase	*A. maculatum*	Decreased native microbial load in midguts and salivary glands	[139]
Rmcystatin3 (cysteine protease inhibitor)	*R. (B.) microplus*	Increased resistance to bacteria	[140]
Pathogen acquisition/ transmission			
Subolesin	*D. variabilis*	Inhibited *Anaplasma marginale* infection in salivary glands	[141, 142]

Target gene	Tick species	RNAi Effect	Refs
	R. (B.) microplus	Decreased *A. marginale* infection level in salivary glands and tick cells	[143]
Salp15	*I. scapularis*	Decreased *Borrelia burgdorferi* transmission to the host	[52]
Salp14	*I. scapularis*	No effect on acquisition of *A. phagocytophilum* and *B. burgdorferi* in nymphs	[49]
Salp16	*I. scapularis*	Reduced *A. phagocytophilum* acquisition	[48]
Salp25D	*I. scapularis*	Decreased acquisition of *B. burgdorferi* after knockdown in salivary glands	[44]
Varisin	*D. variabilis*	Decreased *A. marginale* infection level	[144]
Immunophilin	*R. (B.) microplus*	Decreased hatch, decreased larval survival, increased *B. bovis* infection in larval progeny	[41]
Kunitz-type serine protease inhibitor (Spi)	*R. (B.) microplus*	Inhibition of engorgement, decreased egg weight	[41]
Glutathione S-transferase	*D. variabilis*	Inhibited *A. marginale* infection	[142]
H^+ transporting lysosomal vacuolar proton pump (vATPase)	*D. variabilis*	Inhibited *A. marginale* infection in the midgut after acquisition feeding	[142]
Selenoprotein M	*D. variabilis*	Inhibited *A. marginale* infection and multiplication in salivary glands	[142]
Putative von Willebrand factor (94Will)	*R. (B.) microplus*	Decreased *A. marginale* infection level in salivary glands	[143]
Flagelliform silk protein (100Silk)	*R. (B.) microplus*	Decreased *A. marginale* infection level in salivary glands and tick cells	[143]
Putative metallothionein (93 Meth)	*R. (B.) microplus*	Increased *A. marginale* infection level in tick cells	[143]
Tick salivary lectin pathway inhibitor (TSLPI)	*I. scapularis*	Decreased load of *B. burgdorferi* and transmission to host	[145]
Kunitz-type serine protease inhibitor (DvKPI)	*D. variabilis*	Increased rickettsial infection in the midgut	[146]
Kunitz-type protease inhibitor 5 (KTPI)	*R. annulatus, R. (B.) microplus*	Decreased post-blood meal weight	[126]
Histamine release factor	*I. scapularis*	Decreased post-blood meal weight, decreased *B. burgdorferi* transmission	[147]
TROSPA	*R. annulatus, R. (B.) microplus*	Decreased *B. bigemina* infection level; Decreased post-blood meal weight in *R. microplus*	[126]

Target gene	Tick species	RNAi Effect	Refs
Serum amyloid A	*R. annulatus, R. (B.) microplus*	Decreased *B. bigemina* infection level	[126]
Ricinusin	*R. annulatus, R. (B.) microplus*	Decreased post-blood meal weight in *R. annulatus*	[126]
Calreticulin	*R. annulatus, R. (B.) microplus*	Decreased *B. bigemina* infection level in *R. microplus*; decreased post-blood meal weight in *R. annulatus*	[126]
Chitin deacetylase-like protein (IsCDA)	*I. scapularis*	No significant effect on *B. burgdorferi* acquisition or transmission	[50]
Antifreeze glycoprotein	*I. scapularis*	Decreased survival and mobility of ticks in extremely cold temperature; decreased *A. phagocytophilum* infection level	[148]
x-linked inhibitor of apoptosis protein (E3 ubiquitin ligase, XIAP)	*I. scapularis*	Increased *A. phagocytophilum* infection	[149]
Cytochrome c oxidase subunit III	*R. (B.) microplus*	Failure in transmission of *A. marginale*	[150]

Table 1. Genes functionally characterized through RNAi in different tick species.

Silencing these genes through RNAi greatly reduced the reproductive capacity of female ticks, which showed immature and light-colored oocytes. The uptake of vitellogenin in the oocytes is facilitated by vitellogenin receptor, which has been characterized in *D. variabilis* [34], *H.longicornis* [99], and *A. hebraeum* [100]. Aside from the negative impact in oviposition consistently induced by RNAi in all these studies, silencing of *H. longicornis* vitellogenin receptor also reportedly inhibited the transovarial transmission of *Babesia gibsoni*. Three factors involved in the initiation of vitellogenesis, the GATA factor, S6 kinase [103], and target of rapamycin (TOR) pathway [104], have been also characterized in *H. longicornis* ticks using RNAi. The significance of other proteins to reproduction, such as a tick homologue of the human follistatin-related protein [98] and the engorgement protein voraxin [101] from the male gonad, has been also demonstrated using RNAi.

4.4. Genes related to structural and metabolic functions

Various gene encoding proteins important in cellular structure and metabolism have been characterized using RNAi. Due to their wide distribution and systemic function, knockdown of these proteins caused detrimental effects on different tick physiological functions and some even proved to be lethal (Table 1). Among these proteins is the multifunctional ubiquitin, which has been first targeted based on a homologous gene of *D. melanogaster* in a study investigating the components of tick RNAi pathway [14]. Ubiquitin knockdown in *R. (B.)*

microplus shortened the post-blood meal survival of ticks and impaired egg viability and hatch. In separate studies, ubiquitin has also been the subject in examining off-target effects of RNAi [29] and the feasibility of dsRNA feeding in *R. (B.) microplus* [72]. RNAi-mediated silencing of ribosomal proteins in *A. americanum* [118], and ubiquitin, elongation factor-1 alpha and several other proteins in *R. (B.) microplus* and *R. annulatus* [45] has been employed to screen potential antigens for tick control.

In the hard tick *H. longicornis*, individual knockdown of glutamine:fructose-6-phosphate aminotransferase [105], cyclophilin A [108], the ribosomal protein P0 [109], protein disulphide isomerases [110], and tropomyosin [123] resulted to decreased survival of ticks after engorgement. Two proteins with apparent roles in withstanding long starvation period, lysine-ketoglutarate reductase/saccharopine dehydrogenase (LKR/SDH) [114] and 4E-BP [120], have also been characterized in *H. longicornis*. LKR/SDH mRNA expression is higher in starved ticks than in unfed ticks and knockdown of LKR resulted to high volume of hemolymph after blood feeding, suggesting its role in osmoregulation. Meanwhile, 4E-BP knockdown led to decreased lipid storage in the midguts and fat bodies of ticks during longer starvation period. An interesting report on the application of RNAi in studying tick neurobiology targetedβ-actin and Na^+-K^+-ATPase of *I. scapularis* using fluorescently labeled dsRNAs to monitor the uptake in tick synganglia [106].

The significance of proteins involved in iron metabolism to tick feeding and reproduction has been also demonstrated using RNAi in two hard tick species, *I. ricinus* [111] and *H. longicornis* [112]. Silencing two types of the iron storage protein ferritin greatly reduced the ticks' capacity to engorge and produce eggs, also affecting post-blood meal survival due to occurrence of iron-mediated oxidative stress [113]. An iron regulatory protein responsible for translation of iron binding proteins was characterized in *I. scapularis*, with its knockdown greatly reducing egg hatchability [111]. Two enzymes, spook and shade, were characterized in the soft tick *O. moubata* and were shown to be important in ecdysteroidogenesis through RNAi [53]. Silencing spook protein in nymphs caused arrested development and molting, whereas silencing shade delayed molting and led to abnormal ecdysis.

5. RNAi studies on tick protective antigens and immunity

The immune system of ticks has a vital role of protecting them from harmful substances in the blood, including components of their host's immune system, and from various pathogens that they acquire in their blood feeding activity. Tick protective antigens, therefore, gain wide interest due to their potential as target for tick control. The highly conserved tick protective antigen subolesin, previously known as 4D8, was first identified from *I. scapularis* through cDNA expression library immunization (ELI) [153], after which, it has been also identified in other hard tick species, and using RNAi, was found to be important in the success of blood feeding and reproduction [124]. An ortholog of subolesin has also been characterized in two soft tick species and RNAi demonstrated that subolesin is also important in the reproduction of soft ticks [127]. The function of subolesin is unclear, but a report showed that subolesin knockdown affected the expression of several genes involved in multiple cellular pathways, suggesting a role in gene expression by interacting with regulatory proteins [154]. Aside from being reported as a promising anti-tick vaccine antigen candidate in many studies, it has been also proposed that subolesin may be targeted in ticks that subsequently will be released for sterile acarine technique (SAT) [38].

The membrane-bound glycoprotein Bm86 expressed mainly in the midgut of *R.* (*B.*) *microplus* [155] is the first, and until recently, the only tick antigen that is commercially available as an anti-tick vaccine in some countries. The exact function of Bm86, however, remains unclear yet. RNAi has been employed to knockdown *Bm86* and its homologues in other tick species, including *R. sanguineus, H. longicornis,* and *R. evertsi evertsi,* which in most cases affected the blood feeding and reproduction of adult ticks, except in *R. evertsi evertsi* wherein knockdown of two homologues did not yield significant effects [130]. A study in *R.* (*B.*) *microplus* also showed that knockdown of *Bm86* decreased the blood feeding capacity and survival of ticks after feeding on a *B. bovis*-infected host, suggesting that Bm86 may have a critical role in the fitness of ticks after feeding from an acutely *B. bovis*-infected host [129].

The function of some components of immunity, such as α2-macroglobulin proteins [132, 133], antimicrobial peptides [131], Janus kinase (JAK)-signaling transducer activator of transcription (STAT) pathway [135], dityrosine network [136], and cysteine protease inhibitor in the hemocytes [140] have been analyzed using RNAi. The α2-macroglobulin proteins of *I. ricinus,* related to vertebrate complement system, were shown to be involved in the phagocytic activity of hemocytes against Gram-negative bacteria [132, 133]. In contrast, a cysteine protease Rmcystatin3 identified in *R.* (*B.*) *microplus* was implicated as a negative modulator of tick immune response after its silencing greatly reduced the number of bacterial load in the ticks [140]. The role of a defensin from *H. longicornis,* longicin, in ticks' immune defense against *Babesia* parasites was demonstrated through RNAi, as exhibited by a higher load of *B. gibsoni* in the midgut and ovary of *longicin*-silenced ticks after infestation in an infected host [131]. Meanwhile, JAK-STAT pathway was shown to be important in *Anaplasma phagocytophilum* infection in ticks after its knockdown increased the infection in the salivary glands of nymphs that fed on infected mice [135]. A dual oxidase and a peroxidase, ISCW017368, which together forms a dityrosine network, were separately silenced in *I. scapularis,* both resulting to reduced *Borrelia burgdorferi* persistence in ticks [136].

The obligatory blood feeding lifestyle of ticks exposes them to high levels of pro-oxidants that may trigger oxidative stress. Antioxidant enzymes function to protect them from the harmful effects of oxidative stress. Furthermore, these antioxidant enzymes provide detoxification mechanisms to counteract toxins that they encounter in the environment, such as chemical acaricides. RNAi has been very useful in evaluating the function of these antioxidants. Silencing a selenoprotein in *R.* (*B.*) *microplus* reduced the engorged body weight and egg output [45]. In contrast, a study on *A. maculatum* showed that silencing two selenoproteins did not alter blood feeding, although the egg output was reduced. Interestingly, the total antioxidant capacities of the saliva from knockdowned ticks were higher, indicating that other antioxidant enzymes may have compensated for the absence of selenoproteins [138]. In another study, silencing thioredoxin reductase, another selenoprotein, in *A. maculatum* did not have a negative impact on blood feeding and reproduction. Likewise, variations in transcriptional expression of some antioxidant enzymes were also observed, suggesting compensatory mechanism in the absence of thioredoxin reductase [139]. However, the more interesting finding in that study was the decreased microbiota population following thioredoxin reductase knockdown, possibly because of disturbed redox homeostasis balance. Meanwhile, silencing a glutathione S-transferase (GST) gene affected the attachment of ticks and reduced the post-blood meal bodyweight of *R. (B.) microplus* [45]. It also made *R. sanguineus* ticks more susceptible to permethrin, although no significant effects on tick attachment, feeding and reproductive capacity were observed [137].

6. Understanding tick-pathogen interaction through RNAi

RNAi has undoubtedly paved a way to better understand the different aspects of ticks' association with various pathogens. Numerous tick proteins with different functions have been found to be involved in the acquisition, establishment, and transmission of pathogens. Several proteins have been studied through RNAi to determine their importance in the development cycle of different pathogens. The knockdown of subolesin [142, 156], GST, vATPase, and selenoprotein M [142] in *D. variabilis*, and putative von Willebrand factor, flagelliform silk protein and subolesin in *R. (B.) microplus* [143] decreased the infection level of *A. marginale* in these hard ticks, implying that these proteins are significant in the establishment of infection of this rickettsia.

RNAi also demonstrated that the Lyme disease agent *B. burgdorferi* can utilize several proteins of *I. scapularis* to facilitate its transmission to the host. These include salivary proteins such as tick histamine release factor [147], Salp15 [52], and the lectin complement pathway inhibitor (TSLPI) [145]; the latter two provide protection for *B. burgdorferi* against components of the host immune system. Salivary proteins Salp14 [49], Salp16 [48], and Salp25D [44] have been examined for their function in acquiring *A. phagocytophilum* or *B. burgdorferi* through RNAi. Knockdown of Salp14 did not affect the acquisition of either rickettsiae, whereas the knockdown of Salp16 and Salp25D decreased the infection level of *A. phagocytophilum* and *B. burgdorferi* in the tick, respectively.

An interesting study on *I. scapularis* showed that *A. phagocytophilum* promotes cold tolerance through an antifreeze glycoprotein [148]. In the absence of this antifreeze glycoprotein, the survival rate of ticks after exposure to extremely cold temperature and the infection level of *A. phagocytophilum* following exposure was reduced. Tick defensins, varisin from *D. variabilis* [144], and ricinusin from *Rhipicephalus* ticks [126] have been silenced to examine their functions in pathogen establishment; the former reduced *A. marginale* infection level, while the latter did not have an effect on *B. bigemina* infection.

Several reports also demonstrated the interaction of *Babesia* parasites and tick proteins through RNAi. Knockdown of the immunophilin gene in *R. (B.) microplus* had negative impact on the reproductive performance of the tick and also increased the infection rate of *B. bovis* in larval progeny [41], while knockdown of TROSPA, serum amyloid A, and calreticulin reduced the infection level of *B. bigemina* in *Rhipicephalus* ticks [126]. Silencing a Kunitz-type serine protease inhibitor from *D. variabilis* increased the rickettsial infection in the midgut [146], whereas in *R. (B.) microplus*, silencing a Kunitz-type serine protease inhibitor, Spi, tended to increase the infection rate of *B. bovis* in larval progeny [41], but silencing of another Kunitz-type protease inhibitor 5 (KTPI) did not have any effect on *Babesia* infection [126].

7. Future directions in tick research and application in tick control

Indeed, great progress in understanding tick biology has been already accomplished in the past. However, many aspects of tick physiology and host-tick-pathogen interaction need to be unraveled yet. Moreover, several optimizations can still be done to improve RNAi in tick research. While being the most widely used method of introducing dsRNA, the injection method (particularly microinjection) that requires elaborate equipment may not be accessible to all laboratories. Moreover, injection is mostly applicable to adult and sometimes nymphal stages, and may be injurious to the ticks, especially when performed by an inexperienced researcher. The soaking method is simpler, less invasive, and less laborious. Electroporation has been recently shown to be effective in introducing dsRNA in eggs [66] and may be useful in studying the function of genes that are involved in embryogenesis and physiology of immature tick stages.

RNAi may also prove to be a promising tick control method and not just a research tool. In pest insect management, the possibility of using RNAi as a novel tool of pest control is already being explored by feeding liposome-coated dsRNA or dsRNA expressed in transgenic plants or bacteria [32]. RNAi targeting several genes have been accomplished by feeding plants expressing dsRNA in several species of economically important crop pests [16]. Feeding dsRNA to ticks is still an underdeveloped approach, which has been yet accomplished only by artificial feeding. Coating dsRNAs with liposomes or nanocarriers may increase dsRNA stability that may make it feasible for administration to the host. Genes that are highly conserved across different tick species, and are of importance in tick survival are good candidate targets. These include proteins with structural and metabolic functions, such as ubiquitin, tropomyosin, and ferritin. However, the specificity of dsRNA to the tick gene should be highly considered. Additional consideration would be the establishment of a minimum effective dose, since the synthesis of dsRNA is costly.

Additionally, RNAi has been proposed as an alternative method for the sterile insect technique in blood-sucking mosquitoes that will produce sterile males by feeding dsRNA in mosquito larvae [64]. Quite similarly, the application of RNAi for tick control was also proposed in a single report on *D. variabilis*, wherein the highly conserved subolesin was targeted leading to reproductive incapacity [38]. In conclusion, the authors suggested that RNAi may be used to massively produce sterile ticks (SAT) that may be released in the field. Releasing subolesin-silenced ticks may also aid in the control of *A. marginale*, since it has been reported that subolesin knockdown reduced the infection level of this pathogen [141–143]. Introducing dsRNA to eggs through electroporation described above may be a more convenient way of producing knockdowned ticks.

8. Summary

In this chapter, we have reviewed the application of RNAi in tick research and described the significant contribution of RNAi in advancing our knowledge on tick biology and tick-pathogen interaction. RNAi has revolutionized the advancement of our understanding of various aspects of tick blood feeding and digestion, reproduction, metabolism, and immunity. As a functional analysis tool, RNAi has become very handy in elucidating the functions of different proteins from more than 10 hard tick species and a few soft tick species. It has been particularly helpful in screening potential target antigens for anti-tick and tick-borne pathogen vaccine development [157]. Several methods of introducing dsRNA in ticks have been employed but injection has remained to be the most widely used technique. The number of published research on ticks that involves the application of RNAi has been continuously increasing through the years, and it is expected to continue doing so. A great majority of the published reports focused on hard ticks, but due to some physiological differences, more research using RNAi on soft ticks should be conducted. Finally, with numerous potential target genes already identified, the application of RNAi as a tick control method should be investigated in the future, starting with optimization of dsRNA delivery method for practical use.

Acknowledgements

This work was supported by the Japan Society for the Promotion of Science (JSPS) KAKENHI Grant Numbers 22580335, 25292173, and 26660229. We also thank our colleague, Melbourne R. Talactac, at the Laboratory of Infectious Diseases, Joint Faculty of Veterinary Medicine, Kagoshima University, for his assistance in writing this chapter.

Author details

Remil Linggatong Galay[1,2], Rika Umemiya-Shirafuji[3], Masami Mochizuki[1], Kozo Fujisaki[4] and Tetsuya Tanaka[2*]

*Address all correspondence to: tetsuya@ms.kagoshima-u.ac.jp

1 Department of Veterinary Paraclinical Sciences, College of Veterinary Medicine, University of the Philippines Los Baños, Los Baños, Philippines

2 Laboratory of Infectious Diseases, Joint Faculty of Veterinary Medicine, Kagoshima University, Kagoshima, Japan

3 National Research Center for Protozoan Diseases, Obihiro University of Agriculture and Veterinary Medicine, Inada-cho, Obihiro, Hokkaido, Japan

4 National Agricultural and Food Research Organization, Tsukuba, Ibaraki, Japan

References

[1] Dantas-Torres F, Chomel B, Otranto D. Ticks and tick-borne diseases: A One Health perspective. Trends Parasitol. 2012;28:437-46. doi:10.1016/j.pt.2012.07.003.

[2] Jonjegan F, Uilenberg G. The global importance of ticks. Parasitology 2004;129:S3-S14.

[3] de la Fuente J. The fossil record and the origin of ticks (Acari: Parasitiformes: Ixodida). Exp Appl Acarol. 2003;29:437-46.

[4] Estrada-Peña A, Salman M. Current limitations in the control and spread of ticks that affect livestock: A review. Agriculture. 2013;3:221-35. doi:10.3390/agriculture3020221.

[5] Estrada-Peña A, de la Fuente J. The ecology of ticks and epidemiology of tick-borne viral diseases. Antiviral Res. 2014;108:104-28. doi:10.1016/j.antiviral.2014.05.016.

[6] Kim E, Bauer C, Grevelding CG, Quack T. Improved PCR/nested PCR approaches with increased sensitivity and specificity for the detection of pathogens in hard ticks. Ticks Tick Borne Dis. 2013;4:409-16. doi:10.1016/j.ttbdis.2013.04.004.

[7] Baneth G. Tick-borne infections of animals and humans: A common ground. Int J Parasitol. 2014;44:591-6. doi:10.1016/j.ijpara.2014.03.011.

[8] Guerrero FD, Lovis L, Martins JR. Acaricide resistance mechanisms in *Rhipicephalus* (*Boophilus*) *microplus*. Rev Bras Parasitol Vet. 2012;21:1-6. doi:10.1590/S1984-29612012000100002.

[9] Hannon GJ. RNA interference. Nature. 2002;418:244-51. doi:10.1038/418244a.

[10] Aljamali MN, Sauer JR, Essenberg RC. RNA interference: Applicability in tick research. Exp App Acarol. 2002;28:89-96.

[11] de la Fuente J, Kocan KM, Almazan C, Blouin EF. RNA interference for the study and genetic manipulation of ticks. Trends Parasitol. 2007;23:427-33. doi:10.1016/j.pt.2007.07.002.

[12] Mello CC, Conte Jr. D. Revealing the world of RNA interference. Nature. 2004;431:338-42. doi:10.1038/nature02872.

[13] Whangbo JS, Hunter CP. Environmental RNA interference. Trends Genetics. 2008;24:297-305. doi:10.1016/j.tig.2008.03.007.

[14] Kurscheid S, Lew-Tabor AE, Valle MR, Bruyeres AG, Doogan VJ, Munderloh UG, et al. Evidence of a tick RNAi pathway by comparative genomics and reverse genetics screen of targets with known loss-of-function phenotypes in *Drosophila*. BMC Mol Biol. 2009;10:26. doi:10.1186/1471-2199-10-26.

[15] Barnard AC, Nijhof AM, Fick W, Stutzer C, Maritz-Olivier C. RNAi in arthropods: Insight into machinery and applications for understanding the pathogen-vector interface. Genes. 2012;3:704-41. doi:10.3390/genes3040702.

[16] Aronstein K, Oppert B, Lorenzen MD. RNAi in agriculturally-important arthropods. In: Grabowski P, editor. RNA Processing: InTech; 2011. p. 157-80. doi:10.5772/19768.

[17] Rocheleau CE. RNA interference: Systemic RNAi SIDes with endosomes. Curr Biol. 2012;22:R873-R5. doi:10.1016/j.cub.2012.08.039.

[18] Hunter CP, Winston WM, Molodowitch C, Feinberg EH, Shih J, Sutherlin M, et al. Systemic RNAi in *Caenorhabditis elegans*. Cold Spring Harb Symp Quant Biol. 2006;71:95-100. doi:10.1101/sqb.2006.71.060.

[19] Jose AM, Smith JJ, Hunter CP. Export of RNA silencing from *C. elegans* tissues does not require the RNA channel SID-1. Proc Natl Acad Sci USA. 2009;106:2283-8. doi: 10.1073/pnas.0809760106.

[20] Hinas A, Wright AJ, Hunter CP. SID-5 is an endosome-associated protein required for efficient systemic RNAi in *C. elegans*. Curr Biol. 2012;22:1938-43. doi:10.1016/j.cub. 2012.08.020.

[21] Winston WM, Sutherlin M, Wright AJ, Feinberg EH, Hunter CP. *Caenorhbaditis elegans* SID-2 is required for environmental RNA interference. Proc Natl Acad Sci USA. 2007;104:10565-70. doi:10.1073/pnas.0611282104.

[22] Tijsterman M, May RC, Simmer F, Okihara KL, Plasterk RHA. Genes required for systemic RNA interference in *Caenorhabditis elegans*. Curr Biol. 2004;14:111-6. doi: 10.1016/j.cub.2003.12.029.

[23] Ulvila J, Parikka M, Kleino A, Sormunen R, Ezekowitz RA, Kocks C, et al. Double-stranded RNA is internalized by scavenger receptor-mediated endocytosis in *Drosophila* S2 cells. J Biol Chem. 2006;281:14370-5. doi:10.1074/jbc.M513868200.

[24] Ramet M, Pearson A, Manfruelli P, Li X, Koziel H, Gobel V, et al. *Drosophila* scavenger receptor CI is a pattern recognition receptor for bacteria. Immunity. 2001;15:1027-38. doi:10.1016/S1074-7613(01)00249-7.

[25] Kocks C, Cho JH, Nehme N, Ulvila J, Pearson A, Meister M, et al. Eater, a transmembrane protein mediating phagocytosis of bacterial pathogens in Drosophila. Cell. 2005;123:335-46. doi:10.1016/j.cell.2005.08.034.

[26] Aung KM, Boldbaatar D, Liao M, Umemiya-Shirafuji R, Nakao S, Matsuoka T, et al. Identification and characterization of class B scavenger receptor CD36 from the hard tick, *Haemaphysalis longicornis*. Parasitol Res. 2011;108:272-85. doi:10.1007/ s00436-010-2053-1.

[27] Aung KM, Boldbaatar D, Umemiya-Shirafuji R, Liao M, Xuan X, Suzuki H, et al. Scavenger receptor mediates systemic RNA interference in ticks. PLoS ONE. 2011;6:e28407. doi:10.1371/journal.pone.0028407.

[28] Aung KM, Boldbaatar D, Umemiya-Shirafuji R, Liao M, Tsuji N, Xuan X, et al. HlSRB, a Class B Scavenger Receptor, is Key to the Granulocyte-Mediated Microbial Phagocytosis in Ticks. PloS ONE. 2012;7:e33504. doi:10.1371/journal.pone.0033504.

[29] Lew-Tabor AE, Kurscheid S, Barrero R, Gondro C, Moolhuijzen PM, Valle MR, et al. Gene expression evidence for off-target effects caused by RNA interference-mediated gene silencing of *Ubiquitin-63E* in the cattle tick *Rhipicephalus microplus*. Int J Parasitol. 2011;41:1001-14. doi: 10.1016/j.ijpara.2011.05.003.

[30] Lee YS, Nakahara K, Pham JW, Kim K, He Z, Sontheimer EJ, et al. Distinct roles for *Drosophila* Dicer-1 and Dicer-2 in the siRNA/miRNA silencing pathways. Cell. 2004;117:69-81. doi:10.1016/S0092-8674(04)00261-2.

[31] Hock J, Meister G. The Argonaute protein family. Genome Biology. 2008;9:210. doi: 10.1186/gb-2008-9-2-210.

[32] Xue X, Mao Y, Tao X, Huang Y, Chen X. New approaches to agricultural insect pest control based on RNA interference. In: Zayed A, Kent CF, editors. Advances in insect physiology. 42: Elsevier; 2012. p. 73-117. doi:10.1016/B978-0-12-387680-5.00003-3.

[33] Karim S, Adamson SW. RNA interference in ticks: A functional genomics took for the study of physiology. In: Zayed A, Kent CF, editors. Advances in insect physiology. 42: Elsevier; 2012. p. 120-54. doi:10.1016/B978-0-12-387680-5.00004-5.

[34] Mitchell III RD, Ross E, Osgood C, Sonenshine DE, Donohue KV, Khalil SM, et al. Molecular characterization, tissue-specific expression and RNAi knockdown of the first vitellogenin receptor from a tick. Insect Biochem Mol Biol. 2007;37:375-88. doi: 10.1016/j.ibmb.2007.01.005.

[35] Decrem Y, Beaufays J, Blasioli V, Lahaye K, Brossard M, Vanhamme L, et al. A family of putative metalloproteases in the salivary glands of the tick *Ixodes ricinus*. FEBS J. 2008;275:1485-99. doi:10.1111/j.1742-4658.2008.06308.x.

[36] Karim S, Ramakrishnan VG, Tucker JS, Essenberg RC, Sauer JR. *Amblyomma americanum* salivary glands: Double-stranded RNA-mediated gene silencing of synaptobrevin homologue and inhibition of PGE_2 stimulated protein secretion. Insect Biochem Mol Biol. 2004;34:407-13. doi:10.1016/j.ibmb.2004.01.005.

[37] Mulenga A, Khumthong R, Chalaire KC, Strey O, Teel P. Molecular and biological characterization of the *Amblyomma americanum* organic anion transporter polypeptide. J Exp Biol. 2008;211:3401-8. doi:10.1242/jeb.022376.

[38] de la Fuente J, Almazan C, Naranjo V, Blouin EF, Meyer JM, Kocan KM. Autocidal control of ticks by silencing of a single gene by RNA interference. Biochem Biophys Res Comm. 2006;344:332-28. doi:10.1016/j.bbrc.2006.03.109.

[39] Narasimhan S, Montgometry RR, DePonte K, Tschudi C, Marcantonio N, Anderson JF, et al. Disruption of *Ixodes scapularis* anticoagulation by using RNA interference. Proc Natl Acad Sci USA. 2004;101:1141-6. doi:10.1073/pnas.0307669100.

[40] Kocan KM, Blouin EF, de la Fuente J. RNA interference in ticks. J Vis Exp. 2011;20:2472. doi:10.3791/2474.

[41] Bastos RG, Ueti MW, Guerrero FD, Knowles DP, Scoles GA. Silencing of a putative immunophilin gene in the cattle tick *Rhipicephalus* (*Boophilus*) *microplus* increases the infection rate of *Babesia bovis* in larval progeny. Parasit Vectors. 2009;2:57. doi: 10.1186/1756-3305-2-57.

[42] Nijhof AM, Taoufik A, de la Fuente J, Kocan KM, de Vries E, Jonjegan F. Gene silencing of the tick protective antigens, *Bm86, Bm91* and *subolesin* in the one-host tick *Boophilus microplus* by RNA interference. Int J Parasitol. 2007;2007:653-62. doi:10.1016/j.ijpara.2006.11.005.

[43] Kocan KM, Manzano-Roman R, de la Fuente J. Transovarial silencing of the subolesin gene in three-host ixodid tick species after injection of replete females with subolesin dsRNA. Parasitol Res. 2007;100:1411-5. doi:10.1007/s00436-007-0483-1.

[44] Narasimhan S, Sukumaran B, Bozdogan U, Thomas V, Liang X, DePonte K, et al. A tick antioxidant facilitates the lyme disease agent's successful migration from the mammalian host to the arthropod vector. Cell Host Microbe. 2007;2:7-18. doi:10.1016/j.chom.2007.06.001.

[45] Almazan C, Lagunes R, Villar M, Canales M, Rosario-Cruz R, Jonjegan F, et al. Identification and characterization of *Rhipicephalus* (*Boophilus*) *microplus* candidate protective antigens for the control of cattle tick infestations. Parasitol Res. 2010;106:471-9. doi:10.1007/s00436-009-1689-1.

[46] Merino O, Almazan C, Canales M, Villar M, Moreno-Cid JA, Estrada-Pena A, et al. Control of *Rhipicephalus* (*Boophilus*) *microplus* infestations by the combination of subolesin vaccination and tick autocidal control after subolesin gene knockdown in ticks fed on cattle. Vaccine. 2011;29:2248-54. doi:10.1016/j.vaccine.2011.01.050.

[47] Soares TS, Watanabe RMO, Tanaka-Azevedo AM, Torquato RJS, Lu S, Figueiredo AC, et al. Expression and functional characterization of boophilin, a thrombin inhibitor from *Rhipicephalus* (*Boophilus*) *microplus* midgut. Vet Parasitol. 2012;187:521-8. doi: 10.1016/j.vetpar.2012.01.027.

[48] Sukumaran B, Narasimhan S, Anderson JF, DePonte K, Marcantonio N, Krishnan MN, et al. An *Ixodes scapularis* protein required for survival of *Anaplasma phagocytophilum* in tick salivary glands. J Exp Med. 2006;203:1507-17. doi:10.1084/jem.20060208.

[49] Pedra JOF, Narasimhan S, DePonte K, Marcantonio N, Kantor FS, Fikrig E. Disruption of the salivary protein 14 in *Ixodes scapularis* nymphts and impact on pathogen acquisition. Am J Trop Med Hyg. 2006;75:677-82.

[50] Kariu T, Smith A, Yang X, Pal U. A chitin deacetylase-like protein is a predominant constituent of tick perotrophic membrane that influences the persistence of Lyme disease pathogens within the vector. PLoS ONE. 2013;8:e78376. doi:10.1371/journal.pone.0078376.

[51] Pal U, Li X, Wang T, Montgometry RR, Ramamoothi N, Desilva AM, et al. TROSPA, an *Ixodes scapularis* receptor *Borrelia burgdorferi*. Cell. 2004;119:457-68. doi:10.1016/j.cell.2004.10.027.

[52] Ramamoorthi N, Narasimhan S, Pal U, Bao F, Yang XF, Fish D, et al. The Lyme disease agent exploits a tick protein to infect the mammalian host. Nature. 2005;436:573-7. doi:10.1038/nature03812.

[53] Ogihara MH, Hikiba J, Suzuki Y, Taylor D, Kataoka H. Ovarian ecdysteroidogenesis in both immature and mature stages of an Acari, *Ornithodoros moubata*. PLoS ONE. 2015;10:e0124953. doi:10.1371/journal.pone.0124953.

[54] Clemens JC, Worby CA, Simonson-Leff N, Muda M, Maehama T, Hemmings BA, et al. Use of double-stranded RNA interference in *Drosophila* cell lines to dissect signal transduction pathways. Proc Natl Acad Sci USA. 2000;97:6499-503. doi:10.1073/pnas.110149597.

[55] Blouin EF, Manzano-Roman R, De la Fuente J, Kocan KM. Defining the role of subolesin in tick cell culture by use of RNA interference. Ann NY Acad Sci. 2008;1149:41-4. doi:10.1196/annals.1428.058.

[56] Barry G, Alberdi P, Schnettler E, Weisheit S, Kohl A, Fazakerley JK, et al. Gene silencing in tick cell lines using small interfering or long double-stranded RNA. Exp App Acarol. 2013;59:319-38. doi:10.1007/s10493-012-9598-x.

[57] de Abreu LA, Calixto C, Waltero CF, Noce BPD, Githaka NW, Seixas A, et al. The conserved role of the AKT/GSK3 axis in cell survival and glycogen metabolism in *Rhipicephalus* (*Boophilus*) *microplus* embryo tick cell line BME26. Biochim Biophys Acta. 2013;1830:2574-82. doi:10.1016/j.bbagen.2012.12.016.

[58] Aljamali MN, Bior AD, Sauer JR, Essenberg RC. RNA interference in ticks: A study using histamine binding protein dsRNA in the female tick *Amblyomma americanum*. Insect Mol Biol. 2003;12:299-305. doi:10.1046/j.1365-2583.2003.00416.x.

[59] Karim S, Ramakrishnan VG, Tucker JS, Essenberg RC, Sauer JR. *Amblyomma americanum* salivary gland homolog of nSec1 is essential for saliva protein secretion. Biochem Biophys Res Comm. 2004;324:1256-63. doi:10.1016/j.bbrc.2004.09.189.

[60] Ramakrishnan VG, Aljamali MN, Sauer JR, Essenberg RC. Application of RNA interference in tick salivary gland research. J Biomol Tech. 2005;16:297-305.

[61] Karim S, Miller NJ, Valenzuela J, Sauer JR, Mather TN. RNAi-mediated gene silencing to assess the role of synaptobrevin and cystatin in tick blood feeding. Biochem Biophys Res Commun. 2005;334:1336-42. doi:10.1016/j.bbrc.2005.07.036.

[62] Campbell EM, Budge GE, Bowman AS. Gene-knockdown in the honey bee mite *Varroa destructor* by a non-invasive approach: Studies on a glutathione S-transferase. Parasit Vectors. 2012;3:73. doi:10.1186/1756-3305-3-73.

[63] Kamau LM, Wright HW, Nisbet AJ, Bowman AS. Development of an RNA-interference procedure for gene knockdown in the poultry red mite, *Dermanyssus gallinae*: Studies on histamine releasing factor and Cathepsin-D. Afr J Biothechnol. 2013;12:1350-6. doi:10.5897/AJB12.2693.

[64] Whyard S, Erdelyan CNG, Partridge AL, Singh AD, Beebe NW, Capina R. Silencing the buzz: A new approach to population suppression of mosquitoes by feeding larvae double-stranded RNAs. Parasit Vectors. 2015;8:96. doi:10.1186/s13071-015-0716-6.

[65] Gong H, Umemiya R, Zhou J, Liao M, Zhang H, Jia H, et al. Blocking the secretion of saliva by silencing the *HlYkt6* gene in the tick *Haemaphysalis longicornis*. Insect Biochem Mol Biol. 2009;39:372-81. doi:10.1016/j.ibmb.2009.03.002.

[66] Neumann E, Schaeffer-Ridder M, Wang Y, Hofschneider PH. Gene transfer into mouse lyoma cells by electroporation in high electric fields. EMBO J. 1982;1:841-5.

[67] Karim S, Troiano E, Mather TN. Functional genomics tool: Gene silencing in *Ixodes scapularis* eggs and nymphs by electroporated dsRNA. BMC Biotech. 2010;10:1. doi: 10.1186/1472-6750-10-1.

[68] Ruiz N, de Abreu LA, Parizi LF, Kim TK, Mulenga A, Braz GRC, et al. Non-invasive delivery of dsRNA into de-waxed tick eggs by electroporation. PLoS ONE. 2015. doi: 10.1371/journal.pone.0130008.

[69] Yu N, Christiaens O, Liu J, Niu J, Cappelle K, Caccia S, et al. Delivery of dsRNA for RNAi in insects: An overview and future directions. Insect Sci. 2013;20:4-14. doi: 10.1111/j.1744-7917.2012.01534.x.

[70] Krober T, Guerin PM. *In vitro* feeding assays for hard ticks. Trends Parasitol. 2007;23:445-9. doi:10.1016/j.pt.2007.07.010.

[71] Soares CAG, Lima CMR, Dolan MC, Piesman J, Beard CB, Zeidner NS. Capillary feeding of specific dsRNA induces silencing of the *isac* gene in nymphal *Ixodes scapularis* ticks. Insect Mol Biol. 2005;14:443-52. doi:10.1111/j.1365-2583.2005.00575.x.

[72] Lew-Tabor AE, Bruyeres AG, Zhang B, Valle MR. *Rhipicephalus* (*Boophilus*) *microplus* tick in vitro feeding methods for functional (dsRNA) and vaccine candidate (antibody) screening. Ticks Tick Borne Dis. 2014;5:500-10. doi:10.1016/j.ttbdis.2014.03.005.

[73] Francischetti I, Sa-Nunes A, Mans B, Santos I, Ribeiro J. The role of saliva in tick feeding. Front Biosci. 2010;14:2051-88.

[74] Chmelar J, Calvo E, Pedra J, Francischetti I, Kotsyfakis M. Tick salivary secretion as a source of antihemostatics. J Proteomics. 2012;75:3842-54. doi:10.1016/j.jprot. 2012.04.026.

[75] Kazimirova M, Stibraniova I. Tick salivary compounds: Their role in modulation of host defences and pathogen transmission. Front Cell Infect Microbiol. 2013;3:43. doi: 10.3389/fcimb.2013.00043.

[76] Kaufman WR. Ticks: Physiological aspects with implications for pathogen transmission. Ticks Tick Borne Dis. 2010;1:11-22. doi:10.1016/j.ttbdis.2009.12.001.

[77] Browning R, Karim S. RNA interference mediated depletion of NSF and SNAP-25 results in the inhibition of blood feeding of the Gulf-Coast tick, *Amblyomma maculatum*. Insect Mol Biol. 2013;22:245-57. doi:10.1111/imb.12017.

[78] Villareal AM, Adamson SW, Browning RE, Budachetri K, Sajid MS, Karim S. Molecular characterization and functional significance of the Vti family of SNARE proteins in tick salivary glands. Insect Biochem Mol Biol. 2013;2013:483-93. doi:10.1016/j.ibmb. 2013.03.003.

[79] Anisuzzaman, Islam MK, Alim MA, Miyoshi T, Hatta T, Yamaji K, et al. Longistatin, a plasminogen activator, is key to the availability of bloodmeals for ixodid ticks. PloS Pathog. 2011;7:e1001312. doi:10.1371/journal.ppat.1001312.

[80] Kim TK, Curran J, Mulenga A. Dual silencing of long and short *Amblyomma americanum* acidic chitinase forms weakens the tick cement cone stability. J Exp Biol. 2014;217:3493-503. doi:10.1242/jeb.107979.

[81] Kotsyfakis M, Karim S, Andersen JF, Mather TN, Ribeiro JMC. Selective cysteine protease inhibition contributes to blood-feeding success of the tick *Ixodes scapularis*. J Biol Chem. 2007;282:29256-63. doi:10.1074/jbc.M703143200.

[82] Gao X, Shi L, Zhou Y, Zhang H, Zhou J. Characterization of the anticoagulant protein Rhipilin-1 from the *Rhipicephalus haemaphysaloides* tick. J Insect Physiol. 2011;57:339-43. doi:10.1016/j.jinsphys.2010.12.001.

[83] Chalaire KC, Kim TK, Garcia-Rodriguez H, Mulenga A. *Amblyomma americanum* (L.) (Acari: Ixodidae) tick salivary gland serine protease inhibitor (serpin) 6 is secreted into tick saliva during feeding. J Exp Biol. 2011;214:665-73. doi:10.1242/jeb.052076.

[84] Yu Y, Y.J. C, Zhou Y, Zhang H, Zhou J. Isolation and characterization of two novel serpins from the *Rhipicephalus haemaphysaloides*. Ticks Tick Borne Dis. 2013;4:297-303. doi:10.1016/j.ttbdis.2013.02.001.

[85] Guo X, Booth CJ, Paley MA, Wang X, DePonte K, Fikrig E, et al. Inhibition of neutrophil function by two tick salivary proteins. Infect Immun. 2009;77:2320-9. doi:10.1128/ IAI.01507-08.

[86] Campbell EM, Burdin M, Hoppler S, Bowman AS. Role of an aquaporin in the sheep tick *Ixodes ricinus*: Assessment as a potential control target. Int J Parasitol. 2010;40:15-23. doi:10.1016/j.ijpara.2009.06.010.

[87] Barnard AC, Nijhof AM, Gaspar ARM, Neitz AWH, Jonjegan F, Maritz-Olivier C. Expression profiling, gene silencing and transcriptional networking of metzincin metal-

loproteases in the cattle, *Rhipicephalus* (*Boophilus*) *microplus*. Vet Parasitol. 2012;186:403-14. doi:10.1016/j.vetpar.2011.11.026.

[88] Adamson SW, Browning RE, Chao CC, Bateman Jr. RC, Ching WM, Karim S. Molecular characterization of tick salivary gland glutaminyl cyclase. Insect Biochem Mol Biol. 2013;43:781-93. doi:10.1016/j.ibmb.2013.05.011.

[89] Mulenga A, Kim TK, Ibelli AMG. Deorphanization and target validation of cross-tick species conserved novel *Amblyomma americanum* tick saliva protein. Int J Parasitol. 2013;43:439-51. doi:10.1016/j.ijpara.2012.12.012.

[90] Boldbaatar D, Sikasunge CS, Battsetseg B, Xuan X, Fujisaki K. Molecular cloning and functional characterization of an aspartic protease from the hard tick *Haemaphysalis longicornis*. Insect Biochem Mol Biol. 2006;36:25-36. doi:10.1016/j.ibmb.2005.10.003.

[91] Hatta T, Umemiya R, Liao M, Gong H, Harnnoi T, Tanaka M, et al. RNA interference of cytosolic leucine aminopeptidase reduces fecundity in the hard tick, *Haemaphysalis longicornis*. Parasitol Res. 2007;100:847-54. doi:10.1007/s00436-006-0336-3.

[92] Hatta T, Tsuji N, Miyoshi T, Islam MK, Alim MA, Yamaji K, et al. Leucine aminopeptidase, HlLAP, from the ixodid tick *Haemaphysalis longicornis*, plays vital roles in the development of oocytes. Parasitol Int. 2010;59:286-9. doi:10.1016/j.parint.2010.03.001.

[93] Liao M, Zhou J, Gong H, Boldbaatar D, Shirafuji R, Battur B, et al. Hemalin, a thrombin inhibitor isolated from a midgut cDNA library from the hard tick *Haemaphysalis longicornis*. J Insect Physiol. 2009;55:165-74. doi:10.1016/j.jinsphys.2008.11.004.

[94] Miyoshi T, Tsuji N, Islam MK, Alim MA, Hatta T, Huang X, et al. A set of serine protease paralogs are required for blood-digestion in the ixodid tick *Haemaphysalis longicornis*. Parasitol Int. 2008;57:499-505. doi:10.1016/j.parint.2008.08.003.

[95] Tsuji N, Miyoshi T, Battsetseg B, Matsuo T, Xuan X, Fujisaki K. A Cysteine Protease Is Critical for *Babesia* spp. Transmission in *Haemaphysalis* Ticks. PLoS Pathog. 2008;4(5):e1000062.

[96] Franta Z, Sojka D, Frantova H, Dvorak J, Horn M, Srba J, et al. *Ir*CL1—the haemoglobinolytic cathepsin L of the hard tick, *Ixodes ricinus*. Int J Parasitol. 2011;41:1253-62. doi:10.1016/j.ijpara.2011.06.006.

[97] Yamaji K, Miyoshi T, Hatta T, Matsubayashi M, Alim MA, Anisuzzaman, et al. HlCPL-A, a cathepsin L-like cysteine protease from the ixodid tick *Haemaphysalis longicornis*, modulated midgut proteolytic enzymes and their inhibitors during blood meal digestion. Infect Genet Evol. 2013;16:206-11. doi:10.1016/j.meegid.2013.01.018.

[98] Zhou J, Liao M, Hatta T, Tanaka M, Xuan X, Fujisaki K. Identification of a follistatin-related protein from the tick *Haemaphysalis longicornis* and its effect on tick oviposition. Gene. 2006;372:191-8. doi:10.1016/j.gene.2005.12.020.

[99] Boldbaatar D, Battsetseg B, Matsuo T, Hatta T, Umemiya-Shirafuji R, Xuan X, et al. Tick vitellogenin receptor reveals critical role in oocyte development and transovarial transmission of *Babesia* parasite. Biochem Cell Biol. 2008;86:331-44.

[100] Smith AD, Kaufman WR. Molecular characterization of the vitellogenin receptor from the tick, *Amblyomma hebraeum* (Acari: Ixodidae). Insect Biochem Mol Biol. 2013;43:1133-41. doi:10.1016/j.ibmb.2013.10.002.

[101] Smith A, Guo X, de la Fuente J, Naranjo V, Kocan KM, Kaufman WR. The impact of RNA interference of the subolesin and voraxin genes in the male *Amblyomma hebraeum* (Acari: Ixodidae) on female engorgement and oviposition. Exp App Acarol. 2009;47:71-86. doi:10.1007/s10493-008-9195-1.

[102] Boldbaatar D, Umemiya-Shirafuji R, Liao M, Tanaka T, Xuan X, Fujisaki K. Multiple vitellogenins from the *Haemaphysalis longicornis* tick are crucial for ovarian development. J Insect Physiol. 2010;56:1587-98. doi:10.1016/j.jinsphys.2010.05.019.

[103] Boldbaatar D, Battur B, Umemiya-Shirafuji R, Liao M, Tanaka T, Fujisaki K. GATA transcription, translation and regulation in *Haemaphysalis longicornis* tick: Analysis of the cDNA and an essential role for vitellogenesis. Insect Biochem Mol Biol. 2010;40:49-57. doi:10.1016/j.ibmb.2009.12.009.

[104] Umemiya-Shirafuji R, Boldbaatar D, Liao M, Battur B, Rahman MS, Kuboki T, et al. Target of rapamycin (TOR) controls vitellogenesis via activation of the S6 kinase in the fat body of the tick, *Haemaphysalis longicornis*. Int J Parasitol. 2012;42:991-8. doi: 10.1016/j.ijpara.2012.08.002.

[105] Huang X, Tsuji N, Miyoshi T, Motobu M, Islam MK, Alim MA, et al. Characterization of glutamine:fructose-6-phosphate aminotransferase from the ixodid tick, *Haemaphysalis longicornis,* and its critical role in host blood feeding. Int J Parasitol. 2007;37:383-92. doi:10.1016/j.ijpara.2006.11.012.

[106] Karim S, Kenny B, Troiano E, Mather TN. RNAi-mediated gene silencing in tick synganglia: A proof of concept study. BMC Biotech. 2008;8:30. doi: 10.1186/1472-6750-8-30.

[107] Boldbaatar D, Battsetseg B, Hatta T, Miyoshi T, Tsuji N, Xuan X, et al. Valosin-containing protein from the hard tick *Haemaphysalis longicornis*: Effects of dsRNA-mediated HlVCP gene silencing. Biochem Cell Biol. 2007;85:384-94.

[108] Boldbaatar D, R.M. K, Battur B, Umemiya R, Liao M, Tanaka T, et al. Identification of two forms of cyclophilin from the hard tick *Haemaphysalis longicornis*. Process Biochemistry. 2008;43:615-25.

[109] Gong H, Liao M, Zhou J, Hatta T, Huang P, Zhang G, et al. Gene silencing of ribosomal protein P0 is lethal to the tick *Haemaphysalis longicornis*. Vet Parasitol. 2008;151:268-78. doi:10.1016/j.vetpar.2007.11.015.

[110] Liao M, Boldbaatar D, Gong H, Huang P, Umemiya R, Harnnoi T, et al. Functional analysis of protein disulfide isomerases in blood feeding, viability and oocyte devel-

opment in *Haemaphysalis longicornis* ticks. Insect Biochem Mol Biol. 2008;38:285-95. doi:10.1016/j.ibmb.2007.11.006.

[111] Hajdusek O, Sojka D, Kopacek P, Buresova V, Franta Z, Sauman I, et al. Knockdown of proteins involved in iron metabolism limits tick reproduction and development. Proc Natl Acad Sci U S A 2009;106:1033-8. doi:10.1073/pnas.0807961106.

[112] Galay RL, Aung KM, Umemiya-Shirafuji R, Maeda H, Matsuo T, Kawaguchi H, et al. Multiple ferritins are vital to successful blood feeding and reproduction of the hard tick *Haemaphysalis longicornis*. J Exp Biol. 2013;216:1905-15. doi:10.1242/jeb.081240.

[113] Galay RL, Umemiya-Shirafuji R, Bacolod ET, Maeda H, Kusakisako K, Koyama J, et al. Two kinds of ferritin protect ixodid ticks from iron overload and consequent oxidative stress. PLoS ONE. 2014;9:e90661. doi:10.1371/journal.pone.0090661.

[114] Battur B, Boldbaatar D, Umemiya-Shirafuji R, Liao M, Battsetseg B, Taylor D, et al. LKR/SDH plays important roles throughout the tick life cycle including a long starvation period. PLoS ONE. 2009;4:e7136. doi:10.1371/journal.pone.0007136.

[115] Fabres A, De Andrade CP, Guizzo M, Sorgine MH, Paiva-Silva GO, Masuda A, et al. Effect of GSK-3 activity, enzymatic inhibition and gene silencing y RNAi on tick oviposition and egg hatching. Parasitology. 2010;137:1537-46. doi:10.1017/S0031182010000284.

[116] Mulenga A, Khumthong R. Disrupting the *Amblyomma americanum* (L.) CD147 receptor homolog prevents ticks from feeding to repletion and blocks spontaneous detachment of ticks from their host. Insect Biochem Mol Biol. 2010;40:524-42. doi:10.1016/j.ibmb.2010.04.012.

[117] Mulenga A, Khumthong R. Silencing of three *Amblyomma americanum* (L.) insulin-like growth factor binding protein-related proteins prevents ticks from feeding to repletion. J Exp Biol. 2010;213:1153-61. doi:10.1242/jeb.035204.

[118] de la Fuente J, Manzano-Roman R, Naranjo V, Kocan KM, Zivkovic Z, Blouin EF, et al. Identification of protective antigens by RNA interference for control of the lone star tick, *Amblyomma americanum*. Vaccine. 2010;28:1786-95. doi:10.1016/j.vaccine.2009.12.007.

[119] Alim MA, Islam MK, Anisuzzaman, Miyoshi T, Hatta T, Yamaji K, et al. A hemocyte-derived Kunitz-BPTI-type chymotrypsin inhibitor, HlChl, from the ixodid tick *Haemaphysalis longicornis*, plays regulatory functions in tick blood-feeding processes. Insect Biochem Mol Biol. 2012;42:925-34. doi:10.1016/j.ibmb.2012.09.005.

[120] Kume A, Boldbaatar D, Takazawa Y, Umemiya-Shirafuji R, Tanaka T, Fujisaki K. RNAi of the translation inhibition gene *4E-BP* identified from the hard tick, *Haemaphysalis longicornis*, affects lipid storage during the off-host starvation period of ticks. Parasitol Res. 2012;111:889-96. doi:10.1007/s00436-012-2915-9.

[121] Umemiya-Shirafuji R, Tanaka T, Boldbaatar D, Tanaka T, Fujisaki K. Akt is an essential player in regulating cell/organ growth at the adult stage in the hard tick *Haema-*

physalis longicornis. Insect Biochem Mol Biol. 2012;42:164-73. doi:10.1016/j.ibmb.2011.12.001.

[122] Wang Y, Zhou Y, Gong H, Cao J, Zhang H, Li X, et al. Functional characterization of a cystatin from the tick *Rhipicephalus haemaphysaloides*. Parasit Vectors. 2015;8:140. doi:10.1186/s13071-015-0725-5.

[123] Tian M, Tian Z, Luo J, Xie J, Yin H, Zeng Q, et al. Idenfification of the tropomyosin (Hl-Tm) *Haemaphysalis longicornis*. Vet Parasitol. 2015;207:318-23. doi:10.1016/j.vetpar.2014.10.007.

[124] de la Fuente J, Almazan C, Blas-Machado U, Naranjo V, Mangold AJ, Blouin EF, et al. The tick protective antigen, 4D8, is a conserved protein involved in modulation of tick blood ingestion and reproduction. Vaccine. 2006;24:4082-95. doi:10.1016/j.vaccine.2006.02.046.

[125] de la Fuente J, Almazan C, Naranjo V, Blouin EF, Kocan KM. Synergistic effect of silencing the expression of tick protective antigens 4D8 and Rs86 in *Rhipicephalus sanguineus* by RNA interference. Parasitol Res. 2006;99:108-13. doi:10.1007/s00436-006-0132-0.

[126] Antunes S, Galindo RC, Almazan C, Rudenko N, Golovchenko M, Grubhoffer L, et al. Functional genomics studies of *Rhipicephalus* (*Boophilus*) *annulatus* ticks in response to infection with the cattle protozoan parasite, *Babesia bigemina*. Int J Parasitol. 2012;42:187-95. doi:10.1016/j.ijpara.2011.12.003.

[127] Manzano-Roman R, Diaz-Martin V, Oleaga A, Siles-Lucas M, Perez-Sanchez R. Subolesin/akirin orthologs from *Ornithodoros* spp. soft ticks: Cloning, RNAi gene silencing and protective effect of the recombinant proteins. Vet Parasitol. 2012;185:248-59. doi:10.1016/j.vetpar.2011.10.032.

[128] Liao M, Zhou J, Hatta T, Umemiya R, Miyoshi T, Tsuji N, et al. Molecular characterization of *Rhipicephalus* (*Boophilus*) *microplus Bm86* homologue from *Haemaphysalis longicornis* ticks. Vet Parasitol. 2007;146:148-57. doi:10.1016/j.vetpar.2007.01.015.

[129] Bastos RG, Ueti MW, Knowles DP, Scoles GA. The *Rhipicephalus* (*Boophilus*) *microplus Bm86* gene plays a critical role in the fitness of ticks fed on cattle during acute *Babesia bovis* infection. Parasit Vectors. 2010;3:111. doi:10.1186/1756-3305-3-111.

[130] Nijhof AM, Balk JA, Postigo M, Rhebergen AM, Taoufik A, Jonjegan F. Bm86 homologues and novel ATAQ proteins with multiple epidermal growth factor (EGF)-like domains from hard and soft ticks. Int J Parasitol. 2010;40:1587-97. doi:10.1016/j.ijpara.2010.06.003.

[131] Tsuji N, Battsetseg B, Boldbaatar D, Miyoshi T, Xuan X, Oliver Jr. JH, et al. Babesial vector tick defensin against *Babesia* sp. parasites. Infect Immun. 2007;75:3633-40. doi:10.1128/IAI.00256-07.

[132] Buresova V, Hajdusek O, Franta Z, Loosova G, Grunclova L, Levashina EA, et al. Functional genomics of tick thioester-containing proteins reveal the ancient origin of the complement system. J Innate Immun. 2011;3:623-30. doi:10.1159/000328851.

[133] Buresova V, Hajdusek O, Franta Z, Sojka D, Kopacek P. IrAM-An alpha2-macroglobulin from the hard tick *Ixodes ricinus*: Characterization and function in phagocytosis of a potential pathogen *Chryseobacterium indologenes*. Dev Comp Immunol. 2009;33:489-98. doi:10.1016/j.dci.2008.09.011.

[134] Bowen CJ, Jaworski DC, Wasala NB, Coons LB. Macrophage migration inhibitory factor expression and protein localization in *Amblyomma americanum* (Ixodidae). Exp Appl Acarol. 2010;50:343-52. doi:10.1007/s10493-009-9324-5.

[135] Liu L, Dai J, Zhao YO, Narasimhan S, Yang Y, Zhang L, et al. *Ixodes scapularis* JAK-STAT pathway regulates tick antimicrobial peptides, thereby controlling the agent of human granulocytic anaplasmosis. J Infect Dis. 2012;206:1233-41. doi:10.1093/infdis/jis484.

[136] Yang X, Smith AA, Williams MS, Pal U. A dityrosine network mediated by dual oxidase and peroxidase influences the persistence of Lyme disease pathogens within the vector. J Biol Chem. 2014;289:12813-22. doi:10.1074/jbc.M113.538272.

[137] Duscher GG, Galindo RC, Tichy A, Hummel K, Kocan KM, de la Fuente J. Glutathione S-transferase affects permethrin detoxification in the brown dog tick, *Rhipicephalus sanguineus*. Ticks Tick Borne Dis. 2014;5:225-33. doi:10.1016/j.ttbdis.2013.11.006.

[138] Adamson S, Browning R, Singh P, Nobles S, Villareal A, Karim S. Transcriptional activation of antioxidants may compensate for selenoprotein deficiencies in *Amblyomma maculatum* (Acari: Ixodidae) injected with *selK*- or *selM*-dsRNA. Insect Mol Biol. 2014;23:497-510. doi:10.1111/imb.12098.

[139] Budachetri K, Karim S. An insight into the functional role of thioredoxin reductase, a selenoprotein, in maintaining normal native microbiota in the Gulf Coast tick (*Amblyomma maculatum*). Insect Mol Biol. 2015. doi:10.1111/imb.12184.

[140] Liu S, Soares TS, Vaz Jr. Id, Lovato DV, Aparecida ST. Rmcystatin3, a cysteine protease inhibitor from *Rhipicephalus microplus* hemocytes involved in immune response. Biochimie. 2014;106:17-23. doi:10.1016/j.biochi.2014.07.012.

[141] de la Fuente J, Ayoubi P, Blouin EF, Almazan C, Naranjo V, Kocan KM. Anaplasmosis: Focusing on host-vector-pathogen interactions for vaccine development. Ann NY Acad Sci. 2006;1078:416-23. doi:10.1196/annals.1374.081.

[142] Kocan KM, Zivkovic Z, Blouin EF, Naranjo V, Almazan C, Mitra R, et al. Silencing of genes involved in *Anaplasma marginale*-tick interactions affects the pathogen developmental cycle in *Dermacentor variabilis*. BMC Dev Biol. 2009;9:42. doi: 10.1186/1471-213X-9-42.

[143] Zivkovic Z, Esteves E, Almazan C, Daffre S, Nijhof AM, Kocan KM, et al. DIfferential expression of genes in salivary glands of male *Rhipicephalus* (*Boophilus*) *microplus* in

response to infection with *Anaplasma marginale*. BMC Genomics. 2010;11:186. doi: 10.1186/1471-2164-11-186.

[144] Kocan KM, de la Fuente J, Manzano-Roman R, Naranjo V, Hynes WL, Sonenshine DE. Silencing expression of the defensin, varisin, in male *Dermacentor variabilis* by RNA interference results in reduced *Anaplasma marginale* infections. Exp App Acarol. 2008;46:17-28. doi:10.1007/s10493-008-9159-5.

[145] Schuijt TJ, Coumou J, Narasimhan S, Dai J, DePonte K, Wouters D, et al. A tick mannose-binding lectin inhibitor interferes with the vertebrate complement cascade to enhance transmission of the lyme disease agent. Cell Host Microbe. 2011;10:136-46. doi:10.1016/j.chom.2011.06.010.

[146] Ceraul SM, Chung A, Sears KT, Popov VL, Beier-Sexton M, Rahman MS, et al. A kunitz protease inhibitor from *Dermacentor variabilis*, a vector for spotted fever group Rickettsiae, limits *Rickettsia montanensis* infection. Infect Immun. 2011;79:321-9. doi: 10.1128/IAI.00362-10.

[147] Dai J, Narasimhan S, Zhang L, Liu L, Wang P, Fikrig E. Tick histamine release factor is critical for *Ixodes scapularis* engorgement and transmission of the Lyme diseases agent. PloS Pathog. 2010;6:e1001205. doi:10.1371/journal.ppat.1001205.

[148] Neelakanta G, Sultana H, Fish D, Anderson JF, Fikrig E. *Anaplasma phagocytophilum* induces *Ixodees scapularis* ticks to express an antifreeze glycoprotein gene that enhances their survival in the cold. J Clin Invest. 2010;120:3179-90. doi:10.1172/JCI42868.

[149] Severo MS, Choy A, Stephen sKD, Sakhon OS, Chen G, Chung DD, et al. The E3 ubiquitin ligase XIAP restricts *Anaplasma phagocytophilum* colonization of *Ixodes scapularis* tick. J Infect Dis. 2013;208:1830-40. doi:10.1093/infdis/jit380.

[150] Bifano TD, Ueti MW, Esteves E, Reif KE, Braz GRC, Scoles GA, et al. Knockdown of the *Rhipicephalus microplus* cytochrome c oxidase subunit III gene is associated with a failure of *Anaplasma marginale* transmission. PLoS ONE. 2014;9:e98614. doi:10.1371/journal.pone.0098614.

[151] Sojka D, Franta Z, Horn M, Caffrey C, Mares M, Kopacek P. New insights into the machinery of blood digestion by ticks. Trends Parasitol. 2013;29:276-85. doi:10.1016/j.pt.2013.04.002.

[152] Friesen KJ, Kaufman WR. Quantification of vitellogenesis and its control by 20-hydroxyecdysone in the ixodid tick, *Amblyomma hebraeum*. J Insect Physiol. 2002;48:773-82. doi:10.1016/S0022-1910(02)00107-5.

[153] Almazan C, Kocan KM, Bergman DK, Garcia-Garcia JC, Blouin EF, de la Fuente J. Identification of protective antigens for the control of *Ixodes scapularis* infestations using cDNA expression library immunization. Vaccine. 2003;21:1492-501. doi:10.1016/S0264-410X(02)00683-7.

[154] de la Fuente J, Maritz-Olivier C, Naranjo V, Ayoubi P, Nijhof AM, Almazan C, et al. Evidence of the role of tick subolesin in gene expression. BMC Genomics. 2008;9:372. doi:10.1186/1471-2164-9-372.

[155] Willadsen P, Riding GA, McKenna RV, Kemp DH, Tellam RL, Nielsen JN, et al. Immunologic control of a parasitic arthropod. Identification of a protective antigen from *Boophilus microplus*. J Immunol. 1989;143:1346-51.

[156] de la Fuente J, Blouin EF, Manzano-Roman R, Naranjo V, Almazan C, de la Lastra JMP, et al. Functional genomic studies of tick cells in response to infection with the cattle pathogen, Anaplasma marginale. Genomics. 2007;90:712-22. doi:10.1016/j.ygeno.2007.08.009.

[157] de la Fuente J, Merino O. Vaccinomics, the new road to tick vaccines. Vaccine. 2013;31:5923-9. doi:10.1016/j.vaccine.2013.10.049.

11

Current Status for Application of RNA Interference Technology as Nucleic Acid Drug

Tomoko Takahashi, Yuko Nakano and Kumiko Ui-Tei

Abstract

RNA interference (RNAi) is a convenient and useful gene suppression technology induced by small interfering RNA (siRNA) composed of 21-nucleotide long double-stranded RNA. The successful application of RNAi for clinical use is expected for a long time. Although siRNA drug is categorized into a nucleic acid drug, it has a prominent advantage that genetic function can be suppressed by destroying mRNA at the posttranscriptional level without wounding genomic DNA. Nevertheless, unfortunately there are no siRNA certified as pharmaceuticals passing through clinical trials, since there are several problems, such as gene suppression efficiency, stability in blood stream, or other undesirable effects. Here, we describe the current status and future prospects for clinical application of the siRNA nucleic acid drug.

Keywords: RNA interference, siRNA, off-target effect, thermodynamic property, chemical modification

1. Introduction

In recent years, nucleic acid drugs have attracted attention as a next-generation medicine following low molecular weight drugs and antibody drugs. Research and development of these drugs for clinical application is advanced in major pharmaceutical companies, bio-ventures, or research institutions including universities. Nucleic acid drugs, such as DNA/RNA or their modified molecules, act directly on molecules causing diseases and regulate their functions by administering chemically synthesized nucleic acid to the body by local administration or subcutaneous injection. Unlike the hitherto known gene therapy, the nucleic acid drugs directly act on the target molecules and relieve symptoms of the diseases without manipulating the genomes. Although the effects of various nucleic acid drugs, including antisense RNA, small interfering RNA (siRNA), aptamer, or decoy, are investigated in the clinical trials, only five examples including four antisense oligos and an aptamer are already approved. However, no siRNA drug is certified so far. In this manuscript, we outline the advantages, current status, and problems to be solved in the development of nucleic acid drugs, in particular, focusing on the development of siRNA drug.

2. RNA interference

RNA interference (RNAi) is a highly regulated, evolutionarily conserved mechanism of post-transcriptional gene regulation. siRNA, consists of double-stranded RNA with 19 nucleotides in length with 2 nucleotides overhangs, is the intermediate utilized in this mechanism [1].

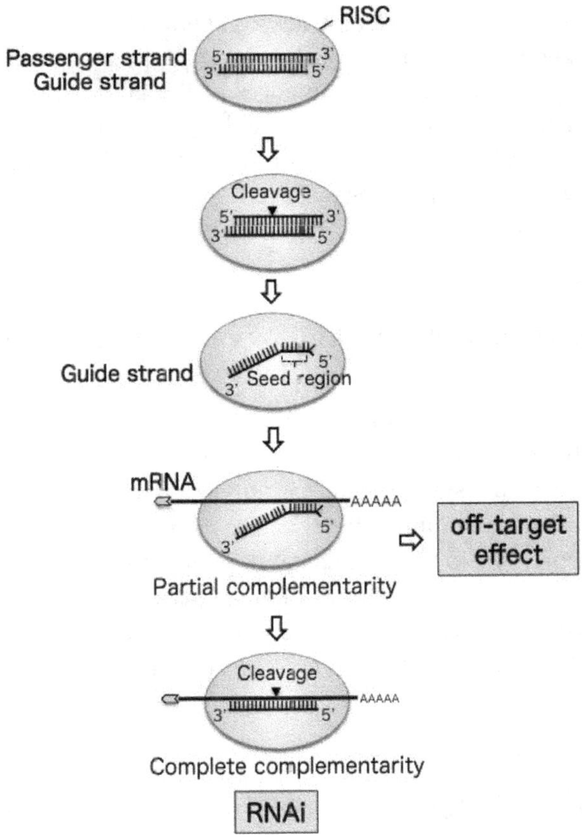

Figure 1. Mechanism of RNA interference. siRNA is the approximately 21-nt double-stranded RNA composed of the guide strand RNA and the passenger strand RNA. siRNA is incorporated into a protein complex called RISC and unwound into single-stranded RNAs. After unwinding, the guide strand is remained on the AGO protein, while the passenger strand is degraded. The mRNAs only with partial complementarities with the seed region of siRNA guide strand are off-target genes and are repressed by siRNA as a mechanism known to be "off-target effect." the mRNA, which has a complete complementary sequence with the guide strand RNA, is cleaved by "RNAi" as an actual target.

When siRNA is introduced into the cells, it is loaded onto the Argonaute (AGO) protein, which is a component of a protein complex called RNA-induced silencing complex (RISC) [2, 3]. In the RISC, siRNA is unwound into single-stranded RNAs, and a functional RNA strand called the guide strand is remained in the RISC and the opposite passenger strand is degraded [4–8]. The activated guide strand RNA-containing RISC binds to the target transcript in a sequence-specific manner. The perfectly complementary target transcript is then cleaved between the 10th and 11th nucleotide relative to the 5′ end of the guide strand [2]. Thus, gene functions of mRNAs which have the complementary nucleotide sequences of the guide strand are suppressed (**Figure 1**) [9]. This elegant, endogenous process has been extensively utilized in functional genomics studies and shows potential as a therapeutic platform [10]. However, although the clinical application of siRNA is expected for a long time, it has not been put into practical use due to some essential problems. For example, the difficult delivery system of siRNA to the target tissues: siRNA is easily degraded by RNA degradation enzymes when it is introduced into the blood, and it is extremely difficult to deliver siRNA to specific tissues. The other severe problem is off-target effects on messenger RNAs (mRNAs) other than the target gene (**Figure 1**). The siRNA often suppresses unintended mRNAs with partial complementarities in nucleotide sequences of the guide strand. The procedures to overcome such problems have been really expected. There is a new candidate method that has overcome the readily degradable property of RNA by enclosing them in lipid nanoparticles (LNP). Although its clinical trial has reached to phase III, there is no example approved as a formal pharmaceutical so far.

3. Advantages for using RNAi technology for nucleic acid medicine

siRNA with complementary nucleotide sequence to the mRNA of target gene can be designed conveniently, if the nucleotide sequence of the target gene is known. In addition, since siRNA can be chemically synthesized, it is not necessary to undergo complicated manufacturing processes, such as immunization of animals or cell culture like synthesis of antibody drugs. Furthermore, due to the complementary binding of siRNA to the target mRNA, its specificity has been considered to be very high, and siRNA can target molecules, such as mRNAs or other noncoding RNAs at the posttranscriptional level that could not be regulated by traditional drugs. These excellent characteristics are reasons to be expected as the future medicine.

4. Problems to be solved for application of siRNA to nucleic acid medicine

Although clinical trials of siRNA application are performed for a long time, there are no authorized siRNA as a clinical drug until now. The current status of the development in RNAi technology and the major problems for its clinical application are discussed in the following section.

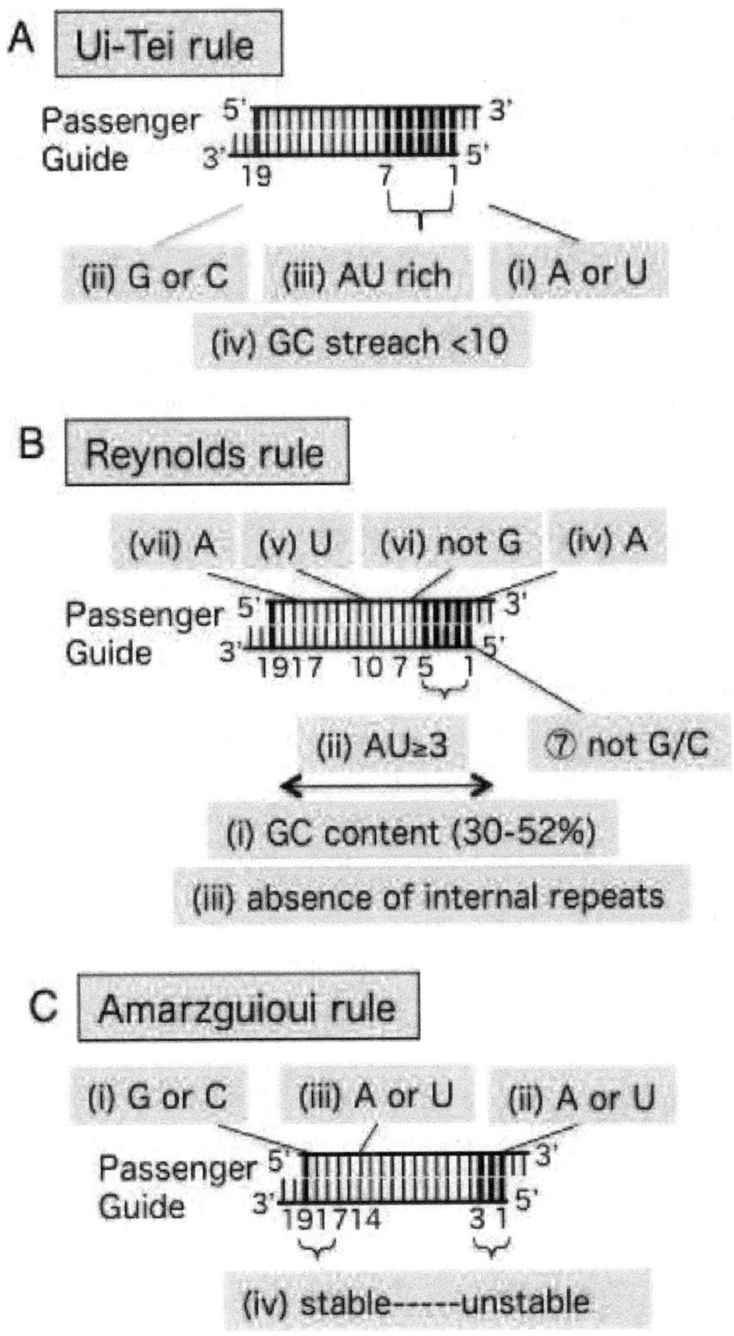

Figure 2. Sequence design algorithms for siRNAs with high RNAi effects. Three widely used siRNA sequence design rules; the Ui-Tei method (A), the Reynolds method (B), and the Amarzguioui method (C). Upper RNA strand indicates the passenger strand, and lower strand indicates the guide strand. The number under the guide strand indicates the nucleotide position measured from the 5′ end of the guide strand. Detailed algorithms are shown in main text.

4.1. Sequence design of highly functional siRNA

The siRNA design is known to define the RNAi efficiency essentially because its effectiveness is dependent on the base-pairing between siRNA and target mRNA. Basic studies so far revealed that the highly efficient RNAi can be induced by almost all siRNAs with any sequences in flies or nematodes, whereas RNAi efficiencies varied greatly depending on the sequences of siRNAs in mammals including human [11]. Among nucleic acid medicines, the nucleotide sequence of aptamer, which specifically acts on a target molecule successfully, is selected by an enormous screening experiment using an artificial nucleic acid library called systematic evolution of ligands by the exponential enrichment (SELEX) method. Such screening requires a great deal of labor and cost. However, the nucleotide sequences of functional siRNAs are designed systematically according to a few reliable algorithms, such as the Ui-Tei rule [11], Reynolds rule [12], or Amarzguioui rule [13] (**Figure 2**). The relationship between siRNA sequence and RNAi was determined by experimental analyses using 62 targets for 4 exogenous and 2 endogenous genes in mammalian cells [11], or 180 siRNAs targeting mRNAs of 2 genes [12], or by the statistical analysis of 49 siRNAs verified by 34 siRNAs [13]. The algorithm of each strategy for the selection of functional siRNA is as follows:

1. Ui-Tei rule
   - **i.** Nucleotide at the 5′ end of the guide strand is A or U.
   - **ii.** Nucleotide at the 5′ end of the passenger strand is preferably G or C.
   - **iii.** A and U are abundant in the region corresponding to the 5′ terminal one-third of the guide strand.
   - **iv.** It is better not to include a long GC stretch over the entire region.
2. Reynolds rule
   - **i.** The content of G and C is 30–5% over the entire region.
   - **ii.** At least three out of five nucleotides at the 3′ end of the passenger strand are preferably A or U.
   - **iii.** Possible inverted repeats that form hairpin structures are absent.
   - **iv.** The third nucleotide from the 5′ end of the passenger strand is A.
   - **v.** The 10th nucleotide from the 5′end of the passenger strand is U.
   - **vi.** The 13th nucleotide from the 5′end of the passenger strand is other than G.
   - **vii.** The 19th nucleotide from the 5′end of the passenger strand is preferably A (other than G or C).
3. Amarzguioui rule
   - **i.** The nucleotide at the 5′ end of the passenger strand is G or C (other than U).
   - **ii.** A or U is preferable at the 5′ end of the guide strand.

iii. The sixth nucleotide from the 5′ end of the passenger strand is A.

iv. The AU content of three nucleotides at the 5′ end of the passenger strand is relatively lower than that of the passenger strand.

The siRNAs with high RNAi effects can be conveniently designed using these three siRNA design algorithms. The application of these algorithms incorporating each of all criteria is shown to improve potent siRNA selection. However, among them, siRNAs designed by the Ui-Tei rule can suppress the target genes with the highest probability of 95% or more. About 15% of all siRNAs complementary for human transcripts satisfy this algorithm, and such siRNA can be designed using siDirect 2.0 (**Figure 3**), which is an open access website [14, 15].

4.2. Avoid the adverse suppression effects on genes other than the target

The siRNA exerts its RNAi effect by binding to the target mRNA via complete complementarity of nucleotide sequence (**Figure 1**). However, its suppression effects are often observed on the genes, other than the target gene, with nucleotide sequences partially complementary to the siRNA. Such phenomenon is known to be "off-target effects," which is an unintended adverse effect of RNAi [16–19]. Especially, the region called "seed" positioned at nucleotides 2–8 from the 5′ terminus of the guide strand contributed to the off-target effects [18, 19] (**Figure 4**), since the seed region loaded on the Argonaute protein in quasi-helical structure and stably form base-pairings with the off-target mRNAs. To avoid such adverse effects, it is desirable to design siRNAs that do not interact with off-target mRNAs other than the target mRNA as much as possible. However, since the off-target effect by siRNA is induced by sequence complementarity of only seven nucleotides sequence in the seed region, it is impossible to select siRNA sequence with no seven nucleotides complementarities with off-target genes. However, such off-target effect was not always observed. It was revealed that the seed-dependent off-target effect is induced only when the base-pairing stability between the guide strand seed region and the off-target mRNA is strong (**Figure 5**). It means that the off-target effect is avoidable when the stability in the seed-target duplex is weak [19, 20]. The melting temperature of RNA–RNA duplex calculated by the nearest-neighbor procedure may be a useful parameter for evaluating the RNA–RNA duplex stability (**Figure 5**).

Thus, the sequence design of siRNA with high specificity for a target gene without off-target effect on the untargeted genes comes to be possible. First, such siRNA satisfies the functional siRNA selection rules, such as Ui-Tei rules. Second, it is preferable to have a lower thermodynamic stability of base-pairing between the siRNA seed region and the target mRNA. The siRNAs simultaneously satisfying these two conditions are considered to show high RNAi effect and reduced off-target effect. However, only 3% of siRNAs, satisfying both conditions simultaneously, is selectable in human. This is relevant to the fact that it is impossible to select any siRNA sequences for about 5000 genes, one quarter of all human genes. Thus, this limitation is inevitable for sequence design of human siRNA [15].

4.3. Reduction of off-target effects using chemical modifications

The off-target effect has been found to depend on the thermodynamic stability of the seed-target duplex, and such thermodynamic property is basically determined according to the nucleotide

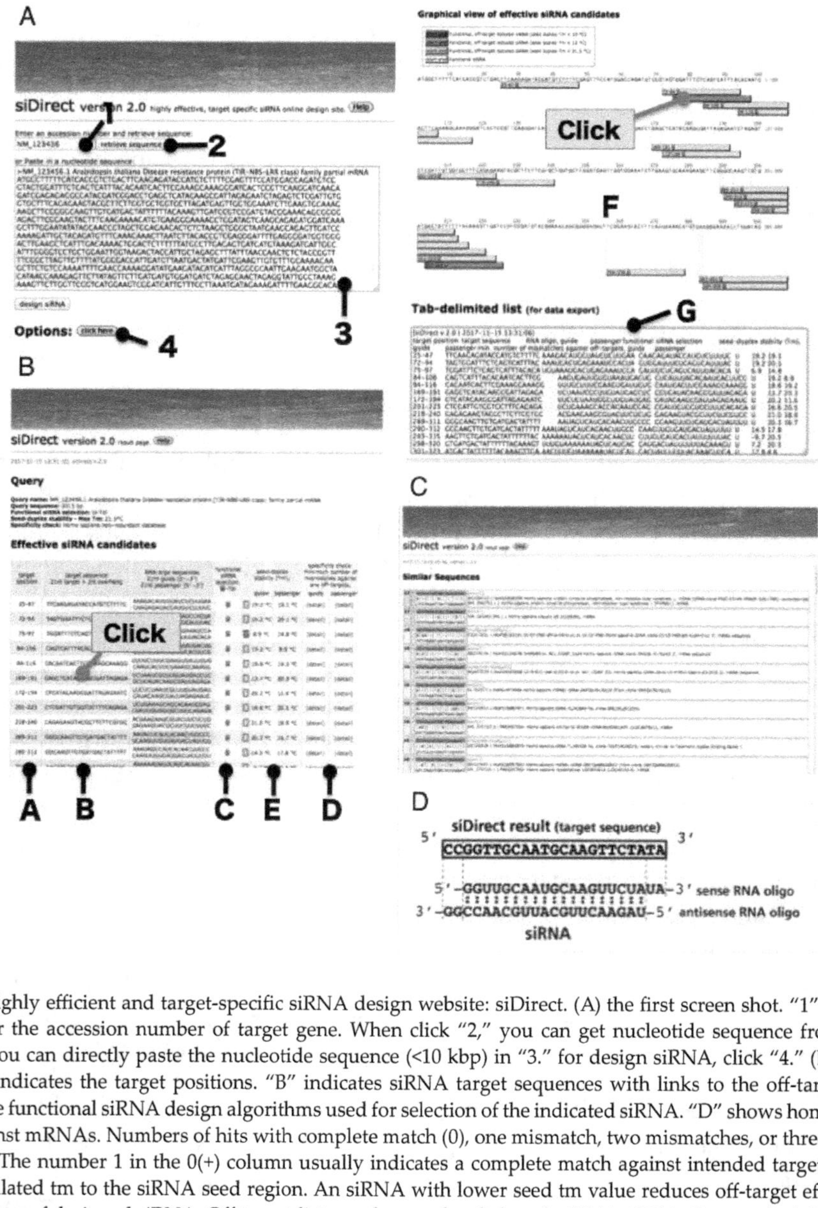

Figure 3. Highly efficient and target-specific siRNA design website: siDirect. (A) the first screen shot. "1" indicates the box to enter the accession number of target gene. When click "2," you can get nucleotide sequence from GenBank. However, you can directly paste the nucleotide sequence (<10 kbp) in "3." for design siRNA, click "4." (B) the second screen "a" indicates the target positions. "B" indicates siRNA target sequences with links to the off-target lists. "C" indicates the functional siRNA design algorithms used for selection of the indicated siRNA. "D" shows homology search results against mRNAs. Numbers of hits with complete match (0), one mismatch, two mismatches, or three mismatches are shown. The number 1 in the 0(+) column usually indicates a complete match against intended target mRNA. "E" shows calculated tm to the siRNA seed region. An siRNA with lower seed tm value reduces off-target effects. "F" is a graphical view of designed siRNA. Off-target lists can be seen by click each siRNA. "G" indicates tab-delimited siRNA list. You can copy and paste the result into excel or text editors, etc. (C) List of off-target candidates for individual siRNA. "6" is siRNA information. "7" shows the alignment between each off-target candidate and each siRNA sequence, clarifying the mismatch positions. (D) Design strategy of guide and passenger strand RNA oligonucleotides based on siDirect result.

sequence. However, the base-pairing stability can be modified by introducing chemical modifications into siRNA. The chemical modifications, including DNA and unlocked nucleic acid (UNA), are known to decrease thermodynamic stabilities. In fact, introduction of DNA molecules into siRNA seed region successfully reduced off-target effects [21, 22], since the DNA-RNA duplex in the seed region shows weak base-pairing stability compared to RNA-RNA duplex.

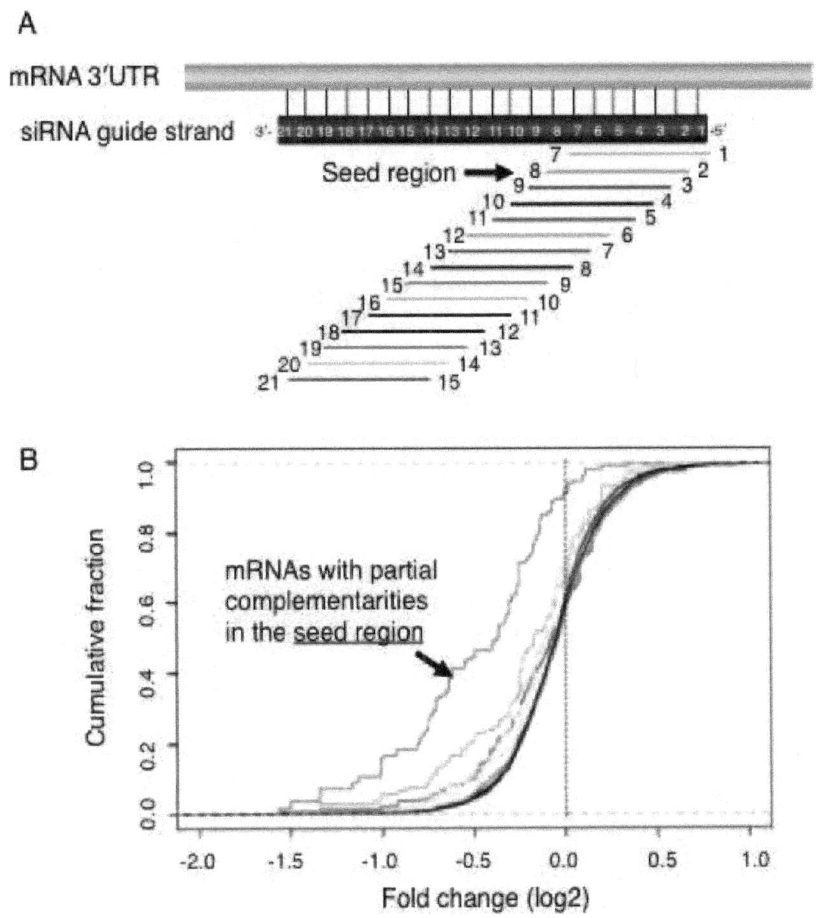

Figure 4. Quantitative analysis of off-target mRNAs by microarray. (A) all of the expressed mRNAs were divided into 15 groups by the region of complementarities with siRNA. (B) Cumulative frequency curve of changes in the expression level of each gene group. When curve shifts to the left, the expression levels of these genes are suppressed. A gene group having a sequence complementary to the siRNA seed region (positions 2–8) in their 3′ UTRs was suppressed.

In contract, the thermodynamic stability of RNA duplex with 2′-O-methyl (2′-OMe) or LNA is known to increase in the protein-free condition. However, we showed that these modifications also reduced the off-target effects [23]. The chemical modification often changes the nucleotide conformation in addition to thermodynamic stability. In RNAi, the guide strand RNA is preloaded on the AGO protein via seed region and form duplex with target mRNA. The 2′-OMe modification in all of the seven nucleotides of siRNA seed region does not disturb the preloading on the AGO protein, but the base-pairing formation with complementary RNA on the AGO protein is apparently disturbed by steric hindrance. As a result, siRNA with 2′-OMe in the guide strand seed region shows weak off-target effect without reduction of RNAi effect [23]. LNA showed more strong effect in the interaction between siRNA and AGO protein or off-target mRNAs. The siRNA modified with LNAs in all of the seven nucleotides in the seed region cannot preload on AGO protein and it cannot base-pair with the complementary RNA. However, siRNA with LNA modifications in three nucleotides among seven

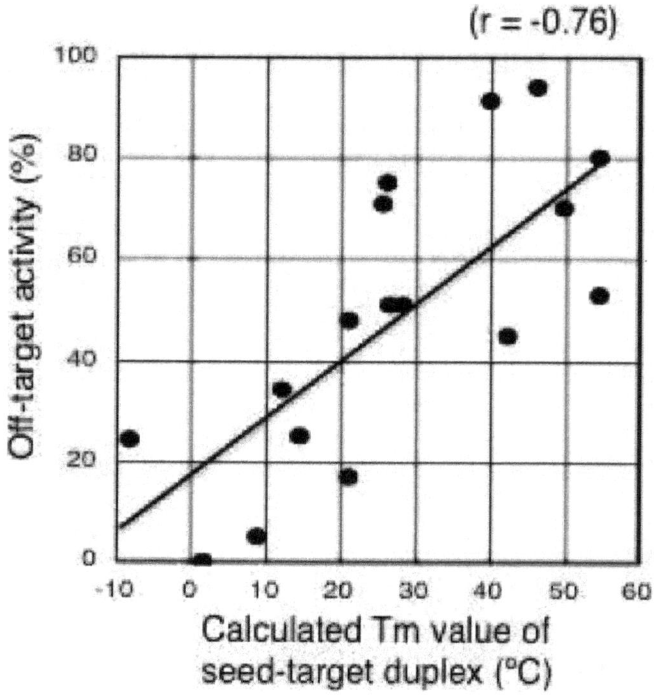

Figure 5. Correlation between thermodynamic stability (Tm value) in the seed-target duplex and off-target effect. siRNAs with low seed tm values in the seed region show low off-target effects, while siRNAs with high seed tm values showed high off-target effects.

can preload on the AGO protein, but it cannot base-pair with the complementary RNA. Thus, siRNA with seven LNA modifications in the seed region has neither RNAi effect nor off-target effect, but siRNA with three LNA modifications shows weak off-target effect without reduction of RNAi effect [23]. Thus, since the chemical modifications can regulate the binding capability of siRNA to the target mRNA depending on the thermodynamic and structural characteristics, the proper application of chemical modifications may be a useful strategy for selection of highly effective and off-target effect-reduced RNAi.

4.4. Increasing stability in blood and efficient transport to the target tissues or cells of siRNA

Nucleic acids are degraded by nucleolytic enzymes when they are released into blood. Fomivirsen is an oligonucleotide used as an antisense antiviral drug that was applied to the treatment of cytomegalovirus retinitis in patients with acquired immunodeficiency syndrome (AIDS). Pegaptanib is a pegylated antivascular endothelial growth factor (VEGF) aptamer and used as an antiangiogenic medicine for the treatment of neovascular age-related macular degeneration (AMD). These nucleic acid drugs are treated by local administration into vitreous bodies. Mipomersen is the second antisense drug used for the treatment of homozygous familial hypercholesterolemia and is administered through subcutaneous injection. The various chemical modifications were introduced into these nucleic acid drugs to increase the stability in the blood. Fomivirsen is involved in the first generation of antisense therapeutics containing phosphorothioate linkages between bases to prevent nuclease digestion. Five 2′-OMe modifications were introduced into mipomersen to allow the resistance to degradation by endonucleases and exonucleases maintaining high affinity and specificity to the target mRNA. Pegaptanib has both modifications of phosphorothioate and 2′-OMe. Incorporation of them greatly improved the aptamer half-life in urine and also improved binding affinity for VEGF. Since it has also reported that siRNAs with chemical modifications, such as 2′-OMe and 2′-fluoro (2′-F), are resistant to degradation by RNA degrading enzymes [24, 25], it is possible to use proper chemical modifications for each siRNA to enhance its stability in blood.

Furthermore, since the nucleic acid has anionic charge, the permeability of the cell membrane is low. Then, the development of drug delivery system (DDS) to transport nucleic acid drugs to target tissues or cells stably using lipid or collagen are also on going. Many trials are performed using lipid nanoparticle (LNP) technology in which pharmacokinetics are indicated to be much better than a naked RNAi approach. Several types of nanoparticles, including LNP, *N*-acetylgalactosamine (GalNAc) conjugates and dynamic polyconjugated (DPCs), are used clinically. The most successful DDS so far is lipid nanoparticle (LNP) developed by Tekmira. LNP, which forms a lipid bilayer membrane similar to the cell membrane, protects siRNA by encapsulation and assists the transport of siRNA to the target tissues. Alnylam has developed a therapeutic agent (ALN-TTR 02) for familial amyloid polyneuropathy by using this LNP, which is currently conducting phase III of clinical trials. In addition, the method for conjugation of atelocollagen and siRNA has also been developed. Atelocollagen makes siRNA less susceptible to degradation by RNase enzymes, which results in a long-lasting RNA silencing effect.

4.5. Suppression of excessive immune response induced by introduction of exogenous nucleic acid

In general, nucleic acid medicine introduces a large amount of artificially synthesized nucleic acids into the body. However, the excessive autoimmune response is often induced by the exogenous introduction of nucleic acids. In mammals, it is well-known that the activation of virus sensor proteins, like Toll-like receptors (TLRs) [26, 27] and RIG-I-like receptors (RLRs) [28], or Protein kinase R (PKR) [29] induces interferon response. Interferon response may upregulate the production of inflammatory cytokines and can possibly cause systemic inflammation. It has been reported that LNA- or 2′-OMe-modified siRNA suppresses the activation of TLR 7/8 and does not induce the excessive immune response without reducing RNAi activity [30, 31]. It was also reported that induction of interferon response was not observed even when a complex of atelocollagen and siRNA was introduced into the cells [32]. By revealing the detailed molecular mechanism of the immune response by introduction of the exogenous nucleic acids, more appropriate chemical modifications to avoid such immune response should be developed.

5. Conclusion

RNAi is a field in which its clinical application is strongly expected, but its first wave for clinical application failed due to the difficulties in the initial stage. However, due to the improvement of its delivery system and the sequence selection method, the new wave has come in 2012. Current clinical trials are applied to targets, including the eye, liver, cancer, blood, gastrointestinal tract, dermis, and others, since it is relatively easy to deliver siRNA to these tissues with currently available nanoparticles [33].

Antibody drugs and low molecular weight drugs were widely used so far. They were synthesized through complicated manufacturing processes, so that mass production at low cost was impossible. However, the nucleic acid drugs can be artificially synthesized by a simple manufacturing process. Then, once a production line is established, it can be synthesized inexpensively in large quantities. In addition, for antibody drugs and low molecular weight drugs, basic data from scratch are required every time when the target changes, but nucleic acid drugs such as siRNA drugs can be designed relatively easily by identifying the nucleotide sequences of target genes. Thus, it is expected that the siRNA is a powerful candidate for nucleic acid therapeutics.

Genome editing techniques such as clustered regularly interspaced short palindromic repeats (CRISPR)/CRISPR-associated proteins 9 (Cas9) system [34] and transcription activator-like effector nucleases (TALEN) [35] can directly modify the genomic DNA that causes disease. Although it is extremely attractive as a potential drug candidate in the future, there are many ethical issues to overcome when the edited genome is transmitted to the next generation. On the other hand, siRNA does not introduce the permanent modification in the genomic DNA and its action is transient, since siRNA knockdown the target mRNA. Then, CRISPR interfering (CRISPRi) system modified from the CRISPR/Cas9 system is developed. CRISPRi inhibit the gene expression without cleavage of genomic DNA by introducing mutations into DNA cleavage domains in Cas9 [36]. Such system may also promote the nucleic acid medicine.

Acknowledgements

We thank Saigo K., Naito Y., Nishi K., Zenno S., Takahashi F., Haraguchi T., Yamato K., Morishita S., Yamada T., Yoshimura J., Juni A., Iribe H., Miyamoto K., Kobayashi Y. and Aida M. to perform the basic studies which serve as foundations of this chapter. This work was mainly supported by grants from the Ministry of Education, Culture, Sports, Science and Technology of Japan (MEXT).

Author details

Tomoko Takahashi, Yuko Nakano and Kumiko Ui-Tei*

*Address all correspondence to: ktei@bs.s.u-tokyo.ac.jp

Department of Biological Sciences, Graduate School of Science, The University of Tokyo, Tokyo, Japan

References

[1] Elbashir SM, Harborth J, Lendeckel W, Yalcin A, Weber K, Tuschl T. Duplexes of 21-nucleotide RNAs mediate RNA interference in cultured mammalian cells. Nature. 2001;**411**:494-498

[2] Hutvagner G, Simard MJ. Argonaute proteins: Key players in RNA silencing. Nature Reviews. Molecular Cell Biology. 2008;**9**:22-32

[3] Doi N, Zenno S, Ueda R, Ohki-Hamazaki H, Ui-Tei K, Saigo K. Short-interfering-RNA-mediated gene silencing in mammalian cells requires dicer and eIF2C translation initiation factors. Current Biology. 2003;**13**:41-46

[4] Matranga C, Tomori Y, Shin C, Bartel DP, Zamore PS. Passenger-strand cleavage facilitates assembly of siRNA into Ago2-containing RNAi enzyme complexes. Cell. 2005;**123**: 607-620

[5] Miyoshi K, Tsukumo H, Nagami T, Siomi H, Siomi MC. Slicer function of *Drosophila* Argonautes and its involvement in RISC formation. Genes & Development. 2005;**19**: 2837-2848

[6] Leuschner PJ, Ameres SL, Kueng S, Martinez J. Cleavage of the siRNA passenger strand during RISC assembly in human cells. EMBO Reports. 2006;**7**:314-320

[7] Kawamata T, Seitz H, Tomari Y. Structural determinants of miRNAs for RISC loading and slicer-independent unwinding. Nature Structural & Molecular Biology. 2009;**16**:953-960

[8] Yoda M, Kawamata T, Paroo Z, Ye X, Iwasaki S, Liu Q, Tomari Y. ATP-dependent human RISC assembly pathways. Nature Structural & Molecular Biology 2009;**17**:117-123

[9] Fire A, Xu S, Montgomery MK, Kostas SA, Driver SE, Mello CC. Potent and specific genetic interference by double-stranded RNA in *Caenorhabditis elegans*. Nature. 1998;**391**: 806-811

[10] Ryther RCC, Flynt AS, Phillips JA, Patton JG. siRNA therapeutics: Big potential from small RNAs. Gene Therapy. 2004;**12**:5-11

[11] Ui-Tei K, Naito Y, Takahashi F, Haraguchi T, Ohki-Hamazaki H, Juni A, Ueda R, Saigo K. Guidelines for the selection of highly effective siRNA sequences for mammalian and chick RNA interference. Nucleic Acids Research. 2004;**32**:936-948

[12] Reynolds A, Leake D, Boese Q, Scringe S, Marchall WS, Khvorova A. Rational siRNA design for RNA interference. Nature Biotechnology. 2004;**22**:326-330

[13] Amarzguioui M, Prydz H. An algorithm for selection of functional siRNA sequences. Biochemical and Biophysical Research Communications. 2004;**316**:1050-1058

[14] Naito Y, Yamada T, Ui-Tei K, Morishita S, Saigo K. siDirect: Highly effective, target-specific siRNA design software for mammalian RNA interference. Nucleic Acids Research. 2004;**32**:W124-W129

[15] Naito Y, Yoshimura J, Morishita S, Ui-Tei K. siDirect 2.0: Updatead software for designing functional siRNA with reduced seed-dependent off-target effect. BMC Bioinformatics. 2009;**10**:392. DOI: 10.1186/1471-2105-10-392

[16] Lin X, Ruan X, Anderson MG, McDowell JA, Kroeger PE, Fesik SW, Shen Y. siRNA-mediated off-target gene silencing triggered by a 7 nt complementation. Nucleic Acids Research. 2005;**33**:4527-4535

[17] Birmingham A, Selfors LM, Forster T, Wrobel D, Kennedy CJ, Shanks E, Santoyo-Lopez J, Dunican DJ, Long A, Kelleher D, Smith Q, Beijersbergen RL, Ghazal P, Sharmu CE. 3′UTR seed matches, but not overall identity, are associated with RNAi off-targets. Nature Methods. 2006;**3**:199-204

[18] Jackson AL, Burchard J, Schelter J, Chau BN, Cleary M, Lim L, Linsley PS. Widespread siRNA "off-target" transcript silencing by seed region sequence complementarity. RNA. 2006;**12**:1179-1187

[19] Ui-Tei K, Naito Y, Nishi K, Juni A, Saigo K. Thermodynamic stability and Watson-crick base pairing in the seed duplex are major determinants of the efficiency of the siRNA-based off-target effects. Nucleic Acids Research. 2008;**36**:7100-7109. DOI: 10.1093/nar/gkn902

[20] Ui-Tei K, Nishi K, Takahashi T, Nagasawa T. Thermodynamic control of small RNA-mediated gene silencing. Frontiers in Genetics. 2012;**3**:101. DOI: 10.3389/fgene.2012.00101

[21] Ui-Tei K, Naito Y, Zenno S, Nishi K, Yamato K, Takahashi F, Juni A, Saigo K. Functional dissection of siRNA sequence by systematic DNA substitution: Modified siRNA with a DNA seed arm is a powerful tool for mammalian gene silencing with significantly reduced off-target effect. Nucleic Acids Research. 2008;**36**:2136-2151. DOI: 10.1093/nar/gkn042

[22] Takahashi T, Zenno S, Ishibashi O, Takizawa T, Saigo K, Ui-Tei K. Interaction between the non-seed region of siRNA and RNA-binding RLC/RISC proteins, ago and TRBP, in mammalian cells. Nucleic Acids Research. 2014;**42**:5256-5269. DOI: 10.1093/nar/gku153

[23] Iribe H, Miyamoto K, Takahashi T, Kobayashi Y, Leo J, Aida M, Ui-Tei K. Chemical modification of the siRNA seed region suppresses off-target effects by steric hindrance to base-pairing with targets. ACS Omega. 2017;**2**:2055-2064. DOI: 10.1021/acsomega.7b00291

[24] Sproat BS, Lamond AI, Beijer B, NEuner P, Ryder U. Highly efficient chemical synthesis of 2′-O-methyloligoribonucleotides and tetrabiotinylated derivatives: Novel probes that are resistant to degradation by RNA or DNA specific nucleases. Nucleic Acids Research. 1989;**17**:3373-3386

[25] Peiken WA, Olsen DB, BEnseler F, Aurup H, Eckstein F. Kinetic characterization of ribonuclease-resistant 2′-modified hammerhead ribozymes. Science. 1991;**253**:314-317

[26] Lemaitre B, Nicolas E, Michaut L, Reichhart JM, Hoffmann JA. The dorsoventral regulatory gene cassette spätzle/toll/cactus controls the potent antifungal response in drosophila adults. Cell. 1996;**86**:973

[27] Medzhitov R, Preston-Hurlburt P, Janeway CA Jr. A human homologue of the drosophila toll protein signals activation of adaptive immunity. Nature 1997;**388**:394-197

[28] Yoneyama M, Kikuchi M, Natsukawa T, Shinobu N, Imaizumi T, Miyagishi M, Taira K, Akira S, Fujita T. The RNA helicase RIG-I has an essential function in double-stranded RNA-induced innate antiviral responses. Nature Immunology. 2004;**5**:730-737

[29] Meurs E, Chong K, Galabru J, Thomas NS, Kerr IM, Williams BR, Hovanessian AG. Molecular cloning and characterization of the human double-stranded RNA-activated protein kinase induced by interferon. Cell. 1990;**62**:379-390

[30] Dahlgren C, Wahlestedt C, Thonberg H. No induction of anti-viral responses in human cell lines HeLa and MCF-7 when transfecting with siRNA or siLNA. Biochemical and Biophysical Research Communications. 2006;**341**:1211-1217

[31] Judge AD, Bola G, Lee AC, MacLachlan I. Design of noninflammatory synthetic siRNA mediating potent gene silencing in vito. Molecular Therapy. 2006;**13**:494-505

[32] Takeshita F, Minakuchi Y, Nagahara S, Honma K, Sasaki H, Hirai K, Teratani T, Namatame N, Yamamoto Y, Hanai K, Kato T, Sano A, Ochiya T. Efficient delivery of small interfering RNA to bone-metastatic tumors by using atelocollagen in vivo. Proceedings of the National Academy of Sciences of the United States of America. 2005;**102**:12177-12182

[33] Bobbin ML, Rossi JJ. RNA interference (RNAi)-based therapeutics: Delivering on the promise ? Annual Review of Pharmacology and Toxicology. 2016;**56**:103-122

[34] Jinek M, Chylinski K, Fonfara I, Hauer M, Doudna JA, Charpentier E. A programmable dual-RNA-guided DNA endonuclease in adaptive bacterial immunity. Science. 2012;**337**:816-821. DOI: 10.1126/science.1225829

[35] Christian M, Cermak T, Doyle EL, Schmidt C, Zhang F, Hummel A, Bogdanove AJ, Voytas DF. Targeting DNA double-strand breads with TAL effector nucleases. Genetics. 2010;**186**:757-761. DOI: 10.1534/genetics.110.120717

[36] Cilbert LA, Larson MH, Morsut L, Liu Z, Brar GA, Torres SE, Stem-Ginossar N, Brandman O, Whitehead EH, Doudna JA, Lim WA, Weissman JS, Qi LS. CRISPR-mediated modular RNA-guided regulation of transcription in eukryotes. Cell. 2013;**154**:442-451. DOI: 10.1016/j.cell.2013.06.044

Permissions

All chapters in this book were first published in RNAI, by InTech Open; hereby published with permission under the Creative Commons Attribution License or equivalent. Every chapter published in this book has been scrutinized by our experts. Their significance has been extensively debated. The topics covered herein carry significant findings which will fuel the growth of the discipline. They may even be implemented as practical applications or may be referred to as a beginning point for another development.

The contributors of this book come from diverse backgrounds, making this book a truly international effort. This book will bring forth new frontiers with its revolutionizing research information and detailed analysis of the nascent developments around the world.

We would like to thank all the contributing authors for lending their expertise to make the book truly unique. They have played a crucial role in the development of this book. Without their invaluable contributions this book wouldn't have been possible. They have made vital efforts to compile up to date information on the varied aspects of this subject to make this book a valuable addition to the collection of many professionals and students.

This book was conceptualized with the vision of imparting up-to-date information and advanced data in this field. To ensure the same, a matchless editorial board was set up. Every individual on the board went through rigorous rounds of assessment to prove their worth. After which they invested a large part of their time researching and compiling the most relevant data for our readers.

The editorial board has been involved in producing this book since its inception. They have spent rigorous hours researching and exploring the diverse topics which have resulted in the successful publishing of this book. They have passed on their knowledge of decades through this book. To expedite this challenging task, the publisher supported the team at every step. A small team of assistant editors was also appointed to further simplify the editing procedure and attain best results for the readers.

Apart from the editorial board, the designing team has also invested a significant amount of their time in understanding the subject and creating the most relevant covers. They scrutinized every image to scout for the most suitable representation of the subject and create an appropriate cover for the book.

The publishing team has been an ardent support to the editorial, designing and production team. Their endless efforts to recruit the best for this project, has resulted in the accomplishment of this book. They are a veteran in the field of academics and their pool of knowledge is as vast as their experience in printing. Their expertise and guidance has proved useful at every step. Their uncompromising quality standards have made this book an exceptional effort. Their encouragement from time to time has been an inspiration for everyone.

The publisher and the editorial board hope that this book will prove to be a valuable piece of knowledge for researchers, students, practitioners and scholars across the globe.

List of Contributors

Wenyi Gu
Australian Institute of Bioengineering and Nanotechnology, University of Queensland, QLD, Australia

Tamara Martínez, Maria Victoria González, Beatriz Vargas, Ana Isabel Jiménez and Covadonga Pañeda
Sylentis SAU, Tres Cantos, Madrid, Spain

Zhaohua Hou
Laboratory of Immunology for Environment and Health, Shandong Analysis and Test Center, Shandong Academy of Sciences, Jinan, China

Qiuju Han, Cai Zhang and Jian Zhang
Institute of Immunopharmaceutical Sciences, School of Pharmaceutical Sciences, Shandong University, Jinan, China

Zhabiz Golkar
Department of Biology, School of Health and Natural Science, Voorhees College, Denmark, SC, USA

Donald G. Pace
School of Humanities & Social Science, Claflin University, Orangeburg, SC, USA

Omar Bagasra
School of Natural Science, Claflin University, Orangeburg, SC, USA

Constanca Figueiredo and Rainer Blasczyk
Institute for Transfusion Medicine, Hannover Medical School, Hannover, Germany

Nidhi Thakur
Plant Molecular Biology Lab, CSIR-National Botanical Research Institute, Lucknow, India
Academy of Scientific and Innovative Research, Anusandhan Bhawan, New Delhi, India

Jaspreet Kaur Mundey and Santosh Kumar Upadhyay
Department of Botany, Panjab University, Chandigarh, India

Thais Barros Rodrigues and Antonio Figueira
Centro de Energia Nuclear na Agricultura (CENA), Universidade de São Paulo, Piracicaba, SP, Brazil

Eduardo C. de Andrade
Embrapa Cassava and Fruits, Rua Embrapa, s/n, Cruz das Almas,BA, Brasil

Wayne B. Hunter
USDA, ARS, U.S. Horticultural Research Laboratory, Fort Pierce, FL, USA

Anna Kourti and Dimitrios Kontogiannatos
Department of Biotechnology, School of Food, Biotechnology and Development, Agricultural University of Athens, Athens, Greece

Luc Swevers
Insect Molecular Genetics and Biotechnology Group, Institute of Biosciences & Applications, National Centre for Scientific Research "Demokritos", Athens, Greece

Remil Linggatong Galay
Department of Veterinary Paraclinical Sciences, College of Veterinary Medicine, University of the Philippines Los Baños, Los Baños, Philippines
Laboratory of Infectious Diseases, Joint Faculty of Veterinary Medicine, Kagoshima University, Kagoshima, Japan

Rika Umemiya-Shirafuji
National Research Center for Protozoan Diseases, Obihiro University of Agriculture and Veterinary Medicine, Inada-cho, Obihiro, Hokkaido, Japan

Masami Mochizuki
Department of Veterinary Paraclinical Sciences, College of Veterinary Medicine, University of the Philippines Los Baños, Los Baños, Philippines

Kozo Fujisaki
National Agricultural and Food Research Organization, Tsukuba, Ibaraki, Japan

Tetsuya Tanaka
Laboratory of Infectious Diseases, Joint Faculty of Veterinary Medicine, Kagoshima University, Kagoshima, Japan

Tomoko Takahashi, Yuko Nakano and Kumiko Ui-Tei
Department of Biological Sciences, Graduate School of Science, The University of Tokyo, Tokyo, Japan

Index

A

Acyrthosiphon Pisum, 97, 104-105, 112-113, 142, 145, 154-157, 167, 184

Adaptive Immunity, 2-3, 6-7, 88-89, 233

Anticoagulant Activity, 94-95, 192-193

Antigen Peptide Transporter, 6-7, 9

Antigen Presentation, 1-7, 9, 54

Antigen Reactivation, 2-3

Argonaute Proteins, 123, 125, 136-137, 161, 231

Autologous Stem Cells, 77

B

Bacillus Thuringiensis, 92-93, 96-97, 106-107, 109, 122-123, 130-131, 139, 176, 183

Bicoid Gene, 94-95

Bio-insecticidal Formulations, 160

Biosynthesis Activator, 95

Biosynthetic Pathways, 93

Blood Pharming, 77, 81

Blood-borne Infections, 81

Bone Marrow Progenitors, 5

C

Cancer Immunotherapy, 2-3, 7, 51-52, 55-56

Chewing Insects, 148-149

Chitin Synthases, 95

Cytotoxic T Lymphocyte, 1-3

D

Dendritic Cells, 5, 9, 39-40, 52-56

Diaphorina Citri, 97, 112-113, 144-147, 153, 156, 182

Drosophila Melanogaster, 92-93, 142-143, 187

Drug Development, 10, 73

Drug Resistances, 2-3

Dsrna Screening, 146-147

E

Endothelial Growth Factor, 12, 43-44, 83, 228

G

Gene Expression, 2-3, 10-12, 22, 27-28, 36, 40-43, 47-48, 58, 63, 80-81, 100-101, 123, 138-139, 141-143, 145, 161, 167, 172, 202-203, 208-209, 219, 230

Gene Region, 127-129, 134-135

Gene Regulation, 7, 10, 49-50, 63, 67, 87, 141, 157, 221

Gene-regulating Roles, 2-3, 5

Gene-silencing, 2-3

Genetic Tool, 91-93, 185

Genetically Modified Plants, 160-161, 171

H

Hox Genes, 94-95, 107

Human Leukocyte Antigen, 43-44, 49-50, 56, 61-62, 77

Human Papillomavirus, 1-3, 8-9, 42

I

Immune Response, 1-7, 12, 16, 39-44, 46, 49-50, 52-54, 59-60, 70-71, 78-81, 93, 101, 136-137, 202-203, 217, 229

Immunity Stimulator, 3

Immunoblotting, 4-5

Immunogenicity, 72-73, 77-81, 87

Immunosuppressive Drugs, 80-81

Immunosuppressive Regimens, 78-81, 88-89

K

Keratoplasty Patients, 87

L

Lentiviral Vector Encoding, 78-79, 81-85

Lentiviral Vectors, 2-3, 80-81

Lepidopteran, 96-97, 102-105, 115, 128-129, 132-133, 145, 175, 177, 181-182, 184

Locomotor Activity Rhythm, 94, 165

M

Megakaryocytes, 81-87

Molecular Silencing, 129

N
Nosema Ceranae, 95

O
Ommochrome, 94-95
Ophthalmology, 10-12, 24-26, 28-29, 32

P
Parasitoids, 150-151, 176
Pest Management, 91-93, 100-103, 105-107, 110-111, 114-115, 117, 134-135, 137, 142-143, 146-147, 150-151, 179, 183-184
Pesticide Detoxifying Gene, 96-97
Platelet Transfusion, 81-83, 88-89
Platelet Transfusion Refractoriness, 81-83
Pluripotency Potential, 82-83
Protein Degradation, 4
Protein Synthesis, 1, 75
Proximodistal Axis, 93, 107-109

R
Ribonucleoprotein Particles, 123
Rna Duplexes, 122-123, 142-143, 160
Rna Interference, 1, 3, 5, 7-10, 12, 18, 20, 22, 28-30, 32, 44, 46, 48, 50, 52, 54-58, 69, 71, 73, 75, 87, 89, 91, 93, 99, 101, 103-119, 121-123, 125, 127, 129, 131, 141, 143, 145, 147, 149-161, 169, 178 189, 191, 197, 203, 231, 233
Rna Precursor, 122-123
Rnai Machinery, 92-93, 95, 101-105, 118-119, 132-133, 136, 175, 184, 188-189
Rnai Therapy, 1-3
Rnai-induced Immunity, 1-3, 5, 7

S
Sensory Information, 11-12
Short Interference Rnas, 10
Silencing Signal, 103-105, 125-127, 188-189
Stem Cell Biology, 77
Subcellular Localization, 12, 182

T
Thrombocytopenia, 80-81
Transcriptional Level, 1, 123, 141
Transgenic Plants, 96-97, 100-101, 103, 121-123, 127, 130-135, 142-143, 146-147, 149, 172-173, 176, 191, 204-205
Translation Inhibition, 141, 215
Transplant Rejection, 77
Tribolium Castaneum, 93, 102-103, 108-109, 125, 142-143, 145, 156-157, 165, 179, 181

V
Viral Genomes, 67, 142